W9-CBF-857

Devices for Cardiac Resynchronization:

Technologic and Clinical Aspects

Devices for Cardiac Resynchronization:
Technologic and Clinical Aspects

Edited by

S. Serge Barold, MD, FRACP, FACP
FACC, FESC, FHRS
Clinical Professor of Medicine
University of South Florida College of Medicine
and Division of Cardiology
Tampa General Hospital
Tampa, Florida, USA

Philippe Ritter, MD
Chairman, Cardiostim
InParys, St Cloud
Clinique Bizet, Paris
Clinique Chirurgicale Val d'Or
St Cloud, Paris, France

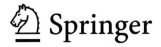 Springer

S. Serge Barold, MD, FRACP, FACP,
FACC, FESC, FHRS
Clinical Professor of Medicine
University of South Florida College of
Medicine and Division of Cardiology
Tampa General Hospital
Tampa, Florida, USA

Philippe Ritter, MD
Chairman Cardiostim
InParys, St. Cloud
Clinique Bizet, Paris
Clinique Chirurgicale Val d'Or
St. Cloud, Paris, France

Library of Congress Control Number: 2007921735

ISBN-13: 978-0-387-71166-9   e-ISBN-13: 978-0-387-71167-6

Printed on acid-free paper

9 8 7 6 5 4 3 2 1

springer.com

Table of Contents

Preface

The last of an ongoing series of Cardiostim monographs all devoted to cardiac pacing, was published four years ago. Since then, cardiac resynchronization for the treatment of heart failure has undergone spectacular progress and has revolutionized device therapy. Many patients have benefited from ventricular resynchronization often combined with an implantable cardioverter-defibrillator. More implantations are likely in the future as the indications continue to evolve with more attention being paid to the primary prevention of heart failure in selected patients and the treatment of earlier stages of left ventricular dysfunction. Thus, we felt it was time for the current Cardiostim monograph to focus exclusively on cardiac resynchronization so as to review the remarkable technologic and clinical advances in the field. We are grateful to the contributors who worked so hard to complete their manuscripts on time and their diligence in presenting new concepts and technical details in an easily understandable fashion.

Working with the Springer publishers, especially Melissa Ramondetta, Executive Editor, Dianne Wuori, Editorial Assistant, and Candace Rosa, Production Editor, was a real pleasure. Their patience, courtesy and efficiency are very much appreciated.

S. Serge Barold
Philippe Ritter

List of Contributors

Christine Alonso, MD
InParys, St Cloud
Clinique Bizet, Paris
Clinique Chirurgicale Val d'Or
St Cloud, France

Juan M. Aranda, Jr., MD
Associate Professor of Medicine
Director Heart Transplant Program
University of Florida
Gainesville, Florida

Shane Bailey, MD, FACC
Department of Cardiovascular Medicine
Cleveland Clinic Foundation
Cleveland, Ohio

S. Serge Barold, MD, FRACP, FACP, FACC, FESC, FHRS
Clinical Professor of Medicine
University of South Florida College of Medicine
Cardiology Division
Tampa General Hospital
Tampa, Florida

Jeroen J. Bax, MD, PhD
Professor of Cardiology
Leiden University Medical Center
Leiden, The Netherlands

Jean-Jacques Blanc, MD
Professor of Cardiology
Head, Department of Cardiology
Hôpital de la Cavale Blanche
Brest University Hospital
Brest, France

Gabe B. Bleeker, MD
Cardiology Department

Leiden University Medical Center
Leiden, The Netherlands

Philippe Castellant, MD
Department of Cardiology
Hôpital de la Cavale Blanche
Brest University Hospital
Brest, France

Serge Cazeau, MD
InParys, St Cloud
Clinique Bizet, Paris
Clinique Chirurgicale Val d'Or
St Cloud, France

Olivier Césari, MD
Département de Cardiologie et Maladies Vasculaires,
Centre Cardio-Pneumologique
Hôpital Pontchaillou
Rennes, France

B. Judson Colley, MD, MPH
Division of Cardiology
Medical University of South Carolina
Charleston, South Carolina

Anne B. Curtis, MD, FACC, FHRS
Professor of Medicine
Chief, Division of Cardiology
University of South Florida College of Medicine
Tampa General Hospital
Tampa, Florida

J. Claude Daubert, MD, FACC, FESC
Professor of Cardiology
Département de Cardiologie et Maladies Vasculaires
Centre Cardio-Pneumologique
Hôpital Pontchaillou
Rennes, France

Yves Etienne, MD
Department of Cardiology
Hôpital de la Cavale Blanche
Brest University Hospital
Brest, France

Marjaneh Fatemi, MD
Department of Cardiology
Hôpital de la Cavale Blanche

Brest University Hospital
Brest, France

Jeffrey Wing-Hong Fung, MBChB (CUHK), FHKCP, FHKAM (Medicine),
FRCP (London)
Division of Cardiology
Department of Medicine and Therapeutics, Prince of Wales Hospital
The Chinese University of Hong Kong
Hong Kong, China

Stéphane Garrigue, MD
Director, Cardiac Pacing and Electrophysiology Department
Clinique Saint Augustin
Bordeaux, France

Safwat A. Gassis, MD
Fellow in Cardiology
Emory University School of Medicine
Atlanta, Georgia

Michael Giudici, MD, FACC, FACP
Division of Cardiology
Genesis Heart Institute
Davenport, Iowa

Michael R. Gold, MD, PhD
Michael E Assey Professor of Medicine
Chief of Cardiology
Director of Heart & Vascular Center
Medical University of South Carolina
Charleston, South Carolina

Bengt Herweg, MD
Associate Professor of Medicine
Director, Electrophysiology and Arrhythmia Services
University of South Florida College of Medicine and Tampa General Hospital
Tampa, Florida

Arzu Ilercil, MD
Associate Professor of Medicine
Director, Non-Invasive Laboratory, University of South Florida College
of Medicine
and Tampa General Hospital
Tampa, Florida

Carsten W. Israel, MD
Associate Professor of Internal Medicine
J. W. Goethe University
Department of Cardiology

Division of Clinical Electrophysiology
Frankfurt, Germany

Gaël Jauvert, MD
InParys, St Cloud
Clinique Bizet, Paris
Clinique Chirurgicale Val d'Or
St Cloud, France

Nadim G. Khan, MD
Assistant Professor of Medicine
Division of Cardiovascular Diseases
University of South Florida College of Medicine
and the James A. Haley VA Hospital
Tampa, Florida

Stéphane Laffitte, MD
Hôpital Cardiologique du Haut Lévêque,
Pessac-Bordeaux, France

Chu-Pak Lau, MD
William M.W. Mong Professor in Cardiology
Chief of Cardiology Division (Academic)
Professor of Medicine
University Department of Medicine
The University of Hong Kong
Hong Kong, China

Arnaud Lazarus, MD
InParys, St Cloud
Clinique Bizet, Paris
Clinique Chirurgicale Val d'Or
St Cloud, France

Christophe Leclercq, MD, PhD, FESC
Professor of Cardiology
Département de Cardiologie et Maladies Vasculaires
Centre Cardio-Pneumologique
Hôpital Pontchaillou
Rennes, France

Angel R. Leon, MD, FACC
The Linton and June Bishop Professor of Medicine
Emory University School of Medicine
Chief of Cardiology

Emory Crawford Long Hospital
Atlanta, Georgia

Philippe Mabo, MD
Professor of Cardiology and Head
Département de Cardiologie et Maladies Vasculaires
Centre Cardio-Pneumologique
Hôpital Pontchaillou
Rennes, France

Chris Madramootoo, BS
Cardiac Sonographer
University of South Florida College of Medicine
and Tampa General Hospital
Tampa, Florida

Sunil T. Mathew, MD
Fellow, Cardiovascular Diseases
University of Oklahoma Health Sciences Center
Oklahoma City, Oklahoma

Arthur J. Moss, MD
Professor of Medicine (Cardiology)
Heart Research Follow-up Program
University of Rochester Medical Center
Rochester, New York

Christina M. Murray, MD
Fellow, Cardiovascular Diseases
University of Oklahoma Health Sciences Center
Oklahoma City, Oklahoma

I. Eli Ovsyshcher, MD, PhD, FESC, FACC, FAHA
Professor of Medicine/Cardiology
Faculty of Health Sciences
Ben Gurion University of the Negev
Beer-Sheva, Israel

Luigi Padeletti, MD
Professor of Cardiology
Director of the Postgraduate School of Cardiology
University of Florence
Florence, Italy

Dwight W. Reynolds, MD, FACC, FHRS
President, Heart Rhythm Society
Professor and Chief, Cardiovascular Section
University of Oklahoma Health Sciences Center
Oklahoma City, Oklahoma

Philippe Ritter, MD
Chairman Cardiostim
InParys, St Cloud
Clinique Bizet, Paris
Clinique Chirurgicale Val d'Or
St Cloud, France

Martin J. Schalij, MD, PhD
Professor of Cardiology
Leiden University Medical Center
Leiden, The Netherlands

Alfons F. Sinnaeve Ing
Emeritus Professor of Electrical Engineering
KHBO University
Ostende, Belgium

Roland X. Stroobandt, MD, PhD
Associate Professor of Medicine
Department of Cardiology
University of Ghent
Ghent, Belgium

Michael O. Sweeney, MD
Cardiac Arrhythmia Service
Brigham and Women's Hospital
Associate Professor of Medicine
Harvard Medical School
Boston, Massachusetts

Hung-Fat Tse, MD
Professor of Medicine
Cardiology Division, Department of Medicine
The University of Hong Kong
Hong Kong, China

Lieselot van Erven, MD, PhD
Department of Cardiology
Leiden University Medical Center
Leiden, The Netherlands

Nico van der Veire, MD
Department of Cardiology
Leiden University Medical Center
Leiden, The Netherlands

Bruce L. Wilkoff, MD, FACC, FHRS
Professor of Medicine
Cleveland Clinic Lerner College of Medicine of Case
Western Reserve University

Director of Cardiac Pacing and Tachyarrhythmia Devices
Department of Cardiovascular Medicine
Cleveland Clinic Foundation
Cleveland, Ohio

Claudia Ypenburg, MD
Department of Cardiology
Leiden University Medical Center
Leiden, The Netherlands

Cheuk-Man Yu, MB ChB(CUHK), MRCP(UK), MD(CUHK), FHKCP,
FHKAM(Medicine), FRACP, FRCP(Edin/London)
Professor and Head of the Division of Cardiology
Department of Medicine and Therapeutics, Prince of Wales Hospital
Director of the Institute of Vascular Medicine (Clinical)
The Chinese University of Hong Kong
Hong Kong, China

Section I

Indications and Implantation for Cardiac Resynchronization Therapy

Do the Official Guidelines for Cardiac Resynchronization Therapy Need to Be Changed?

Nadim G. Khan, Anne B. Curtis, Bengt Herweg, and S. Serge Barold

Heart failure (HF) an ongoing epidemic that shows no signs of abating, despite many advances in medicine. Approximately 5 million Americans and a similar number of Europeans are currently diagnosed with heart failure. More than 500,000 new cases are diagnosed each year in the United States [1, 2]. As our treatment of coronary artery disease, sudden cardiac arrest, and hypertension improves, more patients survive to develop HF. The obesity epidemic, with the accompanying metabolic syndrome, diabetes and hypertension, also contributes to the increasing number of patients with HF. In addition, the advancing age of the population has led to an even further increase in the incidence and prevalence of HF. The incidence of HF approaches 10 per 1,000 population after age 65. HF is the most common Medicare diagnosis-related group, and more dollars are spent in the United States for the diagnosis and treatment of HF than for any other diagnosis.

Over the past 15–20 years, the development of new pharmacologic therapy has lowered mortality by 30–40% in patients with advanced HF. However, despite the use of optimal pharmacologic therapy with beta-blockers, angiotensin converting enzyme inhibitors or angiotensin receptor blockers, and diuretics, many patients still have significant symptoms that affect functional capacity and quality of life. More recently, cardiac resynchronization therapy (CRT) has been added to the armamentarium of HF therapies on the basis of strong evidence from well-designed clinical trials. Patients with evidence of ventricular dyssynchrony by virtue of prolonged QRS durations, typically with left bundle branch block, who have New York Heart Association (NYHA) class III–IV symptoms despite optimal medical therapy have been treated with atrial-synchronous, biventricular pacing using right ventricular leads as well as coronary sinus leads for left ventricular pacing [3]. Clinical trials have shown improvement in exercise capacity, NYHA class, and quality of life with CRT compared with continued medical therapy [4–9]. Landmark clinical trials such as COMPANION [10] and CARE-HF [11] have also shown a survival benefit with CRT. This therapy has opened up a whole new modality in the treatment of HF, focusing on electromechanical assistance to the failing heart.

Clinical Practice Guidelines

Clinical practice guidelines are the result of a rigorous methodologic approach that mandates the review and consideration of the available medical literature in a given field. These guidelines provide an evidence-based standard for effective patient care, weighing results from clinical trials and other studies in order to develop a consensus as to the appropriate indications for different therapeutic modalities and the patients most likely to benefit, with the intention of improving clinical outcomes. They guide clinical practice in the community and have effectively served to unify the practice of medicine.

The process of developing practice guidelines starts with the scientific and clinical documents committees of the major medical societies. Once a decision is made that a guidelines document either needs to be created or revised, a task force is appointed to do so. The document is written and goes through multiple revisions, and then there is a process of several levels of approval, usually including the board of trustees of the society, before the document is published. Often, other societies are asked to review the document and endorse it as well. This process is a time-consuming endeavor, such that it may take 1 to 2 years from the time a decision is made to develop a guidelines document until the actual publication and dissemination occur. The guidelines are then subjected to periodic review based on advances in the area of interest.

Current Guidelines for CRT

The most recent American College of Cardiology (ACC)/American Heart Association and (AHA)/ North American Society of Pacing and Electro-physiology (NASPE) guidelines for pacemakers and antiarrhythmia devices were published in 2002 [3]. These guidelines listed CRT as a class IIA indication with the highest level of evidence, A (data derived from multiple randomized clinical trials or meta-analyses). The indications for CRT in the 2002 guidelines are shown in Table 1.1. In addition, CRT was considered a class III indication (not useful/effective and in some cases harmful) for asymptomatic dilated cardiomyopathy and symptomatic cardiomyopathy that could be treated with drug therapy or revascularization.

The current indications for CRT were classified as class IIA (weight of evidence/opinion is in favor of usefulness/efficacy) and based on a number of randomized clinical trials [4–8]. Since then, there have been several landmark trials that have served to establish CRT even more firmly as an effective therapy, with robust data on more than 4,000 patients in randomized prospective clinical trials [9–12]. In a meta-analysis of CRT trials, HF hospitalizations were reduced by 29% and death from progressive heart failure

Table 1.1 Indications for cardiac resynchronization therapy in the 2002 ACC/AHA/NASPE guidelines.

Symptomatic heart failure
New York Heart Association class III–IV
QRS duration ≥ 130 ms
Idiopathic dilated or ischemic cardiomyopathy with ejection fraction $\leq 35\%$ and left ventricular end diastolic diameter ≥ 55 mm
Refractory symptoms despite optimal medical therapy

Source: Ref. 3.

was reduced by 51% with a positive trend toward reduction of all-cause mortality [13]. This meta-analysis included four randomized trials with 1,634 total patients up to 2002. Subsequently, COMPANION showed hospitalizations were reduced by 32% and all-cause mortality was reduced by 25% [10]. The mortality reduction in COMPANION was found in the group treated with CRT in conjunction with an Implantable cardioverter-defibrillator (ICD). CARE-HF [11] established a significant mortality reduction of 36% and reduction in HF hospitalizations by 52% by the addition of CRT pacemaker therapy without an ICD to optimal medical therapy.

The ACC/AHA 2005 Guideline Update for the Diagnosis and Management of Chronic Heart Failure in the Adult revised the recommendations for CRT [14]. Patients with left ventricular ejection fraction (EF) ≤35%, sinus rhythm, and NYHA functional class III or ambulatory class IV symptoms despite optimal medical therapy who have left ventricular dyssynchrony defined by a QRS duration of greater than 120 ms should receive CRT unless contraindicated (class I recommendation with level of evidence A). These guidelines change the indication from class IIA to class I (evidence and/or general agreement that a given procedure is beneficial, useful, and effective), based on recent clinical trial data.

Current Directions in CRT Research

Having thus firmly established the benefit of CRT in the treatment of HF, research is currently focused on further maturation and refinement of this therapy. Recommended indications for CRT should optimize the proportion of patients who derive significant symptomatic benefit from this therapy on the one hand and should avoid this invasive treatment in patients with a low probability of clinical success of CRT on the other hand. Additional research has also focused on expansion of indications for CRT into the realm of prevention of advanced heart failure by retarding the progression of cardiac remodeling in patients with lesser degrees of HF. Current research is progressing chiefly in the areas outlined in Table 1.2. We will explore

Table 1.2 Areas of current research in cardiac resynchronization therapy.

1. Improvement of preprocedure accuracy in the prediction of response to CRT.
2. Improvement of response rates after implantation.
3. Echo-based techniques for the definition of mechanical dyssynchrony and their correlation with the current standard of prolonged QRS as a surrogate indicator of electrical dyssynchrony.
4. Further mechanistic elucidation of the pathophysiology of cardiac reverse remodeling.
5. Expansion of the current indications to include patient populations with atrial fibrillation, NYHA class I–II, patients with intraventricular conduction defects and right bundle branch block, and patients with significant conduction system disease and structural heart disease without overt heart failure.
6. Improvement in device function, lead performance, and delivery systems.
7. Development of continuous hemodynamic monitoring of heart failure.
8. Telemedicine for device interrogation and management.

Intraventricular dyssynchrony of the LV (septal to inferolateral wall motion delay using tissue Doppler imaging) appears to be most useful in patient selection [19]. These parameters have also been compared with each other to determine the best predictor for response [18]. M-mode measurement is simple and universally available, has been shown to predict reverse remodeling, and has been studied in CARE-HF. Delayed longitudinal contraction predicts response in nonischemic cardiomyopathy. Tissue Doppler imaging–based techniques analyzing multiple segments appear to be more sensitive than those that measure the delay between two segments. The standard deviation of the time to peak myocardial contraction in 12 myocardial segments (Ts-SD-12 or the dyssynchrony index) may have the best predictive value [18]. Studies comparing the various echocardiographic parameters of dyssynchrony are small and usually single center. The identification of a simple, reproducible echocardiographic index for the prediction of response to CRT compared with both clinical and remodeling-based measures would be ideal. The PROSPECT trial may give further direction in this area. It is a prospective study evaluating echocardiographic parameters of systolic dyssynchrony in approximately 700 patients with standard indications for CRT to compare the utility of these different parameters in predicting response to CRT. The primary end points include a clinical composite criterion and a 15% decrease in left ventricular end systolic volume index (LVESVI). Quality of life, NYHA class, 6-min walk test, and EF are secondary end points [20]. The DESIRE trial will enroll 150 patients with NYHA III-IV HF, QRS <150 ms, Left Ventricular Ejection Fraction (LVEF) <40%, in sinus rhythm and left ventricular end diastolic dimension (LVEDD) >2.7 cm/m^2 on optimal medical therapy. This prospective randomized multicenter study will evaluate by echocardiography LV asynchrony and resynchronization and will follow patients for 12 months.

The quest for the best predictor of response to CRT continues. Tissue Doppler–based techniques evaluating intraventricular dyssynchrony show the most promise. In future guidelines, alternative selection criteria, most likely echo-based, are likely to be recommended.

Echocardiography in Patient Follow-up

It has been demonstrated that the response rate to CRT can be improved after implantation of the device by altering the Atrioventricular (A-V) and Interventricular (V-V) timing. The best setting for an individual patient may be determined by using the velocity time integral of the LV outflow tract with various RV–LV timing intervals [21]. The mitral inflow pattern has also been shown to be helpful in optimizing A-V synchrony in patients in sinus rhythm. Upon demonstration of the long-term benefit of postimplant optimization of A-V and V-V timing, these techniques could be added in the guidelines for optimal device management in patients with HF.

Possible Future Expansion of Indications

HF Prevention in NYHA Class II Patients

In the CONTAK CD trial, 33% of patients were in NYHA class II. These patients showed improvement in LVEF and echocardiographic indicators of reverse remodeling. MIRACLE-ICD II was a double-blind, parallel controlled trial that randomized 186 patients with NYHA class II symptoms to CRT and defibrillator versus defibrillator with CRT turned off. This study showed no significant change in the 6-min walk test or quality of life score, but the patient's cardiac structure and function improved [22]. This study raises hope for prevention of HF worsening by halting and reversing the maladaptive cardiac remodeling. A recent study compared the benefit of CRT in patients with NYHA class II HF with patients in NYHA class III and IV HF. The class II patients had EF $\leq 35\%$, QRS >120 ms, and baseline LV dyssynchrony measured by tissue Doppler imaging that was comparable with that found in the patients with NYHA class III and IV symptoms [23]. The magnitude of clinical improvement in NYHA class II patients was significantly less; however, only a minority of patients progressed to class III HF. The mild HF patients had a statistically significant improvement in LVEF and echocardiographic indicators of LV reverse remodeling. As has been discussed earlier, the demonstration of cardiac remodeling better predicts improvement in survival compared with clinical indicators. CRT in NYHA class II HF may be clinically significant in reducing mortality and preventing progression of heart failure.

The REVERSE trial is a prospective, randomized, double-blind parallel study of about 500 patients with NYHA class I–II symptoms, QRS duration ≥ 120 ms, LVEF $\leq 40\%$, and LV end diastolic diameter ≥ 55 mm. This ongoing study will compare optimal medical therapy alone or with CRT $\pm$ ICD in the prevention of progression of HF using both clinical factors and LVESVI as end points at 1 year. The MADIT CRT study is also currently enrolling about 1,800 patients in NYHA class I–II, EF <30%, QRS >130 ms, in sinus rhythm. The primary end point would be a composite of all-cause mortality and HF events by 25%, and a measure of reverse remodeling would be a secondary end point. The results of these studies may expand the indications for CRT into the realm of prevention of HF.

AV Block and Mild HF

Most patients with bradycardia without HF tolerate RV apical pacing. However, in HF, the nonphysiologic effects of RV pacing cause asynchronous electrical activation of the LV, resulting in impaired LV systolic and diastolic function, cardiac remodeling, and HF progression. The MOST trial demonstrated that the risk of HF hospitalization and atrial fibrillation (AF) are directly related to the percentage of cumulative RV pacing [24]. The DAVID trial showed worsening of HF and death in patients with DDDR mode compared with the backup VVI mode [25]. The analysis of MADIT II data also reveals a similar adverse effect of RV pacing on HF. In the era of implantable defibrillators and aggressive beta-blockade, especially in the elderly, it is not uncommon to encounter the coexistence of HF and bradycardia. CRT may mitigate the adverse effects of RV pacing and prevent development or worsening of HF.

A recent study randomized 30 patients with standard indications for permanent ventricular pacing who had LV dysfunction as indicated by LV end diastolic dimension ≥ 60 mm and LV EF $\leq 40\%$ in a prospective crossover design. A 3-month period of RV-only pacing was compared with 3 months of CRT. CRT conferred significant improvement in LV function, quality of life indicators, exercise capacity, and neurohormonal markers [26]. The BLOCK HF trial is currently enrolling patients with AV block (advanced first degree through third degree, provided that pacing is anticipated to be necessary the great majority of the time), NYHA class I–III symptoms, and LV ejection fraction ≤50%. This prospective, multicenter, randomized, double-blind, parallel controlled clinical study compares RV pacing to biventricular pacing. The hypothesis is that CRT may prevent progression to HF compared with conventional RV pacing. The end points include time to first event for all-cause mortality, HF-related urgent care, or a significant change in the LVESVI. The ongoing BIOPACE study is designed to study the benefit of CRT over standard RV pacing, in patients with high degree AV block, regardless of EF and QRS duration. These results may further expand CRT indications into HF prevention.

Atrial Fibrillation

The incidence of AF is directly proportional to heart failure [27]. AF impacts the clinical course of up to 50% of patients with advanced HF who are eligible for CRT with a defibrillator (CRT-D). The likelihood of AF increases with severity of HF, with an annual incidence of approximately 5%. The development of AF doubles the risk of death in patients with HF. Many of the large clinical CRT trials have excluded patients with AF. Small single-center studies have collectively studied a little more than 100 patients and have shown clinical benefit and improvement in reverse remodeling parameters in patients with chronic AF.

The MUSTIC-AF trial studied 59 patients with LVEF <35%, advanced HF, permanent AF (at least 3 months duration), and wide QRS in a prospective randomized controlled trial [28]. Patients adequately treated with CRT showed improvement in 6-min walking distance, quality of life score, NYHA functional class, and HF hospitalizations. This study included patients with a slow ventricular rate that was either spontaneous or induced by AV node ablation. Another study in patients with AV nodal ablation for AF and advanced HF showed improvement in NYHA functional class, LVEF, LV dimensions, and HF hospitalizations [29].

It appears that the response rate to CRT may be lower in patients with chronic AF than in patients in sinus rhythm. However, the response rate is higher in patients with chronic AF who have undergone AV nodal ablation compared with those patients who have not. The PAVE study prospectively randomized patients with chronic AF who received AV nodal ablation to standard RV pacing versus CRT [30]. At 6 months after ablation, the patients in the CRT group showed significant improvement in exercise capacity with preservation of LVEF. This benefit was more prominent in patients with either impaired LV systolic function or symptomatic heart failure. In patients with HF who undergo AV nodal ablation for AF, CRT may become the method of choice for pacing.

A recent study followed approximately 600 HF patients prospectively in two European centers for up to 4 years. More than half of the 114 patients with AF in this study were not able to achieve an arbitrary device-derived cutoff of >85% CRT at 2 months, despite the usual pharmacologic and device programming interventions [31]. These patients were subjected to AV nodal ablation in a nonrandomized format to ensure complete biventricular capture. This study demonstrated long-term improvements in LVEF, reverse remodeling, and functional capacity in both patients in sinus rhythm and AF. However, within the AF group, the patients who received AV nodal ablation and CRT showed statistically significant improvements in LVEF, LV dimensions, and clinical markers compared with patients without AV nodal ablation who had >85% biventricular pacing with standard rate control measures. Among patients with AF, the percentage of responders was threefold higher in the AV nodal ablation group compared with the nonablated group receiving standard pharmacologic rate control. The benefit of AV nodal ablation observed in this study could represent an overestimation of device-based percentage of CRT in the nonablated group due to fusion and pseudofusion, better rate control (and better diastolic function) in the ablated group, and inadvertent effects of rate control medications. The contribution of AV nodal ablation in patients with permanent AF to enhance the benefit of CRT in HF merits further attention in a randomized, adequately powered study.

The ongoing APAF trial is evaluating patients with permanent AF and refractory heart failure. These patients undergo AV nodal ablation and implantation of a biventricular pacemaker. They are then randomized to a strategy of RV pacing based on clinical indications with a strategy of early CRT based on echocardiographic optimization. About 500 patients will be followed for 2 years, with a short-term study involving clinical and echocardiographic indicators of response and a long-term study with a composite end point of HF events and cardiovascular mortality.

CRT in Patients with Narrow QRS

QRS duration >150 ms, especially in association with left bundle branch block, correlates well with LV mechanical dyssynchrony and consequently response to CRT. This relationship does not hold true in HF patients with narrow or mildly prolonged QRS duration. It has been appreciated that LV mechanical dyssynchrony can exist in up to 51% of patients with HF and QRS ≤120 ms [32]. Other studies have demonstrated the presence of left ventricular mechanical dyssynchrony in patients with QRS ≤120 ms, ranging from 27% to 43% depending on the methodology. Sogaard et al. have demonstrated that intraventricular mechanical dyssynchrony is a much better predictor of LV remodeling than QRS duration [33]. Achilli et al. showed response to CRT in patients with narrow QRS, having selected patients based on LV mechanical dyssynchrony [34]. The current CRT guidelines do not appreciate this indication. Future revisions should take into account this patient population, and emphasis on echo-based selection of patients will extend the benefit of CRT to this subpopulation of patients.

Functional (Secondary) Mitral Regurgitation

Up to 30% of patients with severe LV systolic dysfunction also have severe mitral regurgitation (MR). Typically, the valve structure itself is unaffected;

however, a multitude of factors, including change in LV and papillary muscle geometry, mitral annular dilation, regional wall motion abnormalities both due to ischemic heart disease and dyssynchrony, prolonged AV conduction, and LV volume overload, contribute to MR. MR in these patients demonstrates relentless progression and confers an annual survival rate of only 30–40% [35]. Though surgical correction is an option, the operative mortality tends to be high and often these patients are not referred for surgery. CRT has been shown to acutely (30–40% reduction) and chronically (10–20%) reduce the severity of MR [36]. This effect was directly proportional to the closing force on the mitral valve, which is improved by LV synchrony, including papillary muscle activation and reduction of the tethering forces on the mitral valve. With the accumulation of further long-term data, severe functional MR, in patients who are not surgical candidates, could be considered as an indication for CRT

Right Bundle Branch Block and Intraventricular Conduction Delay

The sparse retrospective data from subgroup analysis does not support the use of CRT in Right Bundle Branch Block (RBBB) and Intraventricular Conduction Delay (IVCD). Data from a pooled subset of 61 patients with RBBB from the MIRACLE and CONTAK CD trials did not demonstrate any significant benefit from CRT [37]. On the other hand, coexisting left anterior or left posterior hemiblock may indicate a favorable response to CRT [38]. ECG evidence of anterior wall myocardial infarction and RV dilation may predict lack of response to CRT [39]. Echocardiographic demonstration of significant intraventricular dyssynchrony in patients with RBBB and IVCD may help identify patients who could potentially benefit from CRT.

Upgrade of an RV Pacing System to CRT

RV apical pacing and the attendant LV dyssynchrony may lead in some cases to worsening or appearance of HF symptoms. Long-term RV pacing has been shown to be detrimental to LV function. Upgrading RV pacing systems to biventricular CRT modalities is a theoretically promising option, and small clinical studies seem to indicate such benefit [40]. It is not clear if dyssynchrony induced by RV pacing has the same pathophysiologic effect as left bundle branch block. The clinical benefit in this sometimes complicated procedure is yet to be determined in this situation. Echocardiographic elucidation of mechanical dyssynchrony may be beneficial in determining which patients will benefit from an upgrade to a CRT system. More data is required if this indication is to be included in future guidelines.

Conclusion

The indications for CRT continue to evolve and will expand as further studies identify those most likely to benefit. It is expected that some image-based measure of dyssynchrony will be recommended in addition to or instead of QRS duration in the selection of patients for CRT when the current ACC/AHA/NASPE guidelines are revised. Several new categories of patients

Table 1.4 New patient populations likely to receive at least class II recommendations in revised practice guidelines, pending results of clinical trials.

Heart failure prevention in class II patients
AV block
Atrial fibrillation
Narrow QRS width with echocardiographic indicators of mechanical dyssynchrony

should get at least a class II indication for CRT (Table 1.4). Ongoing trials will provide the level of evidence for these recommendations. The American College of Cardiology in association with the Heart Rhythm Society and the American Heart Association has already initiated the process of revision of guidelines for device-based therapy for heart rhythm abnormalities.

References

1. Lethbridge-Çejku M, Vickerie J. Summary health statistics for U.S. adults: National Health Interview Survey, 2003. National Center for Health Statistics. Washington DC. Vital Health Stat 10 (225). 2005.
2. American Heart Association Statistics Committee and Stroke Statistics Subcommittee. Heart disease and stroke statistic 2006 update. Circulation 2006;113: e85–e151.
3. Gregoratos G, Abrams J, Epstein AE, et al. ACC/AHA/NASPE 2002 guideline update for implantation of cardiac pacemakers and antiarrhythmia devices: A report of the American College of Cardiology/American Heart Association Task Force on Practice Guidelines 2002. Available at: www.acc.org/clinical/guidelines/pacemaker/pacemaker.pdf.
4. Stellbrink C, Breithardt OA, Franke A, et al. Impact of cardiac resynchronization therapy using hemodynamically optimized pacing on left ventricular remodeling in patients with congestive heart failure and ventricular conduction disturbances. J Am Coll Cardiol 2001;38:1957–65.
5. Cazeau S, Leclercq C, Lavergne T, et al. Effects of multisite biventricular pacing in patients with heart failure and intraventricular conduction delay. N Engl J Med 2001;344:873–80.
6. Stellbrink C, Breithardt OA, Franke A, et al. Impact of cardiac resynchronization therapy using hemodynamically optimized pacing on left ventricular remodeling in patients with congestive heart failure and ventricular conduction disturbances. J Am Coll Cardiol 2001;38:1957–65.
7. Abraham WT, Fisher WG, Smith AL, et al. Cardiac resynchronization in chronic heart failure. N Engl J Med 2002;346:1845–53.
8. Butter C, Auricchio A, Stellbrink C, et al. Effect of resynchronization therapy stimulation site on the systolic function of heart failure patients. Circulation 2001;104:3026–9.
9. Linde C, Leclercq C, Rex S, et al. on behalf of the MUltisite STimulation In Cardiomyopathies (MUSTIC) Study Group. Long-term benefits of biventricular pacing in congestive heart failure: Results from the MUltisite STimulation In Cardiomyopathy (MUSTIC) Study. J Am Coll Cardiol 2002;40:111–118.
10. Bristow MR, Saxon LA, Boehmer J, et al. Cardiac-resynchronization therapy with or without an implantable defibrillator in advanced chronic heart failure. N Engl J Med 2004;350:2140–50.
11. Cleland JG, Daubert JC, Erdmann E, et al. for the Cardiac Resynchronization–Heart Failure (CARE-HF) Study Investigators. The effect of cardiac resyn-

chronization on morbidity and mortality in heart failure. N Engl J Med 2005;352:1539–49.

12. McAlister F, Ezekowitz J, Wiebe N, et al. Cardiac resynchronization therapy for congestive heart failure. Evid Rep Technol Assess (Summ.) 2004;106:1–8.

13. Hunt SA, Abraham WT, Chin MH, et al. ACC/AHA 2005 guideline update for the diagnosis and management of chronic heart failure in the adult. A report of the American College of Cardiology/American Heart Association Task Force on Practice Guidelines. Developed in collaboration with the American College of Chest Physicians and the International Society for Heart and Lung Transplantation endorsed by the Heart Rhythm Society. J Am Coll Cardiol 2005;46:1–82.

14. Bradley DJ, Bradley EA, Baughman KL, et al. Cardiac resynchronization and death from progressive heart failure a meta-analysis of randomized controlled trials. JAMA 2003;289:730–40.

15. Yu CM, Bleeker GB, Fung JW, et al. Left ventricular reverse remodeling but not clinical improvement predicts long-term survival after cardiac resynchronization therapy. Circulation 2005;112:1580–6.

16. Ghio S, Constantin C, Klersy C, et al. Interventricular and intraventricular dyssynchrony are common in heart failure patients, regardless of QRS duration. Eur Heart J 2004;25:571–8.

17. Auricchio A, Fantoni C, Regoli F, et al. Characterization of left ventricular activation in patients with heart failure and left bundle-branch block. Circulation 2004;109:1133–9.

18. Bax JJ, Ansalone G, Breithardt OA, et al. Echocardiographic evaluation of cardiac resynchronization therapy: ready for routine clinical use? A critical appraisal. J Am Coll Cardiol 2004;44:1–9.

19. Yu CM, Fung JW, Zhang Q, et al. Tissue Doppler imaging is superior to strain rate imaging and postsystolic shortening on the prediction of reverse remodelling in both ischemic and nonischemic failure after cardiac resynchronization therapy. Circulation 2004;110:66–73.

20. Yu CM, Abraham WT, Bax JJ, et al. Predictors of response to cardiac resynchronization therapy (PROSPECT)-study design. Am Heart J 2005;149:600–605.

21. Sogaard P, Eglebad H, Pedersen AK, et al. Sequential versus simultaneous biventricular resynchronization for severe heart failure evaluation by tissue Doppler imaging. Circulation 2002;106:2078–84.

22. Abraham WT, Young JB, Smith AL et al., Combined cardiac resynchronization and implantable cardioversion defibrillation in advanced chronic heart failure the MIRACLE-ICD trial, Circulation 2004;110:2864–8.

23. Bleeker GB, Schalij MJ, Holman ER, et al. Cardiac resynchronization therapy in patients with systolic left ventricular dysfunction and symptoms of mild heart failure secondary to ischemic or nonischemic cardiomyopathy. Am J Cardiol 2006;98:230–5

24. Sweeney MO, Hellkamp AS, Ellenbogen KA, et al. Adverse effect of ventricular pacing on heart failure and atrial fibrillation among patients with normal baseline QRS duration in a clinical trial of pacemaker therapy for sinus node dysfunction, Circulation 2003;23:2932–7.

25. Wilkoff BL, Cook JR, Epstein AE, et al. Dual-chamber pacing or ventricular backup pacing in patients with an implantable defibrillator the Dual Chamber and VVI Implantable Defibrillator (DAVID) trial. JAMA 2002;288:3115–23.

26. Kindermann M, Hennen B, Jung J, et al. Biventricular versus conventional right ventricular stimulation for patients with standard pacing indication and left ventricular dysfunction: the Homburg Biventricular Pacing Evaluation (HOBIPACE). J Am Coll Cardiol 2006;47:1927–37.

27. Maisel W, Stevenson L. Atrial fibrillation in heart failure epidemiology, pathophysiology and rationale for therapy. Am J Cardiol 2003;91:2D–8D.

28. Leclercq C, Walker S, Linde C, et al. Comparative effects of permanent biventricular and right-univentricular pacing in heart failure patients with chronic atrial fibrillation. Eur Heart J 2002;23:1780–7.

29. Leon AR, Greenberg JM, Kanuru N, et al. Cardiac resynchronization in patients with congestive heart failure and chronic atrial fibrillation: effect of upgrading to biventricular pacing after chronic right ventricular pacing. J Am Coll Cardiol 2002;39:1258–63.

30. Doshi RN, Daoud EG, Fellows C, et al. Left ventricular-based cardiac stimulation post AV nodal ablation evaluation (the PAVE study) J Cardiovasc Electrophysiol 2005;16:1160–5.

31. Gasparini M, Auricchio A, Regoli F. Four-year efficacy of cardiac resynchronization therapy on exercise tolerance and disease progression. The importance of performing atrioventricular junction ablation in patients with atrial fibrillation. J Am Coll Cardiol 2006;48:734–43.

32. Yu CM, Lin H, Zhang Q, et al. High prevalence of left ventricular systolic and diastolic asynchrony in patients with congestive heart failure and normal QRS duration. Heart 2003;89:54–60.

33. Søgaard P, Egeblad H, Kim WY, et al. Tissue Doppler imaging predicts improved systolic performance and reversed left ventricular remodeling during long-term cardiac resynchronization therapy. J Am Coll Cardiol 2002;40:723–30.

34. Achilli A, Sassara M, Ficili S, et al. Long-term effectiveness of cardiac resynchronization therapy in patients with refractory heart failure and "narrow" QRS. J Am Coll Cardiol 2003;42:2117–24.

35. Grigioni F, Enriquez-Sarano M, Zehr KJ, et al. Ischemic mitral regurgitation; long-term outcomes and prognostic implications with quantitative Doppler assessment. Circulation 2001;103:1759–64

36. Yu CM, Chau E, Sanderson JE, et al. Tissue Doppler echocardiographic evidence of reverse remodeling and improved synchronicity by simultaneously delaying regional contraction after biventricular pacing therapy in heart failure. Circulation 2002;105:438–45.

37. Egoavil CA, Ho RT, Greenspon AJ, et al. Cardiac resynchronization therapy in patients with right bundle branch block: Analysis of pooled data from the MIRACLE and Contak CD trials. Heart Rhythm 2005;2:611–5.

38. Aranda JM, Conti JB, Johnson JW, et al. Cardiac resynchronization therapy in patients with heart failure and conduction abnormalities other than left bundle-branch block: Analysis of the Multicenter InSync Randomized Clinical Evaluation (MIRACLE). Clin Cardiol 2004;27:678–82.

39. Reynolds MR, Joventino LP, Josephson ME, et al. Relationship of baseline electrocardiographic characteristics with the response to cardiac resynchronization therapy for heart failure. Pacing Clin Electrophysiol 2004;27:1513–8.

40. Eldadah DA, Rosen B, Hay I, et al. The benefit of upgrading chronically right ventricle-paced heart failure patients to resynchronization therapy demonstrated by strain rate imaging. Heart Rhythm 2006;3:435–42.

Alternative Techniques for Left Ventricular Lead Placement

Shane Bailey and Bruce L. Wilkoff

The standard approach for insertion of left ventricular leads is performed transvenously with fluoroscopic guidance into the cardiac veins that branch from the coronary sinus. The procedure is performed percutaneously and precludes the need for thoracotomy and intubation with general anesthesia, which can lead to prolonged hospitalizations [1, 2]. However, in multiple studies, 8–14% of transvenous attempts to place a lead in a cardiac vein failed [3, 4]. There are multiple reasons for the inability to transvenously insert a left ventricular lead, including inability to cannulate the coronary sinus, small cardiac veins unsuitable to lead placement, stenosis within the coronary sinus or cardiac veins, and coronary sinus perforation. Additionally, long-term complications of left ventricular cardiac vein leads can include increases in pacing thresholds, lead dislodgment, and diaphragmatic stimulation. Within the MIRACLE trial, 6% of patients required repositioning or replacement of the coronary sinus lead within 6 months of the implant [4]. Similarly, in a study comparing epicardial versus coronary sinus leads, 11% of patients with a coronary sinus lead experienced long-term complications at 4 years [3]. Indeed, a learning curve exists for implanting coronary sinus leads, and success with implantation increases with experience and improvement in delivery systems and leads [5].

Surgical Epicardial Approach

Surgical placement of a left ventricular lead is a well-accepted alternative for resynchronization therapy when the transvenous approach fails. Left ventricular stimulation was, in fact, first achieved by the surgical epicardial approach performed by lateral thoracotomy. Recent advances in surgical techniques for left ventricular (LV) lead placement include the minimal thoracotomy approach, video-assisted thoracoscopy, and robotically assisted implantation. These newer techniques reduce wound size and result in shorter hospitalization but require general anesthesia with its inherent risks. Several advantages with surgical placement of left ventricular leads can be appreciated, including less fluoroscopy time, avoidance of intravenous contrast, shorter implant time, and possibly reduced lead-related complications. In a recent study comparing surgically placed left ventricular leads and coronary sinus leads, pacing threshold increases and dislodgment were significantly reduced in the surgically treated patients [3]. Additionally, surgical placement by thoracotomy or endoscopic approach offers the advantage of direct visualization of the left ventricle for optimal lead position.

With the *minimal thoracotomy* approach, a 3- to 5-cm incision is made over the 4th or 5th intercostal space anterior to the midaxillary line [6] (Fig. 2.1). Single-lung ventilation is performed, and the pericardium is opened avoiding the phrenic nerve. Using an epicardial lead implant tool, two screw-in pacing leads are placed on the left ventricular wall. The leads are tested through the analyzer and subsequently tunneled to the pacemaker pocket where the lead with the lowest threshold is connected to the pulse generator. A chest tube is required postoperatively and is typically discontinued within 48 h. This technique is preferred for patients with severely enlarged left ventricles and prior open heart surgery. For these patients, thorascopic techniques are difficult secondary to limited space.

Video-assisted thoracoscopy (VATS) has become a routine endoscopic procedure in thoracic surgery. This approach requires the creation of the two or three ports within the 4th or 5th intercostal space along the anterior and midaxillary line [6, 7]. Similar to the limited thoracotomy approach, single-lung ventilation with a double-lumen tube is used. A camera is inserted through one port with instruments manipulated through the remaining. After the pericardium is opened and the phrenic nerve and marginal arteries are identified, the epicardial lead is screwed in through the instrumentation port (Fig. 2.2). The lead is then tunneled to the device pocket and attached to the generator. Gabor et al. reported on 15 patients who had LV epicardial lead

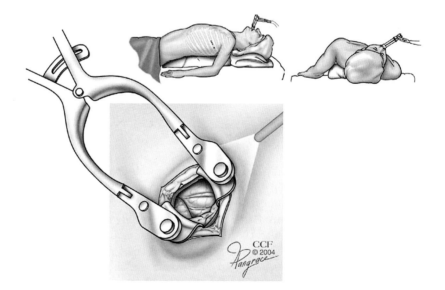

Fig. 2.1 Minithoracotomy approach for insertion of LV epicardial lead, illustrating incision site (upper left), patient position (upper right), and exposure with retractor.

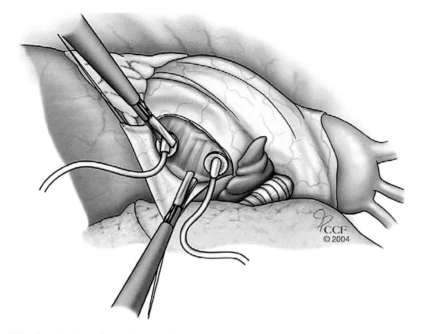

Fig. 2.2 Implantation of two left ventricular epicardial leads using video-assisted thoracoscopy.

placement by VATS after failure with a transvenous attempt. Mean operating time was 55 min with satisfactory pacing thresholds and no lead dislodgments at 7 months [7].

Robotically assisted left ventricular epicardial lead implantation is an emerging technique performed endoscopically. Anesthesia preparation is also performed with single-lung ventilation. Three ports are inserted into the chest cavity along the posterior axillary line through which an endoscope is placed through the center port (Fig. 2.3). Through the outer ports, specialized instruments are used that are capable of 7 degrees of freedom, similar to the human wrist. A fourth port is placed posterior to the camera port for introduction of the epicardial lead. The instruments are controlled by a surgeon located at a console away from the operating table. The robotic arms are then used to fix the lead into a posterobasal location on the left ventricle.

DeRose et al. describe their experience with 13 patients who had LV lead placement using the da Vinci Robotic Surgical System (Intuitive Surgical Inc., Sunnyvale, Calif., USA) [8]. All patients had successful implantation with significant improvements in exercise tolerance and ejection fraction, and no dislodgment or pacing threshold increases were seen. In a similar report, Jansens et al. describe 15 patients who had LV lead placement using the da Vinci robotic system after failure to implant in the cardiac veins [9]. Thirteen patients had successful implant with two requiring a small thoracotomy (one for lung adhesions from prior radiation and the other from epicardial bleeding after fixation of the lead).

Robotic technology provides for visualization of the entire posterolateral left ventricular wall and enables accurate surgical precision in implanting a lead. Other advantages include elimination of tremor and a magnified,

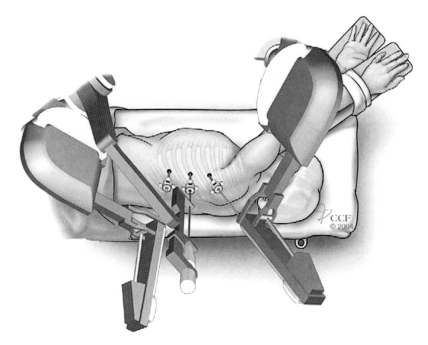

Fig. 2.3 Robotically assisted left ventricular epicardial lead implantation using the da Vinci system.

three-dimensional image that can be viewed through the surgical console. Similar to VATS, minimal incisions are made, and postoperative pain is minimized. Robotics can be helpful in patients with a small cardiothoracic ratio, for which VATS can be very challenging. Additionally, although not contraindicated, reoperations with robotics can be difficult [6].

Transseptal Approach

Left ventricular endocardial pacing has been described using the transseptal approach. This technique has been of interest in patients in whom coronary sinus anatomy is not amenable to placement of a left ventricular lead. As opposed to surgically placed epicardial leads, which require general anesthesia, the transseptal approach can be performed in the same setting as coronary sinus cannulation. Additionally, it has been suggested that endocardial pacing may have benefits in left ventricular contractility and improved synchrony over epicardial pacing, either by cardiac veins or surgically placed epicardial leads [10]. These benefits are contrasted with the risk of thromboembolic events and the transseptal procedure.

Jais et al. described this alternative pacing technique after multiple unsuccessful attempts to enter the coronary sinus in a 73-year-old man with end-stage congestive heart failure [11]. In their technique, transseptal puncture was performed from the right femoral vein through a snare positioned in the right atrium over the fossa ovalis (Fig. 2.4). The snare was introduced from the right internal jugular vein and functioned as a circular retrieval device capable of grasping objects advanced through its body. Once a guide wire

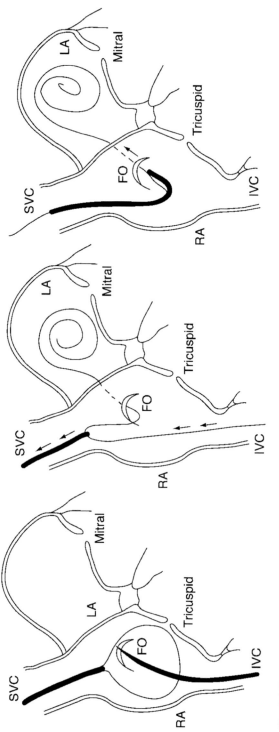

Fig. 2.4 Transseptal puncture is achieved via femoral venous access through which a wire is introduced into the left atrium. The wire is snared via right internal jugular venous access and pulled out the neck access through which the peel-away sheath is advanced across the intraatrial septum for placement of the LV endocardial lead.

was positioned in the left atrium, the sheath was withdrawn back across the septum, and the snare was used to retrieve and exteriorize the proximal portion of the guide wire through the right internal jugular vein. A transseptal sheath was then advanced into the left atrium from the right neck and a lead was able to be advanced into the left ventricle. Leclercq et al. described a modified transseptal catheterization technique in three similar patients [12]. In this approach, the septum was punctured directly from the right internal jugular vein utilizing fluoroscopy and transesophageal echocardiography. After being placed in the left ventricle, the lead was subsequently tunneled from the right neck to the pacemaker pocket. Of interest, in two of the three patients, dislodgment of the left ventricular lead occurred early requiring a second procedure.

In a series of 11 patients who had endocardial left ventricular lead placement via transseptal approach, Jais et al. report on a mean follow-up of 15 months [13]. In this group, seven patients had transseptal puncture with a combined femoral and internal jugular approach, as described above, and the remaining four had transseptal puncture directly from the right internal jugular vein. The procedure was successful in all patients with 10 of the 11 describing functional improvement. All patients were anticoagulated with warfarin. At follow-up, one transient ischemic attack occurred in a patient who interrupted anticoagulation.

The transseptal puncture has also been described from the left axillary vein. A 63-year-old man with severe heart failure requiring upgrade to a cardiac resynchronization therapy defibrillator (CRT-D) device had coronary sinus angiography, which demonstrated poor targets for a left ventricular lead. Surgical placement of an epicardial lead was not possible secondary to a history of tracheal stenosis precluding general anesthesia. Ji et al. describe using a standard transseptal needle shaped to match the contour of the innominate vein and superior vena cava (SVC) [14]. This approach has the advantage of avoiding the need for tunneling the lead as with the transjugular approach.

Epicardial and endocardial pacing has been suggested to result in differences in left ventricular contractility and synchrony. Garrigue et al. studied 15 patients that had epicardial lead placement through the coronary sinus and compared them with 8 patients with endocardial leads placed by transseptal puncture secondary to unsuitable coronary sinus anatomy [10]. Echocardiographic and Doppler characteristics were compared and included amplitude of left ventricular contractility and regional left ventricular electromechanical delay. They reported a significant improvement in the echocardiographic and Doppler variables in the patients that had endocardial pacing, however, no clinical differences were noted.

Pacing endocardially by the transseptal approach offers some advantages over surgical epicardial lead placement, such as obviating the need for general anesthesia and the possible hemodynamic benefits of endocardial pacing. However, this technique should not be routinely attempted in patients. There has not been long-term follow-up on this group of patients who are low in number. The risk of thromboembolic events is not known; however, in a review of patients who inadvertently had left-sided lead placement, the risk of cerebral embolism was more than 20% [15]. Although anticoagulation may reduce the risk of cerebral embolism, it is not negligible [16,17]. Additionally, the transseptal puncture technique may not be routine for many physicians that implant devices and may result in significant complications rates, especially when attempted from the internal jugular approach.

Other Alternative Approaches

A different approach to left ventricular endocardial pacing not requiring a transseptal puncture was described by Grosfeld et al. [18]. *Left interventricular septal pacing* was described in an animal study using a pacemaker lead with a long insulated screw with only the distal two windings electrically active. Using a guiding sheath, the lead is screwed through the right ventricular septum until the endocardium of the left ventricle is paced, as confirmed by injury current and pacing thresholds. Additionally, contrast fluid was given through the guiding sheath to confirm lead position by fluoroscopy and echocardiography. In all animals, the positioning of the electrode was successful as confirmed by necropsy. Pacing thresholds and sensing characteristics were satisfactory, and no perforations were observed.

Percutaneous epicardial left heart pacing lead implantation has been described using a *subxiphoid videopericardioscopic device*. This method was tested in swine using a videopericardioscopic device composed of two parallel lumens, the superior port housing the endoscope and the inferior lumen used to accommodate the lead. The device is inserted through an incision made in the subxiphoid space until the pericardium is visualized (Fig. 2.5). With an endoscopic tool, the pericardium is incised and the device advanced into the pericardial space. The distal portion of the device is placed in angulated

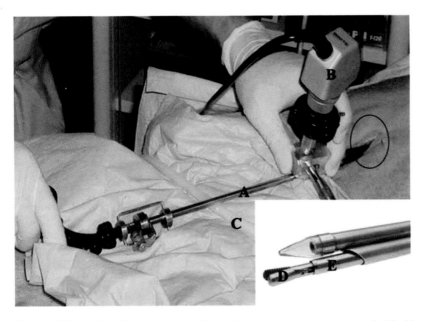

Fig. 2.5 Videopericardioscopic device advanced percutaneously through a subxiphoid incision (circled). A surgical instrument is advanced through the lower port (*A&C*) and the endoscope is seen above (*B*). The inset displays an instrument in the lower port for grasping (*D*) and cutting (*E*).

contact with the myocardium, and the lead is actively fixated. Limitations with this approach include difficultly in positioning the device for lead delivery over the posterolateral left ventricle, inability to maneuver the device through diseased or postoperative pericardium, and finally, the possibility of pericardial inflammation from the epicardial lead.

Conclusion

Various techniques are described to facilitate pacing of the left ventricle to allow for resynchronization in heart failure. The first-line approach remains the transvenous method by way of the coronary sinus. The success rate for this approach remains more than 85% in large series and continues to improve with experienced operators and better delivery systems. Surgical placement of epicardial leads is an acceptable alternative to LV lead placement when the transvenous route fails or is not possible. Several minimally invasive surgical approaches have been described and continue to evolve, allowing precise implantation of LV leads with smaller incisions, less pain, and reduced hospital stays. Transseptal placement of LV endocardial leads has not been thoroughly evaluated and may pose a thromboembolic risk, even with anticoagulation. Additionally, the transseptal puncture, whether from the femoral or jugular approach, may result in a higher rate of complications when not performed by operators routinely familiar with this technique. Other described techniques remain restricted to animal models and require further investigation and technology advancement.

References

1. Daoud EG, Kalbfleisch SJ, Hummel JD, et al. Implantation techniques and chronic lead parameters of biventricular pacing dual-chamber defibrillators. J Cardiovasc Electrophysiol 2002;13(10):964–70.
2. Izutani H, Quan KJ, Biblo LA, et al. Biventricular pacing for congestive heart failure: early experience in surgical epicardial versus coronary sinus lead placement. Heart Surg Forum 2002;6(1):E1–6; discussion E1–6.
3. Mair H, Sachweh J, Meuris B, et al. Surgical epicardial left ventricular lead versus coronary sinus lead placement in biventricular pacing. Eur J Cardiothorac Surg 2005;27(2):235–42.
4. Abraham WT, Fisher WG, Smith AL, et al. Cardiac resynchronization in chronic heart failure. N Engl J Med 2002;346(24):1845–53.
5. Alonso C, Leclercq C, d'Allonnes F, et al. Six year experience of transvenous left ventricular lead implantation for permanent biventricular pacing in patients with advanced heart failure: Technical aspects. Heart 2001;86(4):405–10.
6. Navia JL, Atik FA. Minimally invasive surgical alternatives for left ventricle epicardial lead implantation in heart failure patients. Ann Thorac Surg 2005;80(2):751–4.
7. Gabor S, Prenner G, Wasler A, et al. A simplified technique for implantation of left ventricular epicardial leads for biventricular re-synchronization using video-assisted thoracoscopy (VATS). Eur J Cardiothorac Surg 2005;28(6):797–800.
8. Derose JJ Jr, Belsley S, Swistel D, et al. Robotically assisted left ventricular epicardial lead implantation for biventricular pacing: The posterior approach. Ann Thorac Surg 2004;77(4):1472–4.

9. Jansens JL, Jottrand M, Preumunt N, et al. Robotic-enhanced biventricular resynchronization: An alternative to endovenous cardiac resynchronization therapy in chronic heart failure. Ann Thorac Surg 2003;76(2):413–7; discussion 417.

10. Garrigue S, Jais P, Espil G, et al. Comparison of chronic biventricular pacing between epicardial and endocardial left ventricular stimulation using Doppler tissue imaging in patients with heart failure. Am J Cardiol 2001;88(8):858–62.

11. Jais P, Douard H, Shah DC, et al. Endocardial biventricular pacing. Pacing Clin Electrophysiol 1998;21(11 Pt 1):2128–31.

12. Leclercq F, Hager FX, Macia JC, et al. Left ventricular lead insertion using a modified transseptal catheterization technique: A totally endocardial approach for permanent biventricular pacing in end-stage heart failure. Pacing Clin Electrophysiol 1999;22(11):1570–5.

13. Jais P, Takahashi A, Garrigue S, et al. Mid-term follow-up of endocardial biventricular pacing. Pacing Clin Electrophysiol 2000;23(11 Pt 2):1744–7.

14. Ji S, Cesari D, Swerdww C, et al. Left ventricular endocardial lead placement using a modified transseptal approach. J Cardiovasc Electrophysiol 2004;15(2):234–6.

15. Sharifi M, Sorkin R, Sharifi V, et al. Inadvertent malposition of a transvenous-inserted pacing lead in the left ventricular chamber. Am J Cardiol 1995;76(1):92–5.

16. Warfield DA, Hayes DL, Hyberger LK, et al. Permanent pacing in patients with univentricular heart. Pacing Clin Electrophysiol 1999;22(8):1193–201.

17. Gold MR, Rashba EJ. Left ventricular endocardial pacing: Don't try this at home. Pacing Clin Electrophysiol 1999;22(11):1567–9.

18. Grosfeld MJ, Res JC, Vos DH, et al. Testing a new mechanism for left interventricular septal pacing: The transseptal route; a feasibility and safety study. Europace 2002;4(4):439–44.

3

Importance of the Right Ventricular Pacing Site in Cardiac Resynchronization

Gaël Jauvert, Christine Alonso, Serge Cazeau, Arnaud Lazarus, and Philippe Ritter

Cardiac resynchronization therapy (CRT) has changed the clinical prognosis of patients with heart failure and mechanical ventricular dyssynchrony. Since its introduction in 1994, biventricular pacing has demonstrated a striking functional benefit and more recently a significant reduction of mortality by itself (i.e., with or without the addition of a defibrillator) [1–4]. Yet, 20% to 30% of CRT recipients will not respond to the therapy [2]. This has fostered investigation to better understand the electromechanical disorders that are potentially reversible with multisite pacing. Echocardiography is by far the best noninvasive tool to evaluate the actual significance of intraventricular dyssynchrony (the result of electromechanical disturbances). Various echocardiographic parameters, simple or sophisticated, have been proposed to compensate for the lack of specificity/sensitivity of the QRS configuration and duration for screening of potentially good responders [5,6]. Nevertheless, a potentially good responder cannot receive the full expected hemodynamic benefit of CRT by "simply" pacing the two ventricles either simultaneously or sequentially without meticulous attention to the pacing sites. Therefore, an optimal clinical result requires the establishment of the optimal pacing site(s) and pacing configuration.

Seeking Optimal Pacing Site(s)

In CRT, the search for the best pacing site has focused exclusively on the left side. The midportion of the lateral or posterolateral wall seems to be the segment to target for the best hemodynamic or clinical result. Auricchio et al. showed better acute improvement of left ventricular dp/dt or pulse pressure when the left ventricular (LV) pacing site was located in the midlateral wall [7]. In a MUSTIC substudy, Alonso et al. found that left lateral wall pacing was correlated with a significant decrease of the QRS duration and a significant increase in functional status evaluated by the 6-min walk test [8]. In a retrospective study, Ansalone et al. suggested that improvement in LV end systolic volume (LVESD), LV ejection fraction (LVEF), and exercise

"adverse remodeling" is certainly the underlying mechanical outcome of the "worsened" nonresponders. Thus, to validate a useful method, one must prove that the best pacing configuration determined at implantation (associated with the best initial mechanical result) is correlated with the best mechanical and clinical outcome after the remodeling period.

Is the RV Pacing Site Important?

Why would an RV septal site be less important than the LV free wall pacing site? Does biventricular pacing aim at resynchronizing all the LV segments and not both the LV and RV? The RV pacing site is crucial, because the LV pacing site is more often achieved "where we can" rather than "where we should," whereas it is much easier to place a screw-in lead on a site all over the right interventricular septum on the right side.

Seeking the optimal RV pacing site(s) in CRT is only the beginning of rethinking multisite pacing. Conceptual trials are needed to enhance the hemodynamic response of CRT if the indications are to increase for a wider patient population. New nonsurgical approaches to optimize the LV pacing site is one consideration to determine the possible role of more than two pacing sites.

References

1. Cazeau S, Leclercq C, Lavergne T, et al. Effects of multisite biventricular pacing in patients with heart failure and intraventricular conduction delay. N Engl J Med 2001;344:873–80.
2. Abraham WT, Fisher WG, Smith AL, et al. Cardiac resynchronization in chronic heart failure. N Engl J Med 2002;346:1845–53.
3. Cleland GJF, Daubert J-C, Erdman E, et al. The effect of resynchronization on morbidity and mortality in heart failure. N Eng J Med 2005;352:1539–49.
4. Carson P, Anand I, O'Connor C, et al. Mode of death in advanced heart failure: The comparison of medical, pacing and defibrillation therapy in heart failure (companion) trial. J Am Coll Cardiol 2005;46:2329–34.
5. Garrigue S, Reuter S, Labeque JN, et al. Usefulness of biventricular pacing in patients with congestive heart failure and right bundle branch block. Am J Cardiol 2001;88:1436–41.
6. Sogaard P, Egeblad H, Kim Y, et al. Tissue Doppler Imaging predicts improved systolic performance and reversed left ventricular remodeling during long term cardiac resynchronisation therapy. J Am Coll Cardiol 2002;40:723–30.
7. Auricchio A, Kein H, Tockman B, et al. Transvenous biventricular pacing for heart failure : can the obstacles be overcome? Am J Cardiol 1999;83(suppl):136D–142D.
8. Alonso C, Leclercq C, Victor F, et al. Electrocardiographic predictive factors of long-term clinical improvement with multisite biventricular pacing in advanced heart failure. Am J Cardiol 1999;84:1417–21.
9. Ansalone G, Giannantoni P, Ricci R, et al. Doppler myocardial imaging to evaluate the effectiveness of pacing sites in patients receiving biventricular pacing. J Am Coll Cardiol 2002;39:489–99.
10. Connolly SJ, Kerr CR, Gent M, et al. Effects of physiologic pacing versus ventricular pacing on the risk of stroke and death due to cardiovascular causes. N Eng J Med 2000;342:1385–91.
11. Lamas GA, Lee KL, Sweeney MO, et al. Ventricular pacing or dual-chamber pacing for sinus node dysfunction. N Engl J Med 2002;346:1854–62.

12. Lamas GA, Orav EJ, Stambler BS, et al. Quality of life and clinical outcomes in elderly patients treated with ventricular pacing as compared with dual-chamber pacing. N Engl J Med 1998;338:1097–104.

13. Toff WD, Camm AJ, Skehan JD, et al. Single-chamber pacing versus dual-chamber pacing for high-grade atrioventricular block. N Engl J Med 2005;353:145–55.

14. Link MS, Helkamp AS, Estes NAM III, et al. High incidence of pacemaker syndrome in patients with sinus node dysfunction treated with ventricular-based pacing in the Mode Selection Trial (MOST). J Am Coll Cardiol 2004;43:2066–71.

15. Sweeney MO, Helkamp AS, Ellenbogen KA, et al. Adverse effect of ventricular pacing on heart failure and atrial fibrillation among patients with with a normal baseline QRS in a clinical trial of pacemaker therapy for sinus node dysfunction. Circulation 2003;107:2932–7.

16. Wilkoff BL, Cook JR, Epstein AE, et al. Dual-chamber pacing or ventricular backup pacing in patients with an implantable defibrillator for: The Dual Chamber and VVI Implantable Defibrillator (DAVID) trial. JAMA 2002;288:3115–23.

17. Thambo JB, Bordachar P, Garrigue S, et al. Detrimental ventricular remodelling in patients with congenital complete heart block and chronic right ventricular apical pacing. Circulation 2004;110:3766–72.

18. Karpawitch PP, Rabah R, Hass JE. Altered cardiac histology following apical right ventricular pacing in patients with congenital atrioventricular block. Pacing Clin Electrophysiol 1999;22:1372–7.

19. Spraag DD, Leclercq C, Loghmani M, et al. Regional alterations in protein expression in the dyssynchronous failing heart. Circulation 2003;108(8):929–32.

20. Alonso C, Goscinska K, Ritter P, et al. Upgrading to triple-ventricular pacing guided by clinical outcomes and echo assessment; a pilot study (abstract). Europace 2004;6(suppl 1):195.

21. Sogaard P, Egeblad H, Pedersen AK, et al. Sequential versus simultaneous biventricular resynchronization for severe heart failure. Circulation 2002;106:2078–84.

22. Jauvert G, Cazeau S, Alonso C, et al. Does programmability of the interventricular delay in biventricular pacing improve cardiac asynchrony? [abstract] Europace 2002;3(suppl A):204.

23. De Cock CC, Giudici MC, Twisk JW. Comparaison of the haemodynamic effects of right ventricular outflow-tract pacing with ventricular apex pacing. A quantitative review. Europace 2003;5:275–8.

24. Orchetta E, Bortnik M, Magnani A, et al. Prevention of ventricular desynchronization by permanent para-Hisian pacing after atrioventricular node ablation in chronic atrial fibrillation: A crossover, blinded, randomized study versus apical right ventricular pacing. J Am Coll Cardiol 2006;47:1938–45.

25. Savouré A, Fröhlig G, Galley D, et al. A new dual-chamber pacing mode to minimize ventricular pacing. Pacing Clin Electrophysiol 2005;28:S43–S46.

26. Sweeney MO, Ellenbogen KA, Casavant D, et al. Multicenter, prospective, randomised safety and efficacy study of a new atrial-based managed ventricular pacing mode (MVP) in dual-chamber ICDs. J Cardiovasc Electrophysiol 2005;16:1–7.

27. Kindermann M, Hennen B, Jung J, et al. Biventricular versus conventional right ventricular stimulation for patients with standard pacing indication and left ventricular dysfunction: The Homburg Biventricular Pacing Evaluation (HOBIPACE). J Am Coll Cardiol 2006;16;47:1927–37.

28. Hoijer CJ, Meurling C, Brandt J. Upgrade to biventricular pacing in patients with conventional pacemakers and heart failure: A double-blind, randomized crossover study. Europace 2006;8(1):51–5.

29. Yu CM, Chau E, Sanderson JE, et al. Tissue Doppler echocardiographic evidence of reverse remodelling and improved synchronicity by simultaneously delaying regional contraction after biventricular pacing therapy in heart failure. Circulation 2002;105:438–45.

Alternative Means of Achieving Cardiac Resynchronization

Michael O. Sweeney

Importance of Achieving an Optimal Stimulation Site for Cardiac Resynchronization Therapy

The optimal site for left ventricular (LV) pacing is an unsettled and complex consideration. It is probably true that the optimal site varies between patients and is likely to be modified by venous anatomy, regional and global LV mechanical function, myocardial substrate, characterization of electrical delay, and other factors. In patients with abnormal ventricular conduction due to left bundle branch block and systolic heart failure, the stimulation site influences the response to LV pacing. The success of resynchronization is dependent on pacing from a site that causes a change in the sequence of ventricular activation that translates to an improvement in cardiac performance. Such systolic improvement and mechanical resynchronization does not require electrical synchrony [1] and explains the lack of correlation between change in QRS duration and clinical response to cardiac resynchronization therapy (CRT) [2]. Ideally, the pacing site or sites that produce the greatest hemodynamic effect would be selected.

However, current clinical evidence permits some generalizations regarding LV pacing site selection for optimal acute hemodynamic response. Multiple independent investigations comparing the acute and chronic effects of different pacing sites in similar dilated cardiomyopathy populations have reported concordant evidence that stimulation site is a primary determinant of CRT hemodynamic benefit.

Auricchio et al. [3,4] showed a positive correlation between the magnitude of pulse pressure and LV +dP/dt increases and left ventricular pacing site. The percent increases in pulse pressure and LV +dP/dt averaged over all atrioventricular (AV) delays were significantly larger at midlateral free wall LV epicardial pacing sites compared with any other sample left ventricular region. Furthermore, increases at the midanterior sites were smaller than all other sites.

These observations were extended in an analysis of 30 patients enrolled in the PATH-CHF II trial [5]. Left ventricular stimulation was delivered at the lateral free wall or midanterior wall. Free wall sites yielded significantly larger improvements in LV +dP/dt and pulse pressure than anterior sites. Furthermore, in one third of patients, stimulation at anterior sites worsened acute LV hemodynamic performance, whereas free wall stimulation improved it, and the opposite pattern was never observed. This difference in acute hemodynamic response correlated with intrinsic conduction delays. This may be interpreted as evidence that stimulating a later-activated LV region produces a larger response because it more effectively restores regional activation synchrony. Thus, the negative effect of anterior wall stimulation at all AV delays in some patients may be due to preexcitation of an already relatively early-activated site thereby exaggerating intraventricular dyssynchrony [6].

Stimulation at the latest electrically activated (most delayed) region of the LV is associated with greatest hemodynamic response. This is usually on the posterior or posterolateral-basal wall as demonstrated by endocardial voltage mapping [7–9] and Doppler myocardial imaging [10, 11]. CRT with stimulation at a LV free wall site consistently improves short-term systolic function more than stimulation at an anterior site does. Lateral or posterolateral LV vein lead positions are associated with acute improvements in +dP/dt and pulse pressure [3, 5, 12], significant chronic improvements in functional capacity and ventricular function [13, 14], and possibly mortality compared with anterior vein sites in some [14] but not other studies [13]. However, within a specific coronary vein, the hemodynamic response to LV stimulation at different sites from apex to base is heterogenous, suggesting that optimization of specific pacing sites within a target vein might be necessary for optimal CRT response [12].

It is likely, then, that inadequate LV lead positions contribute significantly to CRT nonresponse. In the MIRACLE study, a lateral or posterolateral vein site was obtained in only 77% of patients, whereas the anterior interventricular vein or middle cardiac vein were used in 19.5% and 4.5% of patients, respectively. A similar situation was reported in the VENTAK CHF/CONTAK CD study where a lateral or posterolateral vein site was obtained in 67% of patients and an anterior interventricular vein site in the remaining 33% [15]. Furthermore, even among patients in whom the transvenous approach failed, necessitating surgical placement of LV leads, a lateral or posterolateral site was obtained in only 34%, whereas the remaining 66% were placed in the anterior or apical LV positions [15]. Thus, even in randomized clinical trials (RCTs) of CRT, as many as 23–33% of patients receive LV stimulation from a suboptimal site. It is conceivable that some of these patients were actually made worse by CRT due to LV pacing in the anterior vein, particularly those with relatively narrow QRSd (less than 150 ms) [5]. These differences in LV stimulation sites may partly account for the varied results and large individual difference observed among clinical studies.

Methods for identifying the best site during implantation are not yet of proven clinical benefit. Furthermore, even if optimal LV pacing sites could be identified a priori, access to such sites is potentially constrained by variations in coronary venous anatomy. The coronary venous circulation demonstrates considerably more variability than the parallel arterial circulation. Careful surveys of retrograde coronary venography have revealed that the anterior interventricular vein is present in 99% of patients and the middle cardiac vein is present in 100% [16, 17]. These veins are generally undesirable for resynchronization therapy because they do not reach the late-activated portion of the LV free wall. Unfortunately, approximately 50% of patients have only a single vein serving the LV free wall [18]. Anatomically, this is a lateral marginal vein in slightly more than 75% and a true posterior vein that ascends the free wall in approximately 50% of patients [17].

Conventional Approach to CRT

Early attempts at LV pacing via the coronary veins were done with conventional endocardial pacing leads and unassisted coronary sinus (CS) cannulation [19]. This was only possible with stylet-driven leads and required considerable technical prowess. Conventional endocardial pacing leads were poorly suited to LV pacing via the coronary veins. The technique mandated selective bending of stylets to achieve a favorable shape of the tip of the lead to permit CS cannulation. Additional stylet shapes were necessary to permit engagement of the ostium of first- and second-order coronary venous branches. The electrodes, particularly the anodal ring of bipolar leads, prevented cornering of tortuous target vein take-offs. Even if the tip of such leads could be manipulated into the ostium of first-order target veins, the cross-sectional diameter of the lead body often exceeded the luminal diameter of the vein and prevented advancement. Ironically, the only relative merit of conventional pacing leads was the larger cross-sectional diameter that assisted with passive fixation within a target vein.

The contemporary conventional approach to CRT uses specially designed delivery sheaths and tools for cannulating the coronary sinus in order to permit delivery of pacing leads into the epicardial coronary venous circulation. Experienced implanters using currently available tools and using techniques and leads specifically designed for coronary veins can achieve optimal LV stimulation in >90% of cases. The techniques for transvenous delivery of CRT have been previously described [20].

Obstacles to Achieving Conventional Transvenous LV Lead Placement

Complex and unpredictable anatomic and technical considerations may preclude successful delivery of the LV lead to an optimal pacing site. These include inability to cannulate the CS and first- or second-order target veins, unacceptably high epicardial pacing thresholds, and a high incidence of lead dislodgment.

Ideally, a suboptimal LV lead position should be identified and rejected at the time of implantation. The most common mistake of the uninformed or uncommitted implanter is to place the LV lead in the anterior vein and "see how the patient does." If a patient is not responding to CRT and the LV lead is in the anterior vein, an attempt to reposition the LV lead (or a different lead) in a lateral vein should be made. If this is not possible due to limitations in coronary venous anatomy or other insuperable technical obstacles (see below), the patient should be referred for surgical placement of the LV lead in an optimal location.

Inability to Localize or Cannulate the CS Ostium

It is difficult to estimate the true percentage of cases in which the coronary sinus cannot be cannulated because this is clearly influenced by operator experience. It is probably in the range of 1–5%. Besides operator inexperience, several anatomic situations may render localization of the CS ostium problematic. These include an unusually high or low position of the CS ostium or, very rarely, absence of the CS orifice. Some implanters advocate bolus contrast injections to visualize the CS ostium. The presence of myocardial staining with visible trabeculations indicates that the CS sheath (and guide catheter) is in the right ventricle (RV), whereas the absence of trabecular staining indicates an atrial position. It is often difficult, however, to achieve adequate opacification of the right atrium (RA) with small volume (10–20 cm^3) hand injections due to swirling of blood within the enlarged RA and torrential competitive flow out of the CS. In this situation, equipment for performing a power injection may be particularly useful.

Cannulation of the CS ostium can be facilitated by a working knowledge of the right heart anatomy. The CS ostium is bounded inferiorly by the Thebesian valve and on the atrial side by the Eustachian ridge. The Thebesian valve is usually thin and crescent-shaped in about one third of hearts but multiple variations have been described, including fibrous bands, strands, filigree network, and large redundant "fishnets" continuous with a Chiari network [21]. In one autopsy study, large membrane-like Thebesian valves almost completely occluded the CS ostium in 25% of specimens [22].

These structures tend to impede forward progress of the CS sheath and coronary guide catheter (or deflectable catheter) when approached from the atrial side. On the other hand, these structures (in particular, the Eustachian ridge) tend to direct the CS sheath and guide catheters into the ostium when approached from the ventricular side. Therefore, in difficult cases, it is useful to advance the tip of the CS sheath and guide catheters into the RV then rotate counterclockwise during gradual withdrawal so as to encounter the CS ostium. If this approach fails, an adaptation of the inferior approach described for complex electrophysiology procedures is often successful in localizing the CS ostium. Alternately, intracardiac ultrasound can be used to assist localization of the CS ostium.

Having localized the CS ostium, it is sometimes very difficult to advance the guide catheter or sheath due to kinking at the neck of the CS. This is most commonly encountered with a "goose neck" proximal CS, which is often associated with massive cardiomegaly. This can result in sheath kinking that prevents LV lead passage. This problem has been virtually eliminated by braided sheath designs (see above discussion of sheaths). Rarely, a combined inferior and superior approach is needed to overcome sheath kinking in the proximal CS. A deflectable electrophysiology catheter is placed in the CS ostium from the inferior approach and downward pressure is applied to "straighten" the "goose neck" segment. This may permit advancement of the CS sheath and guide catheters from the superior approach.

Coronary Venous Anatomy: Absent or Seemingly Inaccessible Target Veins

Despite rapid evolution of implantation techniques including guiding sheaths and catheters and over-the-wire (OTW) delivery systems, a suitable pacing site on the LV free wall cannot be achieved in 20–30% of patients. In many patients, this is simply because of absence of coronary veins reaching the LV free wall. In some instances, target veins are present but too small for cannulation with existing lead systems or paradoxically too large to achieve mechanical fixation with reduced-diameter LV leads that rely primarily on "wedging" the lead tip into a distal site within the target vein for fixation such that the outer diameter of the lead closely approximates the inner luminal diameter of the vein.

Preventing and Overcoming High LV Stimulation Thresholds and Phrenic Nerve Stimulation

The principal limitation of the transvenous approach is that the selection of sites for pacing is entirely dictated by navigable coronary venous anatomy. A commonly encountered problem is that an apparently suitable target vein delivers the lead to a site where ventricular capture can be achieved at only very high output voltages or not at all, rendering potentially optimal target veins unsuitable for use. This presumably relates to the presence of scar on the epicardial surface of the heart underlying the target vein or inadequate contact with the epicardial surface and cannot be anticipated by fluoroscopic examination a priori. Occasionally, mapping of the proximal segment of such veins will yield sites with suitable capture thresholds. Upsizing of the LV lead, or use of a lead with a self-retaining S-shape or cant, may be required to achieve mechanical stability depending on the characteristics of the original lead selected. Similarly, before abandoning such veins, a subselective venogram should be performed because potentially useful tertiary branches are often not visualized during main body CS injection due to low flow and systolic compression. Such tertiary branches may serve a region of myocardium with an acceptable pacing threshold. Depending upon the size of the tertiary branch, downsizing of the LV lead to a purely OTW design may be necessary if not originally used. If this is not successful, surgical placement of LV leads permits more detailed mapping of viable sites in the anatomic region of interest.

A second common problem is that the target vein delivers the lead to a site that results in phrenic nerve stimulation and diaphragmatic pacing. Careful examination of cadaver hearts demonstrates that the phrenic nerve passes over the lateral coronary veins in ~80% of specimens and over the anterior interventricular vein in the remaining ~20% [23]. This presents a high probability of anatomic conflict between the optimal site for LV stimulation and unacceptable phrenic nerve stimulation. Phrenic stimulation can be difficult to demonstrate during implantation when the patient is supine and sedated but may be immediately evident when the patient is later active and changes body positions, even in the absence of lead dislodgment. It is important to recognize that once phrenic nerve stimulation is observed acutely (during implantation), it is almost invariably encountered during follow-up despite manipulation of output voltages, and therefore alternative site LV pacing is sought. As with high LV capture thresholds, phrenic nerve stimulation can often be overcome by repositioning the LV lead more proximally within the target vein. Occasionally, if there is a significant differential in the capture thresholds for phrenic nerve stimulation versus LV capture, this can be overcome by manipulation of LV voltage output in CRT-pacing (CRTP) or CRT-defibrillation (CRTD) devices that permit separate RV and LV outputs. More recently, some LV leads have two electrodes that permit selection of specific LV sites for dual cathodal biventricular stimulation, biventricular stimulation with true bipolar

LV stimulation, or true bipolar LV only univentricular stimulation. It has not been convincingly demonstrated that true bipolar LV stimulation reliably overcomes phrenic stimulation compared with dual cathodal or unipolar LV pacing. On the other hand, selecting alternate LV electrodes for dual cathodal biventricular stimulation may occasionally overcome phrenic stimulation by altering the LV–RV pacing vector. This can be achieved noninvasively using some pulse generators and is referred to as *electronic repositioning*. In either case, the problem of phrenic nerve stimulation is more reliably addressed by LV lead repositioning at implant. If phrenic stimulation during attempted transvenous LV pacing cannot be overcome by any means, surgical placement of LV leads should be considered. Phrenic stimulation can occur with surgically placed epicardial leads if careful visualization of the course of the nerve sheath is not performed prior to fixation. Chronic development of phrenic nerve stimulation results in permanent loss of CRT in about 1–2% of patients [24].

Loss of CRT Due to Differential LV Capture Threshold Rise

There is relatively limited data on long-term pacing thresholds with transvenous or thoracotomy leads for LV pacing. Loss of ventricular capture occurred in 10% of patients in the VENTAK CHF/CONTAK CD study and was the second most common cause of interrupted CRT [24]. Three quarters of these cases were due to gross dislodgment of the LV lead, whereas 23% were due to chronic pacing threshold elevation that was overcome by increasing voltage output in the majority of cases. The reasons for chronic increase in transvenous LV pacing thresholds are not well characterized. Possible explanations include "microdislodgment" not evident by radiographic examination or exit block that occurs as a consequence of inadequate mechanical stability. Hansky et al. [25] have pointed out that an important technique-related factor to postoperative increase in pacing thresholds is an unstable, but not grossly dislodged, lead position. This is based on speculation that repetitive chronic endothelial injuries due to "rocking" of the lead tip may result in progressive fibrotic reorganization of the adjacent vessel wall. It is also possible that late rises in previously acceptable transvenous LV thresholds relate to implantation technique. Aggressive lead manipulations, repeated lead exchanges, or guide-wire maneuvers may traumatize the endothelium of the target vein resulting in a fibrotic reaction, thrombosis, or dissection, all of which may degrade the pacing threshold.

Loss of CRT Due to Lead Dislodgment

Acute dislodgment of right atrial and right ventricular electrodes is uncommon, particularly with active fixation leads, although this is not a specific issue of CRT implantation. The incidence of LV lead dislodgment is considerably higher and has a reported incidence of 5–10% in larger studies [26–28]. This relates to implanter experience and other technical factors such as the lack of fixation mechanisms and stresses placed on the proximal portion of the lead at the junction of the right atrium and CS ostium. Lead dislodgments are readily identified by change in QRS duration and morphology on 12-lead electrocardiogram (ECG) as well as by chest radiography but usually suspected on the basis of device interrogation that discloses a significant decline in local signal amplitude and/or change in pacing capture threshold. Typically, RA leads dislodge onto the floor of the RA, and RV leads dislodge toward the inflow of the RV. LV leads typically dislodge into the main body of the CS and less commonly into the RA.

Several techniques reduce the chance of LV lead dislodgment. Probably of most importance is an optimal match between the diameter of the LV lead and the luminal diameter of the target vein. Support at multiple (>2–3) positions increases mechanical stability. Larger leads with preformed shapes should be advanced sufficiently within the target vein to completely unfold. In the case of the smallest diameter purely OTW leads, it is useful to position the tip in a tertiary branch to achieve support at more than one position and increase mechanical stability.

Nonconventional and Alternative Approaches to CRT

In all of these situations where the conventional coronary venous approach fails due to seemingly insuperable anatomic constraints, nonconventional approaches may be useful to achieve successful LV pacing. A brief survey of these approaches includes (1) left vein pacing using telescoping sheaths, (2) coronary venoplasty and stents to facilitate lead placement and enhance mechanical stability, (3) active fixation leads to achieve mechanical stability, (4) transvenous LV endocardial pacing via transseptal puncture, (5) surgical placement of epicardial LV pacing leads, and (6) transcutaneous or transvenous approaches to the pericardial space for LV pacing. Multisite ("bifocal") RV pacing has been touted as an alternative to LV pacing for CRT; however, this will be discussed separately in view of dubious physiologic rationale and limited clinical exposure.

Left Vein Pacing Using Telescoping Sheaths

Another commonly encountered difficulty in transvenous LV lead placement is tortuosity of the target vessel take-off or main segment. These anatomic constraints can be extremely difficult to overcome and often require the use of multiple LV lead designs and delivery systems not specifically designed for this application. Large-diameter stylet-driven leads are likely to fail in this situation, and most implanters reflexively select the smallest diameter OTW lead upon inspection of the coronary venogram.

One approach uses coronary, renal, or other angiography catheters to selectively cannulate the small and tortuous target vein. Advancement of a percutaneous coronary intervention (PCI) guide wire will often straighten the tortuous segment of the vein permitting navigation with an OTW LV lead. Occasionally, the OTW lead cannot be advanced through the proximal segment despite a straight path of the guide wire. The likely explanation in this situation is that the guide wire has not truly straightened the tortuous segment of the target vein. This is more likely when the target vein has a relatively large diameter. In these conditions, the very-small-diameter guide wire may pursue a straight course through the vessel lumen without exerting any effective straightening pressure on the wall of the vein. Occasionally, this can be overcome by using a stiffer guide wire. However, more often, significant resistance to lead advancement persists despite a stiffer guide wire and a "buddy wire technique" is required. This refers to one or more guide wires placed alongside the first, which may sufficiently straighten the vein to permit lead advancement. After successful placement of the LV lead but before sheath removal, the "buddy wires" are removed.

Despite these techniques, proximal segment tortuosity may persist and prevent advancement of even the smallest diameter OTW leads. An alternative technique that many experienced implanters have adopted as the first-line approach to this situation is the use of telescoping sheaths. Subselection of the target vein with an inner guiding sheath permits straightening of the tortuous proximal segment and direct delivery of the LV lead. This approach often eliminates the use of a guide wire altogether and permits delivery of large-diameter stylet-driven leads if desired, which would otherwise likely fail in this situation.

Telescoping sheaths may require the use of a larger diameter (i.e., 9 F) CS sheath. The target vein is typically cannulated with a stiff PCI guide wire as described above. A smaller diameter straight CS sheath is then advanced over the guide wire into the proximal segment of the target vein. Often, the PCI guide wire does not provide enough support for advancement of the inner straight sheath into the target vein. This can be overcome either by using multiple PCI guide wires or, preferably, a floppy-tipped 0.035-gauge guide wire. Occasionally, the inner straight sheath cannot be advanced into the target vein using any guide-wire technique. In this situation, an angiography catheter can be placed within the inner sheath (triple catheter/sheath approach) (Fig. 4.1). An angiography catheter that closely approximates the shape of the tortuous proximal segment of the target vein should be chosen. A "shepherd's hook" renal angiography catheter is particularly well suited to this requirement. The tip of the angiography catheter is manipulated into the target vein using puffs of contrast if needed. A floppy-tipped 0.035-gauge

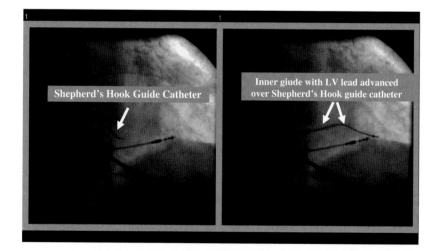

Fig. 4.1 "Triple catheter/sheath" for straightening tortuous proximal coronary veins. *Left:* 5-F shepherd's hook renal angiography catheter has engaged the ostium of a posterolateral vein. *Right:* Inner straight sheath is advanced over the angiography catheter, which was supported distally by an 0.035-gauge floppy-tip guide wire (not shown). Guide wire and angiography catheter are removed, and LV lead is delivered directly through the inner straight sheath.

guide wire is then placed for distal support. The inner straight sheath can then be advanced over the stiff angiography catheter, definitively straightening the tortuous proximal segment. The floppy-tipped guide wire and angiography catheter are then removed, and the LV lead of choice is delivered directly through the inner straight sheath. The inner straight sheath is then cut away using techniques previously described.

Some comments are necessary to reduce complications and increase success of the telescoping sheath technique. First, the patient should be prepped for urgent pericardiocentesis and thoracotomy (which is generally recommended for CRT implantation). Second, excessive force should not be applied to any guide wire or sheath within the coronary veins. Pressure on the vessel wall may causes tension and reduce the normal distensibility of the vein, increasing the probability of perforation. Resistance to advancement of the inner sheath (within or without an inner guide catheter for support) should sponsor a contrast injection to assess the mechanical situation. Third, the inner sheath should have a relatively soft tip segment. Lastly, the telescoping sheath technique should not be applied to small-diameter veins (i.e., <3–3.5 mm).

The telescoping sheath technique may not be ideally suited to lateral coronary veins that arise beyond the proximal one-third of the main body CS. Inability to apply forward axial pressure typically results in failure of this approach, despite the extra support of an 0.035-gauge guide wire or an angiography guide catheter. Additionally, straight LV sheaths are typically not long enough to reach the proximal segments of lateral veins that arise beyond the proximal one-third of the CS.

Therefore, the telescoping sheath technique is most useful for posterolateral veins that arise within 1–3 cm of the CS ostium. This approach is particularly helpful in the situation where the middle cardiac vein and posterolateral vein share a common ostium within the proximal neck of the CS. This anatomic arrangement poses a unique problem for LV lead placement using a single sheath. In order to permit cannulation of the target vein ostium with the LV lead or guide wire, the sheath must be withdrawn to within 1 cm or less of the CS ostium. This commonly results in abrupt dislodgment of the sheath to the floor of the right atrium, pulling the LV lead and guide wire along with it. Occasionally, using a stylet-driven lead and intentionally withdrawing the LV sheath from the CS in a controlled manner can defeat this. The lead is advanced to the midportion of the CS, and the sheath and lead are simultaneously withdrawn while rotating the lead tip into the ostium of the target vein. Attention must be paid to the point when the sheath exits the CS ostium so as to avoid the creation of a redundancy in the LV lead body that could result in prolapse onto the right atrial floor.

Alternatively, a variation of the telescoping sheath approach is often successful in the "common ostium" situation (Figs. 4.2–4.4). An inner guide catheter with a 45- to 60-degree tip angle (i.e., Bern or Berenstein) is advanced through the inner straight sheath (triple catheter/sheath approach) to the mid-CS. The outer LV sheath is withdrawn over the inner straight sheath until it has exited the CS ostium. The inner straight sheath and inner guide catheter are then simultaneously withdrawn while rotating the guide catheter tip until the ostium of the target vein is engaged. A floppy-tipped 0.035-gauge guide wire is advanced into the target vein, followed by the inner guide catheter and the inner straight sheath. The outer LV sheath is essentially irrelevant

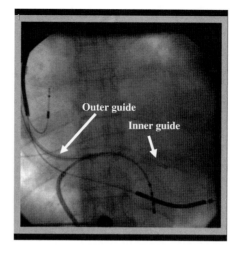

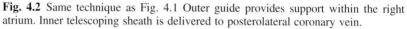

Fig. 4.2 Same technique as Fig. 4.1 Outer guide provides support within the right atrium. Inner telescoping sheath is delivered to posterolateral coronary vein.

at this point and can be withdrawn to the mid right atrium. The inner guide catheter and guide wire are removed, and the LV lead is delivered directly into the target vein through the inner straight sheath. The inner straight sheath and outer sheath are removed in the usual manner. Though these postero-lateral veins present unique challenges to LV lead placement, they often yield mechanically stable positions because of the relatively straight course pursued from the low right atrium through the proximal coronary sinus to the lateral LV wall.

Inner guide catheters specifically packaged for coronary venous application are available. Some of these guide catheters have a deflectable tip to enhance subselection of target veins. These inner guide catheters serve a similar role as the coronary and renal angiographic catheters adapted for this role as described previously. Their primary purpose is to assist with delivery of

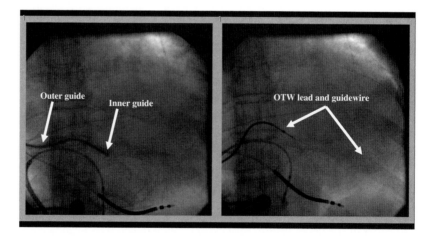

Fig. 4.3 Continuation of technique in Fig. 4.2 *Left:* Inner telescoping sheath in target vein. *Right:* Lead tip and guide wire in target vein.

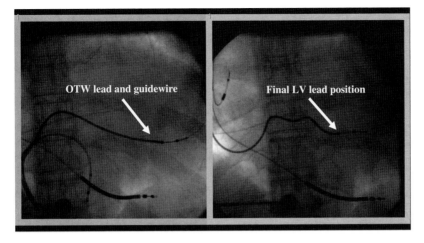

Fig. 4.4 Continuation of technique in Figs. 4.2and 4.3 *Left:* Lead advanced over guide wire. *Right:* Final LV lead placement in posterolateral vein via an inner straight sheath.

a guide wire to the target vein. More recently, inner sheaths of sufficient diameter to deliver LV leads directly have been developed. These have several different distal segment shapes (hockey stick, multipurpose, hook) intended to match patterns of coronary venous take-off anatomy (Figs. 4.5 and 4.6). Such inner sheaths are particularly useful for low-lying posterior and posterolateral veins but typically do not provide sufficient for use with mid and high lateral veins.

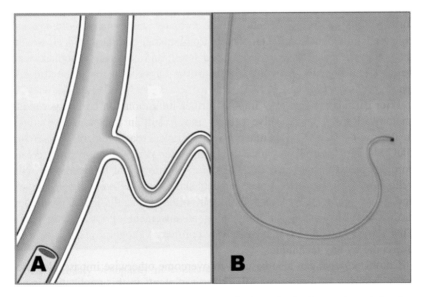

Fig. 4.5 Hockey stick preformed inner sheath for subselecting and straightening tortuous proximal target veins. *Left:* Tortuous proximal segment of target vein. *Right:* Hockey stick inner sheath.

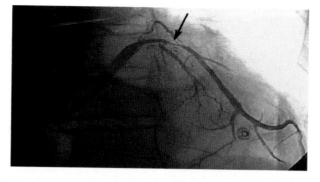

Fig. 4.9 Coronary stenting to obtain access to primary target vessel for LV lead placement [30]. Stenotic segment in proximal target vein (*arrow*).

This approach should be considered with great cautious as stent struts may damage lead insulation and probably render nonsurgical extraction of chronic coronary venous leads impossible due to the danger of vessel rupture.

Active Fixation Leads in the Coronary Venous System

More recently, enhancements to lead design have been directed at combining the maneuverability of smaller-diameter leads with the mechanical stability of large leads. This is achieved by incorporating reversible, self-retaining S- or pigtail-shaped curves at the lead tip, which increase the "effective" diameter of smaller leads for mechanical stability without degrading maneuverability.

The use of true active fixation pacing leads to achieve mechanical stability in the coronary venous system when all other approaches fail has recently been described. In one technique, a 4-F lumenless, catheter-delivered, fixed helix activation fixation pacing lead designed for endocardial use has been successfully and safely used in the coronary venous system. (B. Hansky, personal communication). The lead is delivered through a Judkins right coronary guide catheter within a conventional CS sheath (Figs. 4.14–4.16). The tip of the coronary guide catheter is used to deliver the lead only to the epicardial circumference of the vein in large-caliber veins and proximal segments. A key matter appears to be the choice of active fixation lead. Stiffer leads with preformed bends may be less desirable because they may adapt the distal vein

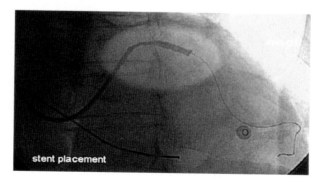

Fig. 4.10 Coronary stenting to obtain access to primary target vessel for LV lead placement [30]. Successful deployment of stent across stenotic segment in target vein.

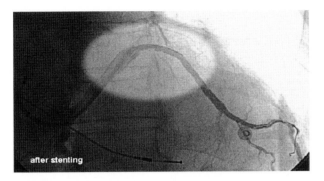

Fig. 4.11 Coronary stenting to obtain access to primary target vessel for LV lead placement [30]. Post-stenting contrast flow in target vein.

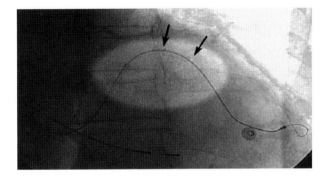

Fig. 4.12 Coronary stenting to obtain access to primary target vessel for LV lead placement [30]. Successful placement of LV lead across stent (*arrows*) in target vein.

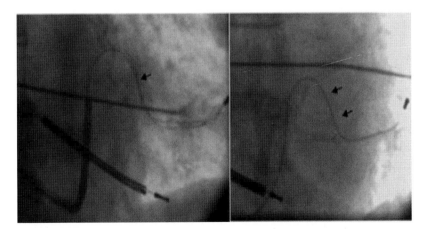

Fig. 4.13 Coronary stenting (*arrows*) to achieve mechanical stability in the coronary venous system [31].

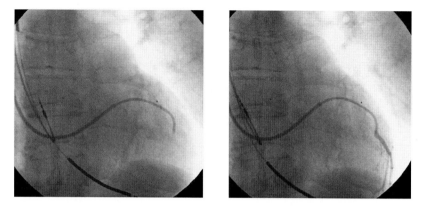

Fig. 4.14 Active fixation leads in the CS (B. Hansky, personal communication). *Left:* Right coronary guide catheter in target vein. *Right:* Venogram of target vein via right coronary guide.

to the lead, resulting in pericardial stimulation without ventricular capture or poor ventricular pacing thresholds. Many obvious questions regarding safety, long-term performance, and approach to removal will arise. Only the most experienced implanters should attempt such exotic approaches to coronary venous pacing.

Transvenous Endocardial LV Pacing

Transvenous left ventricular endocardial pacing via transseptal puncture has been described in the rare circumstance where neither the transvenous epicardial nor surgical options are viable. This was originally described using a right superior approach via the internal jugular vein. A conventional active fixation lead was placed across the mitral valve and on the LV endocardium, and the lead body was tunneled over the clavicle to the pectoral pocket [32–34]. More recently, a technique for a left superior approach entirely within the subclavicular venous system has been described Similar to the right

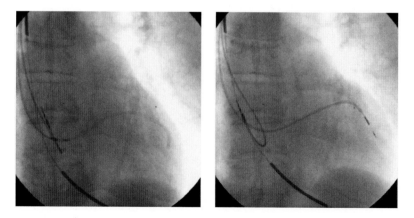

Fig. 4.15 Active fixation leads in the CS (B. Hansky, personal communication). *Left:* Right coronary guide catheter in target vein. *Right:* Delivery of active fix lead through coronary guide catheter.

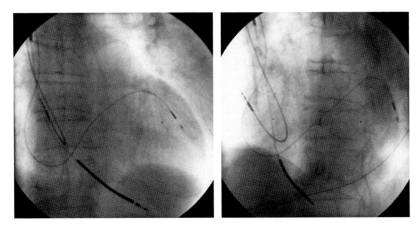

Fig. 4.16 Active fixation leads in the CS (B. Hansky, personal communication). Anterior-posterior (*left*) and left oblique (*right*) view of active fix lead in coronary vein.

superior approach, a standard transseptal puncture via the right femoral vein is performed first [35]. This serves to mark the site for a second transseptal puncture using a peel-away sheath via the left axillary vein. This approach requires manual reshaping of the transseptal needle (with the stylet inside the needle) to allow passage through the innominate vein, superior vena cava–right atrial junction, and then engage the fossa ovalis (Fig. 4.17).

Obviously, both approaches are suitable only in the hands of the most skilled implanters. Although there is some suggestion that LV endocardial pacing may have some physiologic advantages relative to epicardial pacing during CRT [32], there is insufficient experience to comment on the relative risks and benefits of this approach. Major concerns with this approach include thromboembolism and mitral valve disruptions related to the permanent presence of a pacing lead in the LV.

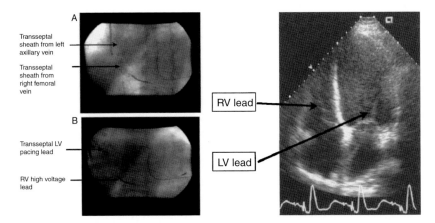

Fig. 4.17 LV endocardial pacing via transseptal puncture [35]. *Left:* Anterior-posterior view. *Right:* Apical four-chamber view of LV endocardial lead via transseptal puncture.

Cardiac Surgical Approach for LV Lead Placement

Left ventricular pacing lead placement can also be achieved under direct visualization using a cardiac surgical approach. The first clinical trial of CRT used a hybrid epicardial LV, endocardial RV pacing lead configuration for multisite ventricular stimulation simply because the technique for transvenous epicardial LV pacing had not been developed [36]. Currently, the cardiac surgical approach is almost exclusively confined to the situation where all other available approaches fail.

Because LV lead placement by the cardiac surgical approach is not limited by the coronary venous anatomy, the ability to achieve an optimal LV pacing site is often touted as a technical advantage. However, even using minimally invasive approaches, the surgical trauma is quite significant and far greater than that associated with the transvenous epicardial LV pacing. The physical stress of this approach on the patient with advanced systolic heart failure should not be underestimated. One critical difference in patient preparation for surgical versus transvenous LV lead placement is that it is better to have the patient a little "dry" (well diuresed) in the former and a little "wet" (diuretics withheld) in the latter. In the case of the transvenous approach, adequate hydration may minimize the risk of contrast-induced renal failure (see above). In contrast, during the surgical approach, volume overload may increase lung volume. This increases the hemodynamic consequences of single-lung ventilation, particularly on right heart function, and may limit LV visualization if complete left lung deflation cannot be achieved. Acute right heart failure complicated by ventricular arrhythmias and requiring cardiopulmonary resuscitation can occur during single-lung ventilation in the decompensated patient.

The approach to surgical implantation of epicardial LV leads depends on whether the reason is planned cardiothoracic surgery (i.e., coronary revascularization, valve repair/replacement) or because of failed transvenous approach for any reason. Epicardial lead placement during surgical procedures that use a standard sternotomy may be compromised by an inability to guarantee sufficient surgical exposure to the posterobasal LV wall. Epicardial lead placement during mitral valve repair from a right para-sternotomy approach may be impossible. In either situation, the surgeon must be willing to lift and rotate the heart to expose the posterobasal LV. The relative relationship of the phrenic nerve and LV pacing sites may be difficult to evaluate visually, and careful stimulation testing with the lungs inflated and heart filled while still on cardiopulmonary bypass is necessary to exclude extracardiac stimulation.

The surgical approach to de novo epicardial LV lead placement is quite different. Many surgeons still use a full left lateral thoracotomy, which permits full visualization of the posterobasal LV wall but results in significant postoperative pain and an extended recovery period. Using a limited left lateral thoracotomy can reduce these consequences. In this approach, the patient is prepped lying on his or her right side with left arm suspended over their head. A 4- to 5-cm incision is made in the left axillary space for access to the posterobasal LV wall (Figs. 4.18 and 4.19). Two epicardial LV leads are typically placed using the obtuse marginal branches of the circumflex coronary artery as regional landmarks, approximately 1 cm apical to the mitral annulus. After the leads are placed, the capped terminal pins are tunneled to a provisional pocket on the chest wall. The patient is then reprepped and draped on his or

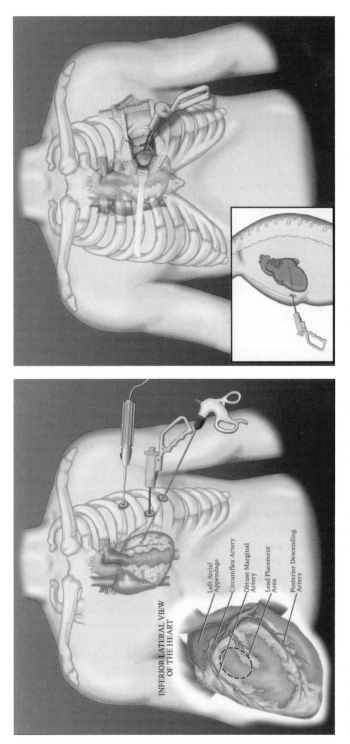

INFERIOR LATERAL VIEW
OF THE HEART

Left Atrial
Appendage

Circumflex Artery

Obtuse Marginal
Artery

Lead Placement
Area

Posterior Descending
Artery

Fig. 4.18 Cardiac surgical approach to LV lead placement. *Left:* "Porthole" approach. *Right:* Limited left lateral thoracotomy approach.

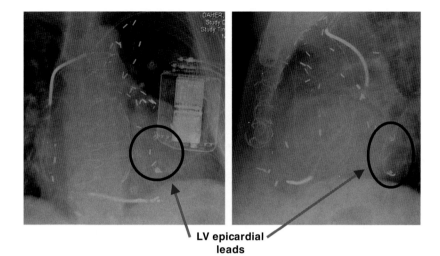

LV epicardial leads

Fig. 4.19 Chest radiograph of LV epicardial leads.

her back; the provisional pocket is opened, and terminal pins are tunneled to the pectoral pocket.

In either of these approaches, muscle relaxants should be temporarily reversed to perform testing for phrenic stimulation. Some cardiac surgeons have touted even more minimally invasive approaches using two or three "porthole" incisions and fiberoptic visualization or robotic assistance. The potential disadvantage to this approach is limited visualization and access to the posterobasal LV that might compromise optimal lead placement.

A particularly difficult problem with chronic epicardial leads is exit block, which in some instances results in voltage thresholds that exceed pulse generator output and results in permanent loss of CRT. Though this is infrequent, it is a devastating problem for the patient, because the epicardial approach is usually taken only when the transvenous approach fails. Several factors contribute to this problem relating to lead design and surgical technique. The most commonly used epicardial pacing lead yielding typically poor long-term performance is a fixed helix mechanism without steroid, and chronic doubling of the implant threshold is common. Furthermore, this situation is made worse by multiple applications of the helix and incautious use of suturing, which increase local tissue trauma and the subsequent inflammatory response.

Therefore, regardless of the cardiac surgical approach, it is imperative that excessive local tissue trauma due to myocardial suturing techniques be avoided. Otherwise, this may result in acute edema and chronic fibrosis causing rapid, significant, and sustained threshold rises or even exit block exceeding the output capacity of the pulse generator. This undesirable outcome would appear to be more likely attending the use of epimyocardial "steroid dot" electrodes, which must be sutured in multiple locations to achieve mechanical stability. An undesirable local inflammatory response due to poor suturing technique could eliminate the otherwise anticipated chronic threshold advantages of local steroid delivery. Screw-in electrodes are more commonly used, particularly in the patient who has had prior surgery where the chronic pericardial inflammatory response limits identification and exposure of viable epimyocardium.

A comparison of thoracotomy and transvenous lead system performance in 87 patients who received CRTD systems between 1998 and 2001 reported no significant differences in chronic thresholds with either approach, which on average were between 1.5 and 2.0 V up to 30 months after implant [37]. Similarly, there were no chronic threshold differences between transvenous lead designs (over-the-wire versus preformed shape). An interim progress report of the InSync Registry Post-Approval Study [38] in 903 patients showed similar range and stability of LV thresholds (mean, 1.88 ± 1.44 V) with two different preformed transvenous lead designs at 6 months that was retained at 36 months. In this same report, epicardial voltage thresholds were similarly stable but slightly higher (2.42 ± 0.74 V) at 12 months, though data were available on a much smaller number of patients.

Finally, it is critically important that the electrophysiologist attend cardiac surgical placement of LV epicardial leads. The cardiac surgeon is often uninformed about the requirements for adequate sensing and pacing thresholds, the need for minimally traumatizing suture techniques, and critical importance of LV lead positioning for optimal CRT response. In one report, a high incidence of anterior LV sites by cardiac surgical implantation was associated with a trend toward increased mortality due to progressive heart failure compared with posterobasal locations by the transvenous approach [14].

Transcutaneous or Transvenous Access to the Pericardial Space for LV Pacing

An alternative approach for delivering pacing leads to the epicardial surface of the LV could incorporate direct pericardial access without thoracotomy. This has been demonstrated to be feasible and safe during catheter ablation for ventricular tachycardia in the electrophysiology laboratory [39,40]. In one approach, percutaneous needle access to the pericardial space is obtained, and ablation sheaths are inserted into the pericardial space over a guide wire. This approach is more likely to be successful among patients who have not had prior cardiac surgical procedures. In the latter case, fibrous adhesions often prevent direct needle access of the pericardial space and limit sheath maneuverability. A limited subxiphoid incision and pericardiotomy is useful in this situation and similarly permits sheath and ablation electrode manipulation within the pericardial space (Fig. 4.20) [41]. Either of these approaches could easily be adapted for delivery of pacing leads to the epimyocardium. An alternate nonsurgical approach to the pericardial space for delivery of pacing leads has been demonstrated in animals. Direct puncture of the right atrium or superior vena cava is performed with a conventional transseptal needle and catheter [42]. The guide wire is advanced into the pericardial space, and a delivery sheath is advanced over the guide wire (Figs. 4.21–4.23). This approach has far less appeal in humans due to obvious safety concerns. Regardless of the technique for obtaining nonsurgical access to the pericardial space, current LV leads are not suitable for permanent pacing due to lack of fixation. Most likely, a new lead design with a deployable fixation mechanism would be required to prevent movement of the lead tip [42].

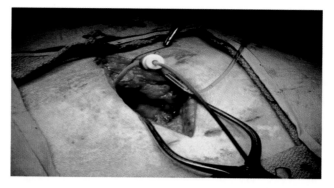

Fig. 4.20 Subxiphoid access to the pericardial space [41]. Diaphragmatic surface of pericardium is exposed by direct surgical visualization via subxiphoid approach. Pericardium is opened with scalpel. Electrophysiology catheter is delivered into pericardial space via 9-F sheath.

Dual Site RV Pacing as an Alternative to CRT

There is a small anecdotal literature that proposes dual-site ("bifocal") RV pacing as an alternative to conventional CRT when LV pacing cannot be achieved. Of course, LV pacing can almost always be achieved using various nonconventional approaches discussed above, and it is more accurate to state that the questionable justification for this approach is an unwillingness of the physician to sponsor the patient for cardiac surgery. Many of these reports are unaccompanied by any meaningful physiologic measures and are presented as "testimonials" of patient improvement without a comparison group [43–48].

More problematic is a fundamental misunderstanding or neglect of the physiologic basis of ventricular conduction, with particular attention to selective site pacing. For example, Vlay has repeatedly stated, "Restoring

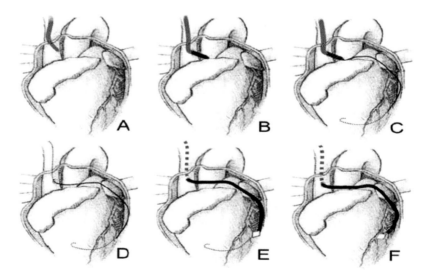

Fig. 4.21 Transvenous access to the pericardial space [42]. Schematic of LV pacing lead entering pericardial space via puncture of superior vena cava.

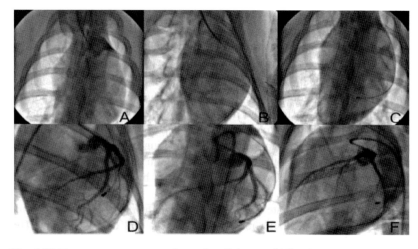

Fig. 4.22 Transvenous access to the pericardial space [42]. Fluoroscopic images of LV pacing lead in pericardial space via puncture of superior vena cava (**A–C**) and concomitant coronary angiography (**D–F**).

the origin of depolarization to the high ventricular septum, restores a more favorable contraction pattern. In addition, since the highest part of the septum is the thinnest, the impulse travels through the septum to depolarize the LV. This route may be an alternative way to achieve earlier LV depolarization" [44, 45]. This physiologically incorrect thinking has appeared in other related publications (see Fig. 2 in Mateos et al. [43]).

Normal activation of ventricular muscle occurs from apex to base, not from base to apex, an error that is repeatedly committed in the "bifocal" RV literature [43–45]. Myerburg [49] demonstrated more than three decades ago that impulse propagation from the normal myocardium can only enter the Purkinje system at the apical sites where impulses exit the specialized conduction system during normal conduction (reviewed in Ref. 50). This corresponds with the lower one-quarter of the RV septum and the lower

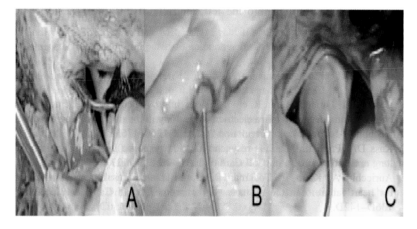

Fig. 4.23 Transvenous access to the pericardial space [42]. Appearance of healed puncture site in superior vena cava (**A**, acute; **B**, 17 days; **C**, 46 days).

24. Knight BP, Desai A, Coman J, et al. Long-term retention of cardiac resynchronization therapy. J Am Coll Cardiol 2004;44:72–77.
25. Hansky B, Schulte-Eistrup S, Vogt J, et al. Lead selection and implantation technique for biventricular pacing. Eur Heart J Suppl 2004;6:D112–116.
26. Abraham WT, Fisher WG, Smith AL, et al., for the MIRACLE Study Group. Cardiac resynchronization in chronic heart failure. N Eng J Med 2002;346(24): 1845–1853.
27. Bristow MR, Saxon LA, Boehmer J, et al., the Comparison of Medical Therapy P, and Defibrillation in Heart Failure (COMPANION) Investigators. Cardiac-resynchronization therapy with or without an implantable defibrillator in advanced chronic heart failure. N Engl J Med 2004;350(21):2140–2150.
28. Young JB, Abraham WT, Smith AL, et al., Multicenter InSync ICD Randomized Clinical Evaluation (MIRACLE ICD) Trial Investigators. Combined cardiac resynchronization and implantable cardioversion defibrillation in advanced chronic heart failure: the MIRACLE ICD Trial. JAMA 2003;289(20):2685–2394.
29. Hansky B, Lamp B, Minami K, et al. Coronary vein balloon angioplasty for left ventricular pacemaker lead implantation. J Am Coll Cardiol 2002;40(12): 2144–2149.
30. Van Gelder BM, Meijer A, Basting P, et al. Successful implanation of a coronary sinus lead after stenting of a coronary vein stenosis. Pacing Clin Electrophysiol 2003;26:1904–1906.
31. Cesario DA, Shenoda M, Brar R, Shivkumar K. Left ventricular lead stabilization using a coronary stent. Pacing Clin Electrophysiol 2006;29:427–428.
32. Garrigue S, Jais P, Espil G, et al. Comparison of chronic biventricular pacing between epicardial and endocardial left ventricular stimulation using Doppler tissue imaging in patients with heart failure. Am J Cardiol 2001;88: 858–862.
33. Jais P, Takahashi A, Garrigue S, et al. Mid-term follow-up of endocardial biventricular pacing. Pacing Clin Electrophysiol 2000;23(11 Pt 2):1744–1747.
34. Leclercq C, Hager FX, Macia JC, et al. Left ventricular lead insertion using a modified transseptal catheterization technique: A totally endocardial approach for permanent biventricular pacing in end-stage heart failure. Pacing Clin Electrophysiol 1999;22(11):1570–1575.
35. Sen J, Cesario DA, Swerdlow CD, Shivkumar K. Left ventricular endocardial lead placement using a modified transseptal approach. J Cardiovasc Electrophysiol 2004(15):234–236.
36. Auricchio A, Stellbrink C, Sack S, et al., Pacing Therapies in Congestive Heart Failure (PATH-CHF) Study Group. Long-term clinical effect of hemodynamically optimized cardiac resynchronization therapy in patients with heart failure and ventricular conduction delay. J Am Coll Cardiol 2002;39(12):2026–2033.
37. Daoud E, Kalbfleisch FJ, Hummel JD, et al. Implantation techniques and chronic lead parameters of biventricular pacing dual-chamber defibrillators. J Cardiovasc Electrophysiol 2002;13(10):964–970.
38. Storm C, Harsch M, DeBus B. InSync Registry: Post Market Study. Progress Report Number Seven. Minneapolis, MN: Medtronic, Inc.; 2005.
39. Sosa E, Scanavacca M, d'Avila A, Oliveira F, Ramires JA. Nonsurgical transthoracic epicardial catheter ablation to treat recurrent ventricular tachycardia occurring late after myocardial infarction. J Am Coll Cardiol 2000;35:1442–1449.
40. Sosa E, Scanavacca M, d'Avila A, Pilleggi F. A new technique to perform epicardial mapping in the electrophysiology laboratory. J Cardiovasc Electrophysiol 1996;7:531–536.
41. Soejima K, Couper G, Cooper JM, et al. Subxiphoid surgical approach for epicardial catheter-based mapping and ablation in patients with prior cardiac surgery or difficult pericardial access. Circulation 2004;110(10):1197–1201.

42. Mickelsen SR, Ashikaga H, Desilva R, et al. Transvenous access to the pericardial space: an approach to epicardial lead implantation for cardiac resynchronization therapy. Pacing Clin Electrophysiol 2005;28:1018–1024.
43. Mateos JCP, Albornoz RN, Materos EIP, et al. Right ventricular bifocal stimulation in the treatment of dilated cardiomyopathy with heart failure. Arq. Bras. Cardiol. 1999;73(6):492–498.
44. Vlay SC. Alternatives when coronary sinus pacing is not possible. Pacing Clin Electrophysiol 2003;26:4–7.
45. Vlay SC. Alternate site biventricular pacing: BiV in the RV—Is there a role? Pacing Clin Electrophysiol 2004;27:567–597.
46. O'Donnell D, Nadurata V, Hamer A, et al. Bifocal right ventricular cardiac resynchronization therapies with unsuccessful percutaneous lateral left ventricular venous access. Pacing Clin Electrophysiol 2005;28:S27–S30.
47. Satish OS, Yeh K-H, Wen M-S, Wang C-C. Cardiac resynchronisation therapy versus dual site right ventricular pacing in a patient with permanent pacemaker and congestive heart failure. Europace 2005;7:380–384.
48. Vlay SC, Kort S. Biventricular pacing using dual-site right ventricular stimulation: is it placebo effect? Pacing Clin Electrophysiol 2006;29(7):779–783.
49. Myerburg RJ, Nilsson K, Gelband H. Physiology of canine intraventricular conduction and endocardial excitation. Circ Res 1972;30:217–243.
50. Prinzen FW, Peschar M. Relation between the pacing induced sequence of activation and left ventricular pump function in animals. Pacing Clin Electrophysiol 2002;25(4 Pt 1):484–498.
51. De Cock CC, Giudici MC, Twisk J. Comparison of the haemodynamic effects of right ventricular outflow-tract pacing with right ventricular apex pacing: a quantitative review. Europace 2003;5:275–278.
52. Peschar M, de Swart H, Michels KJ, et al. Left ventricular septal and apex pacing for optimal pump function in canine hearts. J Am Coll Cardiol 2003;41(7):1218–1226.
53. Schwaab B, Frohlig G, Alexander C, et al. Influence of right ventricular stimulation site on left ventricular function in atrial synchronous ventricular pacing. J Am Coll Cardiol 1999;33:317–323.
54. Sweeney MO, Hellkamp AS. Heart failure during cardiac pacing. Circulation 2006;113:2082–2088.

(CRT-D, CRT-P, and pharmacologic therapy) [5] and the two-arm CARE-HF study published in 2005 (CRT-P, pharmacologic therapy) [15]. A comparison of the baseline clinical characteristics and the outcome of the patients enrolled in these two studies is presented in Table 5.1. Although the baseline characteristics of patients in the two studies are similar, a direct comparison of the two study populations reveals that the patients in the COMPANION study had more severe heart disease with a greater percentage having NYHA class IV heart failure and a lower ejection fraction than those in the CARE study. Furthermore, patients randomized to pharmacologic therapy in the COMPANION study had a higher 2-year mortality and 2-year mortality or hospitalization rate than pharmacologically treated patients in the CARE-HF study.

The fact that heart disease was more severe in the COMPANION than in the CARE-HF study makes a direct comparison of the efficacy of CRT-D versus CRT-P between the two studies difficult. Within the three-arm COMPANION study, the comparative effectiveness for mortality reduction was somewhat better in the CRT-D arm (hazard ratio 0.64, p < 0.01) than in the CRT-P arm (hazard ratio 0.76, p = 0.06) when compared with the pharmacologically treated patients.

Table 5.1 Clinical characteristics of patients enrolled in COMPANION and CARE-HF.

Characteristic	COMPANION CRT-D arm* (N = 595)	CARE-HF CRT-P arm† (N = 409)
Baseline		
Age	66	67
Male sex (%)	67	74
NYHA class IV (%)	14	6
Ischemic cardiomyopathy	55	40
Left ventricular ejection fraction	0.22	0.25
QRS duration (ms)	160	160
Heart rate (beats/min)	72	69
Blood pressure (mmHg)		
Systolic	112	110
Diastolic	68	70
Pharmacologic therapy (%)		
ACE inhibitor or angiotensin-receptor blocker	90	95
Beta-blocker	68	70
Outcome		
Two-year mortality (%)		
Medical therapy group	38	25
Device therapy	26	20
Hazard ratio for death (device:medical Rx)	0.64	0.64
Two-year mortality or hospitalization (%)		
Medical therapy group	80	50
Device therapy group	75	35
Hazard ratio for death or hospitalization (device:medical Rx)	0.80	0.63

*Source: Ref. 5.
†Source: Ref. 15.

Severity of Heart Disease

A recent observational study by Desai et al. provides useful information about the predictors of appropriate defibrillator therapy among patients receiving a CRT-D device [16]. The population of 501 patients was remarkably similar to those in the COMPANION study with mean age 66 years, 83% males, 67% NYHA class III–IV, QRS width 158 ms, and ejection fraction 0.21. NYHA class IV and a history of sustained ventricular arrhythmias are independent predictors of appropriate ICD therapy in the CRT-D population. Heart failure etiology and drug therapy had no significant impact on the rate of appropriate defibrillator therapy. These findings are in good alignment with the recent experience from MADIT-II in which time-dependent interim development of heart failure requiring hospitalization after enrollment was the only factor significantly associated with appropriate ICD firing for ventricular tachycardia and ventricular fibrillation.

Cardiac patients with low ejection are at increased risk for the development of atrial fibrillation, and this arrhythmia frequently exacerbates the development of heart failure and is also a marker for more severe heart disease. Almost all of the CRT-P trials to date have excluded patients with atrial fibrillation. In the recent publication by Gasparini et al. involving more than 600 patients treated with CRT-P, there were 114 patients with atrial fibrillation [17]. Most patients with atrial fibrillation did not receive adequate biventricular capture due to the rapid ventricular response rate from atrial fibrillation. Many of these patients underwent atrioventricular junctional ablation, and this combined therapy was associated with evidence of reverse remodeling and functional improvement. Clinical trials to evaluate CRT-D versus CRT-P in heart failure patients with atrial fibrillation with and without combined atrioventricular nodal ablation are likely to be initiated in the near future.

Clinical Recommendations

In cardiac patients with advanced left ventricular function, there is a high likelihood that cardiac dysfunction will progress over time despite optimal medical management. We cannot accurately predict who will develop life-threatening or fatal ventricular tachyarrhythmias, but we do know that the development of heart failure is a major factor contributing to arrhythmic instability. Furthermore, the available evidence indicates that appropriate ICD therapy for ventricular tachyarrhythmias in high-risk patients identifies subjects at increased risk for subsequent heart failure. At the present time, risk stratification studies have not been able to identify which cardiac patients will die from heart failure and which from sudden cardiac death. This being the case, then current logic favors the use of the CRT-D device in patients with advanced left ventricular dysfunction, especially in those with NYHA class III and IV heart failure and evidence of dyssynchrony. Although the CARE-HF study has shown impressive reduction in mortality and heart failure with CRT-P only in this high-risk group, this is not to say that we cannot achieve better results with CRT-D. The available evidence would favor the latter approach. At the present time, ICD-only is indicted for NYHA class I,

Upgrading Conventional Pacemakers to CRT: Indications and Technical Considerations

Safwat A. Gassis and Angel R. León

Indications and Clinical Implications of Upgrade to CRT

Introduction: CRT Utility and Current Guidelines

Cardiac resynchronization therapy (CRT) has been shown in numerous trials to improve symptoms, ventricular function, and survival in patients with left ventricular (LV) systolic dysfunction and left conduction delay or block [1–9]. The detrimental effects of a wide native QRS have been adequately documented [10, 11]. A large number of patients with previously implanted devices, however, develop or continue to have progression of heart failure. In a study of patients followed at a routine pacemaker clinic, one third of patients receiving dual or ventricular pacing were identified to have reduced ejection fraction (EF) <40%, 88% of whom were symptomatic at the time of clinic follow-up [12]. The upgrade to CRT devices emerges as an effective strategy to overcome native and iatrogenic dyssynchrony in patients with heart failure and chronic pacing.

Current guidelines for CRT include sinus rhythm with reduced EF <35%, marked heart failure symptoms, New York Heart Association (NYHA) class III and ambulatory class IV, and dyssynchrony demonstrated by a QRS >120 ms [13]. The current guidelines do not specifically address pacing-induced dyssynchrony as a criterion for CRT implantation or upgrade. However, a strong body of evidence is accumulating that supports upgrade to CRT in patients who do not fulfill criteria set for the implantation of CRT devices. The benefit of CRT in clinical trials has been demonstrated predominately in patients without antibradycardia indications for atrial and/or ventricular pacing. Patients with indications for antibradycardia pacing due to sinus node dysfunction, atrioventricular conduction abnormalities, or bradycardia in the setting of atrial arrhythmias require particular attention for choice of pacing device, pacing mode, and programmable parameters. This chapter addresses the indications and technical aspects for upgrading conventional pacing devices to CRT or CRT–implantable cardioverter defibrillator (CRT-ICD).

Detrimental Effects of Right Ventricular Pacing

The primary question raised is whether right ventricular (RV) pacing–induced left bundle branch block (LBBB) morphology is equivalent to intrinsic or native LBBB? If so, is congestive heart failure (CHF) associated with RV pacing–induced LBBB ameliorated with CRT in the same way as it is with intrinsic LBBB? Answers to these questions help us understand the utility of upgrading pacing devices to CRT systems.

RV pacing creates an activation pattern similar to LBBB and is characterized by worsened systolic and diastolic function [14–16]. Abnormal contractility patterns have been noted by magnetic resonance imaging during RV pacing in dog studies [17]. Studies of chronic RV pacing in humans with congenital atrioventricular (AV) block have shown histopathologic alteration and remodeling of atrial and ventricular myocardium [18]. These pathologic changes have mirrored clinical and echocardiographic deterioration of atrial and LV dimensions and function [19]. The deleterious effects of chronic right ventricular pacing on hemodynamics and cardiac function have clearly been documented in clinical trials [19–33].

Not all studies support the notion that a paced QRS is equivalent to native LBBB. In a report by Xiao et al., RV pacing–induced widening of the QRS was shown to exhibit different characteristics from native LBBB with respect to electromechanical delay, contraction and relaxation times, and extent of uncoordinated regional ventricular wall motion [34]. Cazeau et al. studied echocardiographic parameters as a guide to selection of patients for CRT. Almost half of the CRT recipients were upgrades from chronic RV pacing. Although the majority noted a clinical response, the mechanism of improved dyssynchrony after CRT was different between the upgrade patients and those receiving de novo CRT devices [35]. In a small study by Garrigue et al. evaluating the acute effects of RV pacing in the presence or absence of LBBB, 10 patients with heart failure and sinus node dysfunction (SND) underwent radionuclide ventriculography comparing single-chamber atrial pacing (AAI) and dual-chamber pacing (DDD) modes [36]. In patients with normal QRS, ventriculography demonstrated better global and regional contractility and less electromechanical dyssynchrony with AAI pacing. Conversely, the patients with LBBB demonstrated better global and regional contractility with DDD pacing than with AAI pacing [36]. The small study did not compare CRT with RV pacing in relation to presence or absence of underlying LBBB. It however demonstrated a difference between RV pacing–induced QRS prolongation and native LBBB that should be taken into consideration as a confounding factor in trials measuring the response to CRT upgrade. Despite these differences, iatrogenic LBBB morphology is similarly associated with progression of LV dysfunction.

One of the first randomized trials comparing rate modulated single-chamber atrial pacing (AAIR) with rate modulated dual-chamber pacing (DDDR) modes by Nielsen et al. showed that DDD modes resulted in a higher atrial fibrillation occurrence rate and increased left atrial diameter. With AV delay shortened to "physiologic" duration, there was a significant increase in percentage ventricular paced beats (90%) associated with a reduction in LV fractional shortening [33]. Data from the MOST trial, which compared dual-chamber versus single-chamber ventricular pacing in patients with SND and normal QRS duration, DDDR mode resulted in a median of 90% cumulative ventricular pacing and rate modulated single chamber ventricular pacing (VVIR) mode in a median of 58% cumulative ventricular paced beats [25]. In the DDDR group, cumulative ventricular pacing up to 40% was associated with an increased risk for heart failure hospitalization (Hazard ratio (HR) = 1.54, p = 0.046). For every 10% increase in RV pacing, there was a 54% increase in heart failure hospitalization until RV pacing reached 40%. Despite maintenance of AV synchrony, the MOST trial showed only a modest benefit to dual-chamber pacing. The incremental benefit also included reduced incidence of atrial fibrillation with dual-chamber pacing. A moderate benefit in heart failure symptoms, also seen in other similar trials of RV pacing [37–39], may have been mitigated by the increased risk of ventricular dysfunction from chronic RV pacing.

A recent analysis from the MADIT II study population showed a remarkable difference in rate of new or worsened heart failure that was dependent on the frequency of RV pacing [31]. In contrast with the MOST trial and other studies of RV pacing, this analysis focused on patients with already reduced LV function, predominately symptomatic, and is therefore more representative of the patients who would be considered for CRT therapy with native LBBB. There was a bimodal distribution of percentage RV pacing at either extreme. Patients with >50% pacing (median percentage pacing = 95.6%) had a 30% incidence of new or worsened heart failure versus 17% in the group with <50% pacing (median percentage pacing = 0.2%). The association was also significant for increased rates of death and ventricular tachyarrhythmia requiring ICD therapy. This association remained significant even after controlling for presence of LBBB and prolonged QRS in the native rhythm.

Does the Duration of the Paced QRS Matter?

There has been conflicting evidence whether the extent of paced QRS prolongation closely tracks the degree of dyssynchrony produced. An echocardiographic study measuring indices of dyssynchrony in RV-paced patients with heart failure versus a control set of RV pacing but no heart failure showed that QRS duration alone with RV pacing does not predict dyssynchrony [40]. Rather, the authors suggest that interventricular or intraventricular electromechanical delays of >50 ms are superior to paced QRS duration for predicting dyssynchrony to guide the decision to upgrade to CRT. Whether echocardiographic parameters are reliable at identifying dyssynchrony in RV pacing ameliorated with CRT remains to be demonstrated in clinical trials.

The duration of the paced QRS complex has been correlated to increased heart failure hospitalization in an analysis of the MOST trial population [41]. This was subsequently illustrated in a study that showed a paced QRS duration >190 ms at implantation, or prolongation of the paced QRS over time, is a strong predictor of subsequent heart failure [30]. From a recent analysis of the MOST study population, Sweeney et al. described the risk of heart failure hospitalization with percentage ventricular pacing while considering potential confounding factors [28]. The analysis showed that prolonged QRS was a predictor of increased CHF hospitalization regardless of the etiology of QRS widening (intrinsic or RV pacing induced) at cumulative ventricular pacing >40% in DDDR mode or >80% in VVIR mode (i.e., relative increased risk remained the same). However, they noted that native QRS prolongation was consistently associated with a twofold higher absolute risk of heart failure hospitalization over RV pacing–induced QRS prolongation. The incremental risk incurred by RV pacing was most pronounced in patients with structural heart disease (low EF, prior infarction and conduction abnormalities). Although the relative risk doubles with RV pacing, the absolute risk of CHF hospitalization in patients with no other structural disease increases from approximately 2% to 4%, whereas in patients with structural disease the risk increases from approximately 20% to 40%. Interestingly, the risk of heart failure increased incrementally with increasing QRS duration—both in the paced and nonpaced groups. Furthermore, patients with reduced EF showed an exaggerated increase in heart failure as the QRS duration increased. This latter effect was seen up until a QRS duration of 200 ms, at which interval both low EF and normal EF patients demonstrated equivalent rates of heart failure hospitalization [28]. This data suggest that a very wide QRS duration with RV pacing may serve as a stronger impetus to upgrade to CRT in select patients.

A change in QRS duration after biventricular pacing in patients with native left ventricular conduction delay or block is now not considered to be a sensitive marker for successful resynchronization. Multiple studies of CRT upgrade have noted a reduction in QRS duration from RV pacing, however, the prognostic value of the extent to which it is altered is yet unclear [40, 42–48].

Strategies to Consider Prior to Deciding to Upgrade to CRT

Patients with indications for antibradycardia pacing and narrow baseline QRS duration present a unique challenge. Chronic RV pacing as discussed above has been shown to be harmful particularly in patients with symptomatic CHF, therefore, every effort should be made to minimize ventricular pacing. Strategies to prevent frequent RV pacing include atrial-based pacing (AAI modes), atrial nontracking (DDI mode), programming a long AV interval delay, ventricular rate support set at low rates (VVI) [24], automated intrinsic AV adjustments [49], and managed ventricular pacing (MVP) mode [50]. These strategies are an appealing alternative to upgrading to CRT in select patients with symptomatic heart failure and with pacing indications.

To illustrate the effect of pacing mode choices, 225 patients with SND randomized to atrial-based pacing versus single-chamber VVIR ventricular-based pacing were followed [51]. After a mean follow-up of 5.5 years, mortality, atrial fibrillation, severity of CHF, and thromboembolic events were lower in the group randomized to atrial pacing. Atrial pacing conferred more favorable outcomes with a relative risk for survival of 0.66 (p = 0.45), cardiovascular mortality of 0.47 (p = 0.0065), atrial fibrillation of 0.54 (p = 0.012), freedom from thromboembolic events of 0.47 (p = 0.023), and lower NYHA class (p = 0.01). The higher frequency of atrial fibrillation and, therefore, higher thromboembolic risk, in the ventricular group probably stems from anatomical and electrical remodeling of the atria due to the AV dyssynchronous activation. The study demonstrated a low risk of heart block (0.6%) and, therefore, supports the idea that single-chamber atrial pacing is a viable treatment option for patients with SND and normal AV conduction. The presence of right bundle branch block (RBBB), however, was associated with increased risk for CHB that was consistent with prior studies [52]. In a more recent study, Nielsen et al. in a study comparing AAI versus DDD pacing reported 3 of 51 patients programmed to AAI developed high-grade AV block (1.9% per year) requiring reprogramming to DDD modes [33].

Patients with CHF frequently have concomitant atrioventricular and intraventricular conduction abnormalities that may prolong the PR interval to a degree greater than would native AV conduction with dual-chamber devices. Furthermore, beta-blocker use in these patients may produce chronotropic and dromotropic incompetence such that frequent ventricular pacing becomes inevitable. In patients considered for upgrade to CRT on such basis, a careful evaluation of the patient's native AV conduction should be performed. Examination of the patient's underlying rhythm may reveal a prolonged AV interval only during rapid atrial rates in which case reprogramming to alternate modes (AAI or VVI at low backup rates) may present a viable option. Increasing atrial pacing rate alone may result in AV nodal Wenckebach at relatively low atrial rates. However, exercise invokes sympathetic enhancement of AV nodal conduction such that AV nodal Wenckebach may be reached at higher atrial rates than would be demonstrated with atrial pacing alone. Therefore, the evaluation should include the effect of activity on the overall heart rate and PR interval. The atrial rate at which ventricular pacing would become inevitable requires individualized assessment. For example, patients who are not active due to other comorbid conditions and thus do not elevate their sinus rates substantially may never reach their AV nodal Wenckebach rate and thus may not require continuous RV pacing. It should be determined, however, whether their reduced activity is due to lack of heart rate support or other limiting comorbid conditions. Studies involving extension of the programmed delay have been inconsistent in showing a significant reduction of ventricular pacing [33, 53]. Studies of dual-chamber pacing for Sick sinus syndrome (SSS) showed that a significant percentage of ventricular beats were paced despite programming a fixed long AV interval [53]. This observation was also demonstrated in a subsequent study involving long and short AV intervals in DDDR modes, which revealed an incidence of 17% of ventricular-paced beats using a programmed AV delay of 300 ms [33]. Furthermore, programming a long fixed AV delay interval limits the programmable upper heart rate and is associated with a high incidence of pacemaker syndrome and pacemaker-mediated tachycardia [53]. Newer algorithms for ventricular pacing management have shown superior efficacy in reducing ventricular pacing in dual-chamber devices in patients without AV block [49, 50].

The data demonstrating the detrimental effects of right ventricular apical pacing is abundant, but recent interest in alternative pacing sites in the RV may permit chronic pacing RV without the associated deterioration of LV function [54]. Right ventricular outflow tract (RVOT) or para-Hisian pacing allows stimulation of the septum and utilization of the native conduction system and, therefore, better mimics the natural activation of the ventricles. Whether dyssynchrony is reduced to the point of making future upgrade to CRT procedures unnecessary, or a viable alternative to CRT, has yet to be determined.

Detrimental Effects in Patients with Atrial Fibrillation Who Require Chronic Pacing

The issue of chronic ventricular pacing is encountered most frequently in patients with chronic atrial fibrillation who require ventricular pacing due to medication or junctional ablation. Although excluded from most of the

Table 6.1 Selected studies of upgrade from chronic RV pacing to CRT demonstrating feasibility and response to the upgrade procedure.

Study	Design/patient characteristics	No. patients	Follow-up	End points	Main findings
Witte et al. 2006 [64]	Comparison in CRT recipients: upgrade vs. de novo CRT implant	32 upgrade from RVP,39 de novo CRT	3 months	Echocardiographic, NYHA, symptoms score	De novo and upgraded patients showed equivalent benefit to CRT; upgrade and de novo group had similar baseline dyssynchrony
Hoijer et al. 2006 [65]	CRT vs. RVP in single-blind double-crossover design	10 patients (4 VVIR and 6 DDDR)	2-month crossover periods	6-min walked distance, NYHA, symptom score, proBNP	Symptom score and 6-min walked distance higher during CRT period; proBNP lower during CRT; 6 patients demanded early crossover to CRT; 9 of 10 patients preferred CRT pacing mode (1 undecided)
Leon et al. 2002 [44]	Chronic AF, prior AV ablation, NYHA III/IV, mean RVP period 26 months.	20 patients, all with atrial fibrillation	3–6 months	Echo, NYHA class, 6-min walked distance, no. hospitalizations	Improvement in all end points: NYHA 29% (p < 0.001), EF 44% (p < 0.001), LV dimensions, no. hospitalizations by 81% (p < 0.001), MLHF by 33% (p < 0.01)
Horwich et al. 2004 [45]	NYHA III/IV, low EF	15 upgrade to CRT (13 sinus, 2 atrial fibrillation)	Acute study	Echocardiographic indices, QRS duration	CRT reduced paced QRS duration, electromechanical delay, ejection time, and LV dimensions. EF and myocardial performance index improved.
Gronda et al. 2005 [46]	Patients from Insync/Insync ICD registries	243 upgraded to CRT and 989 de novo CRT implants	16 ±14 months	Clinical and echocardiographic indices	Clinical, mitral regurgitation and EF improvement in both groups. 71% in upgrade vs. 67% in de novo CRT groups were responders.

Study	Indication/Population	No. of patients	Follow-up	Endpoints	Results
Eldadah et al. 2006 [66]	NYHA III, low EF	12 (9 sinus, 3 atrial fibrillation)	4–6 weeks	Echocardiographic, QRS duration, NYHA class	CRT reduced NYHA class, QRS duration, LV dimensions, peak systolic strain, and coefficient of variation from strain imaging. EF increased (30.7% to 35.8%)
Baker et al. 2002 [43]	Feasibility of upgrade from PPM to CRT	60	3 months	Success and complication rate, NYHA class, echo	Improved symptom score, NYHA (3.4 to 2.4, $p < 0.0001$), EF 23% to 29% ($p < 0.0003$). Low complication rate 8.3%.
Cazeau et al. 2003 [35]	NYHA III/IV with echocardiographic indices of dyssynchrony	35 de novo CRT and 31 upgrades	Acute echo study	Multiple echo indices, NYHA	Improved intraventricular electromechanical delay (EMD) in both groups mirroring clinical improvement; upgrade group showed more interventricular EMD improvement
Valls-Bertault et al. 2004 [47]	Chronic atrial fibrillation with prior junctional ablation	16 consecutive patients for CRT upgrade	6 months	NYHA class, echocardiographic data	Improved NYHA, LV dimensions, pulmonary pressure, mitral regurgitation, and fractional shortening. EF showed trend for improvement ($p = 0.11$). No change in 6-min walked distance.

MLHF, Minnesota Living with Heart Failure score

hematoma, and three pocket infections. The upgrade procedure was found to be feasible and safe and with favorable clinical effects despite that the study was performed at a time when the current commercial CRT devices, leads, and lead delivery tools were not available. CRT upgrade was achieved using Y-adapters to connect the RV and LV leads. In patients with persistent atrial fibrillation, a conventional pacemaker was used and the LV lead was plugged into the atrial port and AV delay was programmed to a minimum (10 ms). At 18 months after upgrade, there was a significant improvement in functional capacity (NYHA 3.4 ± 0.5 to 2.4 ± 0.7, p = 0.0003) and EF ($23 \pm 8\%$ to $29 \pm 11\%$, p = 0.0003). By 18 months, 10 (16.7%) patients had died, two of whom had failed the initial upgrade attempt. The paced QRS duration in this study showed a 17% decrease from RV pacing to biventricular pacing (206 ± 36 to 170 ± 34 ms).

An earlier study of upgrade of conventional pacemakers to CRT in heart failure patients chronically paced due to atrial fibrillation and prior AV junctional ablation was described in 20 patients [44]. The presence of atrial fibrillation in all patients in this study allowed evaluation of the site of pacing without the confounding influence of atrial transport function. All patients had advanced heart failure symptoms (NYHA class III or IV), reduced EF, and wide paced QRS duration (mean 213 ms). RV pacing had been present for 26 ± 12 months prior to upgrade. In this study, EF increased by 40%, from a mean of 21.5% to 30.9%, and the response was associated with improvement in functional status, LV dimensions, reduction in paced QRS duration, and reduction in heart failure hospitalizations. Other studies performed in similar patient populations showed similar improvement [47].

Witte et al. recently described the effects of CRT upgrade in patients with chronic RV pacing to patients with intrinsic LBBB receiving their first CRT device [64]. Patients with prior pacemakers were enrolled if >50% of the ventricular beats were paced. The authors reported that both groups of patients, who had similar functional limitations and echocardiographic indices, were equally as likely to respond to CRT. Although patients in the upgrade group had wider QRS complexes during RV pacing and higher proportion of patients with atrial fibrillation than in the intrinsic LBBB group, both groups had similar echocardiographic measures of dyssynchrony. The EF, along with other echocardiographic measures, improved in both groups (20% to 30% in the upgrade group and 20% to 27% in the native LBBB group, difference between groups p = 0.1). Clinical status also improved to the same extent in both groups (54% in the upgrade group and 57% in the native LBBB group showed >1 NYHA class improvement, difference p = 0.73). The study demonstrated that a widened QRS duration due to RV pacing was equally as likely to lead to dyssynchrony correctable with CRT as that produced by intrinsic LBBB. This was in contrast with other studies that showed that CRT upgrade, while leading to an improved contractility pattern acutely, induces different echocardiographic changes in patients upgraded to CRT from those receiving a de novo CRT system [35].

In a double-blind crossover design study of 10 patients with symptomatic CHF (NYHA class III and IV) who had no underlying LBBB but required chronic right ventricular pacing, upgrade to CRT was performed [65]. Although the percentage RV pacing was not reported, the patients had diagnosis of high-grade AV conduction disease or bradycardia (SND or atrial fibrillation with a slow ventricular response) such that their rhythm was predominately ventricular paced. The median time from the initial pacemaker implantation to CRT upgrade was 5.7 years. After a 1-month run-in period after the upgrade, patients were randomized to receive biventricular or RV pacing in a 2-month crossover design. Upgrade to CRT was associated with a significant improvement in functional status and symptom score. The mean 6-min walked distance, which was 315 m at baseline, became 240 m (p = NS from baseline) with RV pacing and 400 m (p = 0.03 from baseline) with biventricular pacing. During the RV-pacing period, 6 of 10 patients requested an early crossover to biventricular pacing, whereas none in the CRT group requested crossover to RV pacing. Nine of the 10 patients blinded to the pacing modality preferred biventricular pacing and none preferred RV pacing (one patient was undecided). The study also showed a statistically significant decrease in proBNP after the biventricular pacing period compared with the patient's baseline and after the RV-pacing period. There were no measurable differences in echocardiographic parameters in this study.

In an echocardiographic study by Horwich et al., 15 patients with NYHA class III and IV systolic dysfunction and prolonged QRS who were chronically RV paced underwent upgrade to CRT [45]. Upgrade to CRT was associated with a reduction in QRS duration as well as improvement in echocardiographic measurements of dyssynchrony including intraventricular electromechanical delay, EF (decrease in diastolic and systolic dimensions), myocardial performance index, and ejection time. Only a trend to improved interventricular synchrony (p = NS) was observed. The average increase in EF was 7% and the degree of improvement correlated directly with the magnitude of QRS prolongation during RV pacing.

Eldadah et al. described upgrade to CRT in 12 patients with CHF who received a previous RV-pacing device (>90% ventricular paced) [66]. After 4–6 weeks of biventricular pacing, the mean EF improved from 30.8% to 35.8%, and 75% of the patients improved at least one NYHA class. The investigators also compared tissue Doppler and strain rate imaging to measure time to peak systolic strain and the coefficient of variation, both of which showed a significant improvement after the upgrade. The strain rate was unchanged with CRT, which was in contrast with prior studies of CRT for native LBBB [67], suggesting a possible difference in substrate between pacing-induced and native dyssynchrony. The study demonstrated amelioration of CHF symptoms at a magnitude similar to the de novo CRT trials, demonstrating that irrespective of the etiology of dyssynchrony (pacing-induced or intrinsic LBBB), CRT offers a superior therapeutic alternative to RV pacing.

There has been recent interest in use of CRT for the prevention of deterioration of heart failure in mildly symptomatic patients [68, 69]. In a review of patients from the Insync/Insync ICD registries, CRT upgrade recipients were compared with de novo CRT recipients [46]. Both groups demonstrated significant improvement in clinical and echocardiographic outcomes (71% and 67% were responders in the upgrade and de novo groups, respectively). Additionally, there was also a demonstrated benefit in patients with lower NYHA class symptoms, thus suggesting a possible prophylactic role for upgrading to CRT in chronically paced asymptomatic or mildly symptomatic patients for purposes of preventing progression of heart failure.

This concept, however, requires randomized prospective clinical study before being advocated further.

Technical Aspects of the Upgrade Procedure

Evaluation for Venous Stenosis

Endovascular upgrade to CRT obviously requires central venous access for the delivery of the LV lead. Venous stenosis presents perhaps the greatest obstacle to the upgrade procedure. It is frequently characterized by development of a collateral circulation draining the ipsilateral side via the internal jugular vein or chest wall vessels. Incidence of symptomatic venous obstruction after pacemaker implantation is estimated at 1–2% [70]. However, asymptomatic venous obstruction, which may still pose an obstacle for CRT upgrade, is estimated to occur at a much higher rate [71]. The overall incidence of venous obstruction after pacemaker lead implantation (symptomatic and asymptomatic) has been estimated at 23–45% [71–75]. These reported incidences, however, include obstructions that are not severe enough to prevent use of the affected vein for CRT upgrade but may make the procedure more challenging. The incidence of more severe yet asymptomatic obstruction (>75%) in ICD recipients is also not infrequent (7–14%) [76,77].

In a study evaluating the incidence of venous obstruction before and after pacemaker lead implantation, 131 patients had digital subtraction angiography (DSA) where >60% narrowing was defined as obstruction [78]. In the patients without prior obstruction, follow-up DSA showed 32.9% of patients had developed venous obstruction at a mean of 44 months after implantation (a third of which were complete occlusions). There was no significant association with age, gender, left atrial size, ejection fraction, underlying heart disease, or number and size of leads implanted, which was corroborated in other studies [76, 79, 80]. An increased incidence of stenosis, however, is observed in patients with dual-coil ICD leads [77]. The presence of venous collateral flow does not separate complete from partial obstruction as a substantial number of patients with partial obstruction show development of a collateral circulation [71, 74, 78]. Most often, venous obstruction occurs at the level of the left innominate vein [74, 75, 78]. As such, it is important to visualize adequate flow of contrast not only through the subclavian vein but also proximally to opacify the innominate and superior vena cava before proceeding with the upgrade procedure.

Modalities for detection of asymptomatic venous obstruction primarily employ fluoroscopy. Other modalities include ultrasonography and computed tomography (CT) angiography. Magnetic resonance imaging (MRI) is not currently recommended as a screening modality because of the contraindication in patients with implanted pacemakers or ICDs. Ultrasonography, although it effectively identifies subclavian vein occlusion, is still of limited value as it fails to examine the more proximal venous segments at the level of the innominate vein and superior vena cava [75, 81].

Although studies have failed to document an association between number of chronically implanted leads and venous obstruction [74, 75, 78, 82], the implantation of a CRT device requires insertion of at least one additional lead, and frequently a high-voltage lead with dual coils that theoretically could further crowd a partially obstructed vein. Furthermore, the LV lead delivery system uses a large-caliber catheter that requires significant maneuvering, which can be hindered by a partially obstructed vein. Because the majority of partial obstructions are associated with an already developed collateral circulation, even though CRT upgrade can lead to occlusion of a partially obstructed vein, it is unlikely that this will produce symptoms and edema.

Strategies When Venous Stenosis Is Encountered

Obstruction of the venous system as a result of a previous device and lead implantation presents a challenge that can be overcome in most cases. Careful venography of the ipsilateral veins prior to the procedure permits formulation of a strategy to allow successful upgrade of the system. At our institution, patients presenting for upgrade undergo venography under high-resolution fluoroscopy prior to sedation or draping to allow discussion with the patient about alternative upgrade options should there be a limiting obstruction. The venography film can also be used as a guide for venipuncture when traditional landmarks are obscured by the prior implant, although the older leads also serve as a guide for access to the subclavian vein. Frequently, obstruction occurs at the junction of the subclavian and innominate veins. A venogram obtained by injection of contrast solution from a peripheral intravenous site on the ipsilateral arm not only screens for central venous obstruction but also identifies patency of the cephalic vein, which can be used as a conduit for lead delivery (Figs. 6.1–6.6). When the veins are patent, upgrade can proceed without difficulty. Strictures and partial stenosis may limit manipulation of the catheters and lead delivery systems to cannulate the CS orifice. Use of a larger sheath that traverses a stenosis may enable catheter manipulation to the CS. If severe stenosis is present, extraction of one or more of the older leads may be necessary so as to bore a tract through which the upgrade leads can be delivered [83]. It is important in these situations to maintain access to the venous system as the extraction procedure may disrupt fibrotic tissue and completely obstruct the vein. If the region of luminal narrowing permits, a guide wire should be advanced past the stenosis and used to regain venous access after other leads are extracted. Alternatively, the sheath used to extract the older lead can be used as a conduit to advance a guide wire and maintain venous access before removal of the sheath from the vein. This may not always be feasible because in many situations both the extraction sheath and lead are removed from the body simultaneously.

When the ipsilateral vein is completely obstructed and flow is present only through small-caliber and tortuous vessels of a collateral circulation, the decision becomes whether to remove the old device and implant an entirely new system on the contralateral side, extract one or more of the older leads, or subcutaneously tunnel the required leads. Implanting an entirely new system is preferable when multiple leads for the upgrade are to be inserted. Tunneling the lead can be advantageous when the upgrade involves only one lead. A small incision is made overlying the contralateral delto-pectoral groove to implant the LV lead using standard techniques. The LV lead can then be either directly tunneled across the chest through the presternal tissue to the existing device pocket or connected to an extender, which is then tunneled across. The advantage of using a lead extender for the tunneled portion is

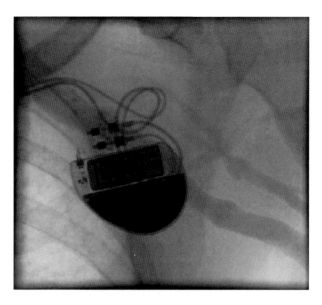

Fig. 6.1 Patent subclavian vein by contrast venography from an ipsilateral peripheral vein. Assessment of central venous patency guides formulation of an alternate upgrade strategy should significant obstruction be identified. This venogram also identifies a large patent cephalic vein, which can also be used for delivery of one or more leads.

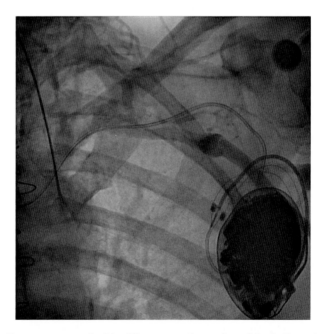

Fig. 6.2 Contrast venography identifies severe obstruction of the ipsilateral vein with well-developed collateral circulation. Identification of such obstruction prior to initiating the upgrade procedure prompts decision to use the contralateral vein or extraction of the old leads. In this situation, the patient elected to have implantation of a complete system via the right pectoral region.

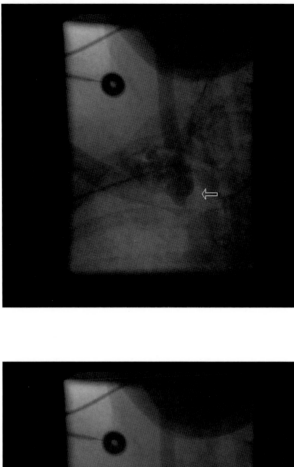

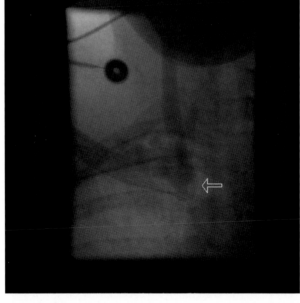

Fig. 6.3 Contrast venogram via sheath in the right subclavian vein showing sequential flow of contrast (**A** to **B** to **C**). Occlusion of the right brachiocephalic vein (*open arrow*) due to prior transvenous leads. Removal of the leads in this situation failed to restore flow through the brachiocephalic vein. Instead, blood flow was retrograde in the right jugular veins leading to collaterals (**B**) that ultimately drained into an enlarged azygous system (**C**) (*filled arrow.*)

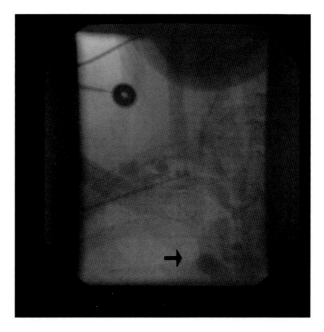

Fig. 6.3 *(Continued)*

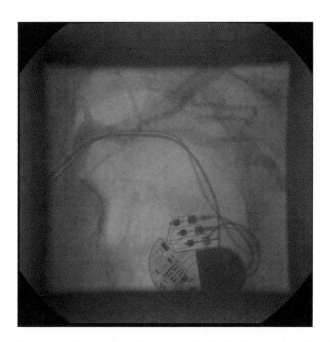

Fig. 6.4 A focal area of stenosis at the proximal left subclavian vein is identified by presence of extensive collaterals in this patient presenting for upgrade to a biventricular defibrillator. The area of stenosis was poorly visualized initially due to an inadequate volume of contrast, but the extent of collateralization is a useful marker to alert for presence of stenosis.

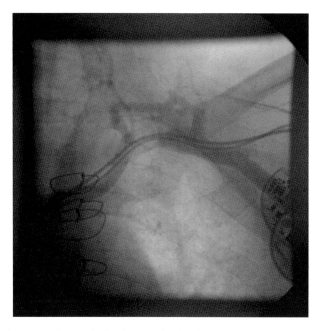

Fig. 6.5 An area of stenosis in the proximal subclavian vein was identified. The reconstituted (from collateral flow) proximal portion, however, was accessible by medial venipuncture that traversed the occluded region. Use of a larger diameter sheath allowed manipulation of the guiding catheter to the CS without significant friction. More medial venipunctures must be performed with caution. In this particular case, atherosclerotic calcification identified the location of the arterial structures—note the proximity of a calcified brachiocephalic artery coursing medial to the reconstituted vein (*arrow*).

that it permits opening of only one surgical site (the site of insertion into the vein) in cases where future repositioning of the lead becomes necessary due to dislodgment.

Venoplasty has been suggested as an option for opening a chronically occluded vein. The technical limitation here is that venoplasty may not preserve patency of the vein for long enough to allow use of the affected vein, probably due to the presence of a collateral circulation and reduced flow in the vein. Furthermore, venoplasty with stenting of the vein, although theoretically feasible, risks damage to the leads and may make future extraction of the jailed leads, should an infection develop, almost impossible. For patients with abdominal devices presenting for upgrade, it is rather cumbersome to attempt tunneling of multiple leads to the distant existing device pocket. These patients should almost always undergo explantation of the old system and implantation of an entirely new system.

When the combination of venous obstruction and poor candidacy for extraction, tunneling, or reimplanting a new system on the contralateral side are present, surgical implantation of an epicardial lead is another alterative. This is also a reasonable option in situations where placement of a stable LV lead position via the coronary sinus while obtaining adequate capture thresholds without extra cardiac stimulation is not possible. Thorascopic and minimally invasive techniques are continually developing to enhance this option for upgrade to CRT.

7. Cazeau S, Ritter P, Lazarus A, et al. Multisite pacing for end-stage heart failure: early experience. Pacing Clin Electrophysiol 1996;19:1748–57.

8. Leclercq C, Cazeau S, Le Breton H, et al. Acute hemodynamic effects of biventricular DDD pacing in patients with end-stage heart failure. J Am Coll Cardiol 1998;32:1825–31.

9. Cazeau S, Leclercq C, Lavergne T, et al. Effects of multisite biventricular pacing in patients with heart failure and intraventricular conduction delay. N Engl J Med 2001;344:873–80.

10. Baldasseroni S, Opasich C, Gorini M, et al. Left bundle-branch block is associated with increased 1-year sudden and total mortality rate in 5517 outpatients with congestive heart failure: A report from the Italian network on congestive heart failure. Am Heart J 2002;143:398–405.

11. Grines CL, Bashore TM, Boudoulas H, Olson S, Shafer P, Wooley CF. Functional abnormalities in isolated left bundle branch block. The effect of interventricular asynchrony. Circulation 1989;79:845–53.

12. Thackray SD, Witte KK, Nikitin NP, Clark AL, Kaye GC, Cleland JG. The prevalence of heart failure and asymptomatic left ventricular systolic dysfunction in a typical regional pacemaker population. Eur Heart J 2003;24:1143–52.

13. Hunt SA, Abraham WT, Chin MH, et al. ACC/AHA 2005 Guideline Update for the Diagnosis and Management of Chronic Heart Failure in the Adult: A report of the American College of Cardiology/American Heart Association Task Force on Practice Guidelines (Writing Committee to Update the 2001 Guidelines for the Evaluation and Management of Heart Failure): Developed in collaboration with the American College of Chest Physicians and the International Society for Heart and Lung Transplantation: Endorsed by the Heart Rhythm Society. Circulation 2005;112:e154–235.

14. Tanabe A, Mohri T, Ohga M, et al. The effects of pacing-induced left bundle branch block on left ventricular systolic and diastolic performances. Jpn Heart J 1990;31:309–17.

15. Verbeek XA, Vernooy K, Peschar M, Van Der Nagel T, Van Hunnik A, Prinzen FW. Quantification of interventricular asynchrony during LBBB and ventricular pacing. Am J Physiol Heart Circ Physiol 2002;283:H1370–8.

16. Vernooy K, Verbeek XA, Peschar M, Prinzen FW. Relation between abnormal ventricular impulse conduction and heart failure. J Interv Cardiol 2003;16: 557–62.

17. Prinzen FW, Hunter WC, Wyman BT, McVeigh ER. Mapping of regional myocardial strain and work during ventricular pacing: experimental study using magnetic resonance imaging tagging. J Am Coll Cardiol 1999;33:1735–42.

18. Karpawich PP, Rabah R, Haas JE. Altered cardiac histology following apical right ventricular pacing in patients with congenital atrioventricular block. Pacing Clin Electrophysiol 1999;22:1372–7.

19. Thambo JB, Bordachar P, Garrigue S, et al. Detrimental ventricular remodeling in patients with congenital complete heart block and chronic right ventricular apical pacing. Circulation 2004;110:3766–72.

20. Lee MA, Dae MW, Langberg JJ, et al. Effects of long-term right ventricular apical pacing on left ventricular perfusion, innervation, function and histology. J Am Coll Cardiol 1994;24:225–32.

21. Rosenqvist M, Isaaz K, Botvinick EH, et al. Relative importance of activation sequence compared to atrioventricular synchrony in left ventricular function. Am J Cardiol 1991;67:148–56.

22. Leclercq C, Gras D, Le Helloco A, Nicol L, Mabo P, Daubert C. Hemodynamic importance of preserving the normal sequence of ventricular activation in permanent cardiac pacing. Am Heart J 1995;129:1133–41.

23. Rosenqvist M, Bergfeldt L, Haga Y, Ryden J, Ryden L, Owall A. The effect of ventricular activation sequence on cardiac performance during pacing. Pacing Clin Electrophysiol 1996;19:1279–86.

24. Wilkoff BL, Cook JR, Epstein AE, et al. Dual-chamber pacing or ventricular backup pacing in patients with an implantable defibrillator: The Dual Chamber and VVI Implantable Defibrillator (DAVID) Trial. JAMA 2002;288:3115–23.

25. Sweeney MO, Hellkamp AS, Ellenbogen KA, et al. Adverse effect of ventricular pacing on heart failure and atrial fibrillation among patients with normal baseline QRS duration in a clinical trial of pacemaker therapy for sinus node dysfunction. Circulation 2003;107:2932–7.

26. Tse HF, Lau CP. Long-term effect of right ventricular pacing on myocardial perfusion and function. J Am Coll Cardiol 1997;29:744–9.

27. Nielsen JC, Andersen HR, Thomsen PE, et al. Heart failure and echocardiographic changes during long-term follow-up of patients with sick sinus syndrome randomized to single-chamber atrial or ventricular pacing. Circulation 1998;97:987–95.

28. Sweeney MO, Hellkamp AS. Heart failure during cardiac pacing. Circulation 2006;113:2082–8.

29. Saad EB, Marrouche NF, Martin DO, et al. Frequency and associations of symptomatic deterioration after dual-chamber defibrillator implantation in patients with ischemic or idiopathic dilated cardiomyopathy. Am J Cardiol 2002;90:79–82.

30. Miyoshi F, Kobayashi Y, Itou H, et al. Prolonged paced QRS duration as a predictor for congestive heart failure in patients with right ventricular apical pacing. Pacing Clin Electrophysiol 2005;28:1182–8.

31. Steinberg JS, Fischer A, Wang P, et al. The clinical implications of cumulative right ventricular pacing in the multicenter automatic defibrillator trial II. J Cardiovasc Electrophysiol 2005;16:359–65.

32. Tse HF, Yu C, Wong KK, et al. Functional abnormalities in patients with permanent right ventricular pacing: the effect of sites of electrical stimulation. J Am Coll Cardiol 2002;40:1451–8.

33. Nielsen JC, Kristensen L, Andersen HR, Mortensen PT, Pedersen OL, Pedersen AK. A randomized comparison of atrial and dual-chamber pacing in 177 consecutive patients with sick sinus syndrome: Echocardiographic and clinical outcome. J Am Coll Cardiol 2003;42:614–23.

34. Xiao HB, Brecker SJ, Gibson DG. Differing effects of right ventricular pacing and left bundle branch block on left ventricular function. Br Heart J 1993;69:166–73.

35. Cazeau S, Bordachar P, Jauvert G, et al. Echocardiographic modeling of cardiac dyssynchrony before and during multisite stimulation: a prospective study. Pacing Clin Electrophysiol 2003;26:137–43.

36. Garrigue S, Barold SS, Valli N, et al. Effect of right ventricular pacing in patients with complete left bundle branch block. Am J Cardiol 1999;83:600–4, A8.

37. Lamas GA, Orav EJ, Stambler BS, et al. Quality of life and clinical outcomes in elderly patients treated with ventricular pacing as compared with dual-chamber pacing. Pacemaker Selection in the Elderly Investigators. N Engl J Med 1998;338:1097–104.

38. Lamas GA, Lee KL, Sweeney MO, et al. Ventricular pacing or dual-chamber pacing for sinus-node dysfunction. N Engl J Med 2002;346:1854–62.

39. Kerr CR, Connolly SJ, Abdollah H, et al. Canadian Trial of Physiological Pacing: Effects of physiological pacing during long-term follow-up. Circulation 2004;109:357–62.

40. Bordachar P, Garrigue S, Lafitte S, et al. Interventricular and intra-left ventricular electromechanical delays in right ventricular paced patients with heart failure: implications for upgrading to biventricular stimulation. Heart 2003;89:1401–5.

41. Shukla HH, Hellkamp AS, James EA, et al. Heart failure hospitalization is more common in pacemaker patients with sinus node dysfunction and a prolonged paced QRS duration. Heart Rhythm 2005;2:245–51.

42. Ritter O, Koller ML, Fey B, et al. Progression of heart failure in right univentricular pacing compared to biventricular pacing. Int J Cardiol 2006;110:359–65.

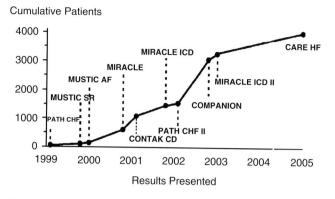

Fig. 7.1 Cumulative enrollment in randomized controlled trials of cardiac resynchronization therapy. (Reproduced with permission from Abraham WT. Cardiac resynchronization therapy. Prog Cardiovasc Dis 2006;48(4): 232–8).

months (by far the longest follow-up to date in trials involving CRT patients) and evaluated for mortality, morbidity, quality of life, and clinical changes in cardiac function. The primary end point was all-cause mortality or unplanned hospitalization for a cardiovascular event, and the principal secondary end point was all-cause mortality alone. The primary end point was reached by 159 patients in the CRT group compared with 224 patients in the medical-therapy group [39% vs. 55%; hazard ratio (HR), 0.63; 95% confidence interval (CI), 0.51–0.77; p < 0.001].

Previous trials were relatively short-term (3–6 months) except the COMPANION trial (12 months) and the MUSTIC trial where the surviving patients remained stable with sustained improvement 1 and 2 years after the initial crossover phases [4, 7] (Fig. 7.2)

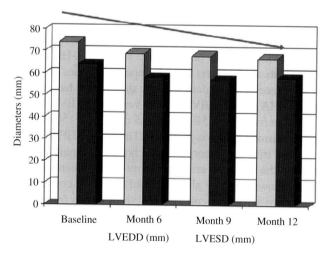

Fig. 7.2 Graphical representation of the progressive decrease in LV dimensions from baseline to the 12th month of follow-up after CRT device implantation in the MUSTIC trial. No control group is displayed as MUSTIC was a crossover study. LVEDD = left ventricular end-diastolic diameter, LVESD = left ventricular end-systolic diameter. (Reproduced with permission from Donal E, Leclercq C, Linde C, Daubert JC. Effects of cardiac resynchronization therapy on disease progression in chronic heart failure. Eur Heart J 2006:1018–25).

Table 7.1 CARE-HF: Primary and main secondary end points.

	Control (n = 404)	CRT (n = 409)	HR	95% CI	P
Primary end point:					
All-cause mortality or unplanned hospitalization for a CV event (%)	224 (55%)	159 (39%)	0.63	0.51–0.77	< 0.001
Secondary end points:					
All-cause mortality	120 (30%)	82 (20%)	0.64	0.48–0.85	< 0.002
All-cause mortality or unplanned hospitalization for worsening HF (%)	191 (47%)	118 (29%)	0.54	0.43–0.68	< 0.001

CI, confidence interval; CRT, cardiac resynchronization therapy; CV, cardiovascular; HF, heart failure; HR, hazard ratio.

At the end of the CARE-HF study, patients in the CRT group demonstrated the unequivocal benefit of CRT and confirmed its safety (Table 7.1). The results of the study remained consistent across various subgroups, including patients with and without ischemic heart disease. (1) Primary end point: A 37% relative risk reduction in the combined all-cause mortality or unplanned cardiovascular hospitalization in the CRT group (HR, 0.63; p < 0.001) (Fig. 7.3A). (2) Secondary end point: 36% relative risk reduction in all-cause mortality (HR, 0.64; p = 0.002) (Fig. 7.3B). The mortality was 20% in the CRT group (n = 82) versus 30% in the control group (n = 120). CARE-HF did not compare CRT-P (pacemaker only) with CRT-D (with defibrillator) directly. Nonetheless, it provided strong evidence in support of the potential for CRT-P alone to reduce mortality of HF patients significantly. CARE-HF was the first study to demonstrate a survival benefit attributable to CRT alone. The results were similar to the reduction of all-cause mortality found in COMPANION in the CRT-D arm. (3) Other secondary end points: The CARE-HF trial also found in that CRT significantly reduced end points of all-cause mortality combined with HF hospitalization by 46% and HF hospitalization alone by 52%. The effect on mortality was mainly attributable to a marked reduction in HF-related deaths. It is, however, noteworthy that the absolute number of sudden cardiac deaths was lower in the CRT group (n = 29) than in the control group (n = 38). (4) Reverse remodeling: Echocardiographic evidence of remodeling was seen at 18 months with improved left ventricular ejection fraction (LVEF), mitral regurgitation, and LV end-systolic volumes (Figs. 7.4 to 7.7). Furthermore, changes in LVEF were more pronounced in CRT patients with nonischemic versus ischemic disease (Fig. 7.8). Similar findings were also noted in the CRT group with respect to changes in LV end-systolic volume. These results confirm the reverse remodeling findings in the MIRACLE trial [8, 9]. The study also showed that CRT improves myocardial performance progressively over time. (5) Biochemical profile: CARE-HF was the first study to show that biochemical neurohormonal measures (e.g., N-terminal pro-brain natriuretic peptide) improve dramatically with CRT.

Cardiac resynchronization therapy in the CARE-HF trial thus showed significant improvement in survival, reduction in morbidity, and improvement

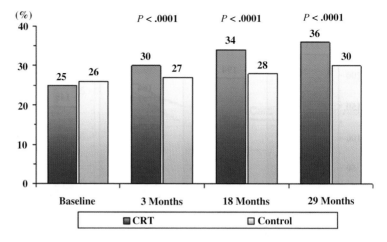

Fig. 7.7 CARE-HF trial. LV ejection fraction.

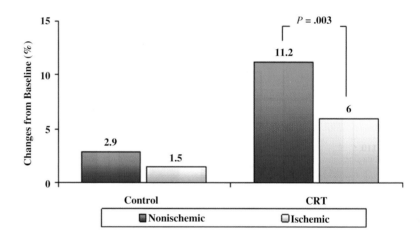

Fig. 7.8 CARE-HF trial. Change in LV ejection fraction from baseline: ischemic versus nonischemic etiology.

in cardiac function and heart failure symptoms in patients with moderate to severe heart failure. The trial demonstrated convincingly that CRT saves lives, slows the progression of heart failure, and improves symptoms and morbidity. A defibrillator might have reduced the risk of sudden death, as 7% of patients in the CRT group died suddenly in the CARE-HF trial.

Extension Phase of CARE-HF

The mean follow-up by the end of the CARE-HFP extension phase had increased from 29.4 months (range, 18.0–44.7) to 37.4 months [median, 37.6; interquartile range (IQR), 31.5–42.5; range, 26.1–52.6 months] [10]. There were 120 deaths in the main study and a further 34 in the extension phase leading to a total of 154 deaths (38.1, or 12.2% per annum) in 404 patients assigned to medical therapy. There were 82 deaths in the main study and

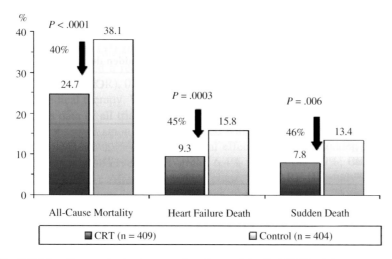

Fig. 7.9 Mortality results in the extension phase of the CARE-HF trial.

a further 19 in the extension phase leading to a total of 101 deaths (24.7, or 7.9% per annum) in 409 patients assigned to CRT (HR, 0.60; 95% CI, 0.47–0.77; p < 0.0001). Reductions in the risk of death due to HF (64 vs. 38 deaths, or 5.1% vs. 3.0% per annum; HR, 0.55; 95% CI, 0.37–0.82, p = 0.003) and sudden death were observed (54 vs. 32, or 4.3% vs. 2.5% per annum; HR, 0.54; 95% CI, 0.35–0.84, p = 0.005) (Fig. 7.9). Of 19 sudden deaths in the extension phase, 16 occurred in the control group.

The use of CRT compared to the control group was associated with a 40% reduction in the risk of all-cause mortality, a 45% reduction in the risk of heart failure mortality, and a 46% reduction in sudden death (Fig. 7.9). Thus, the CARE-HF extended trial provides overwhelming evidence that CRT reduces all-cause mortality and that CRT reduces sudden death and death due to worsening HF. CRT-P therapy may reduce the incidence of sudden cardiac death by slowing the progression of HF, improving the autonomic milieu, and causing anatomic remodeling.

Comparison of Mortality in the CARE-HF Versus COMPANION Trials

Although the predominant mode of death after CRT is progressive pump dysfunction, sudden death still accounts for a third of all deaths [5, 11, 12]. Furthermore, for those who benefit most from CRT, sudden death risk after CRT may actually increase proportionately compared with the risk of a pump death. The relative mortality reduction with CRT alone in the CARE-HF study was approximately the same as with CRT-D in the COMPANION trial [13] (Table 7.2). Figure 7.10 shows the percentage of deaths that were sudden in these two studies. In the COMPANION trial, 36% of the deaths in the CRT-P arm were sudden, very similar to the 35% in the CARE-HF study [13]. As one-third of the deaths in the CARE-HF study were sudden, a back-up defibrillator (i.e., CRT-D), might have prevented many of these sudden deaths. As seen in Figure 7.10, the CRT-D arm of the COMPANION trial reduced the sudden cardiac death incidence to 16%, a 55% relative risk

Table 8.2 Morbidity and mortality comparison.

Study(n randomized)	Follow-up	Treatment	Relative risk reduction with CRT or CRT + ICD				
			Mortality and hospitalization	Mortality and HF hospitalization	Mortality	HF mortality	HF hospitalization
COMPANION [10] (n = 1,520)	12 to 16 months (median)	CRT + ICD	20%*	40%*	36%*		
		CRT	20%*	34%*	24%		
MIRACLE [6] (n = 453)	6 months (protocol)	CRT			27%		50%*
CARE-HF [4]	29.4 months (mean >18 months per protocol)	CRT		40%*	36%*	40%	52%*
Bradley et al. [31] (meta-analysis) (n = 1,634)	3–6 months (protocol)	CRT			23%	51%*	29%*
McAllister et al. [32] (meta-analysis) (n = 3,216)	6 months (protocol)	Pooled: CRT and CRT + ICD			21%*	40%	32%

HF, heart failure.

*p < 0.05.

et al. [33], with cohort characteristics similar to CRT trials already reported, attempted to provide information about the long-term efficacy of CRT. This study followed patients for at least 24 months and had a mean follow-up of 36 months. These authors reported that among the cohort receiving CRT, no sudden death occurred and that survival and freedom from death or transplantation at 3 years were 63% and 58%, respectively.

Nonresponders Versus Responders

Despite the high rates (70% to 80%) of clinical improvement after CRT frequently cited, not all patients receive a sustained clinical benefit after the implantation of a CRT device [34]. Defining CRT success as a reduction of at least one NYHA functional class over 6 months, MIRACLE found that a net rate of positive CRT response was 30% after 6 months (68% of patients assigned to active therapy and 38% of control subjects responded to CRT). Other studies [35–38] defining CRT response based on objective improvement (i.e., left ventricular volumes or ejection fraction) reported that approximately 50% of patients with NYHA class III or IV symptoms, an ejection fraction of 0.35 or less, and a QRS duration of 130 ms or longer respond to CRT.

CRT nonresponse may be explained by a lack of baseline mechanical dyssynchrony, suboptimal placement of the left ventricular lead, or other less tangible factors [34, 36, 39, 40]. The major limitation is that lead placement options with transvenous implants are governed largely by the patient's venous anatomy, which shows considerable interindividual variability [41]. In addition, left phrenic nerve stimulation and high stimulation thresholds may occur. In up to 15% of cases, it may not be possible to achieve what is considered to be satisfactory left ventricular pacing position. These factors underscore the intricacies of the underlying complexities of heart failure, its coexisting illnesses, and the potential morbidity of the invasive procedure required for biventricular pacing.

Implantable Cardioverter Defibrillators Versus Cardiac Resynchronization Therapy

Most randomized trials have evaluated CRT pacemaker devices. However, the relative incremental benefit of resynchronization therapy with defibrillator backup in patients who are CRT candidates is the subject of ongoing studies such as Resynchronization/defibrillation for Advanced Heart Failure Trial (RAFT). Despite this, the Sudden Cardiac Death in Heart Failure Trial (SCD-HeFT) [42] has provided evidence that implantation of a defibrillator in addition to optimal medical therapy is an effective long-term (5-year) treatment compared with conventional optimal therapy alone or with the addition of amiodarone to prolong life in heart failure patients. COMPANION, unique in combining CRT with and without implantable cardioverter defibrillator (ICD) therapy, as well as comparing to optimal medical therapy, demonstrated marked reduction in combined measures of morbidity and mortality with both CRT alone and with CRT plus defibrillator backup with a similar 1-year event-free survival rate. However, when comparing the benefit of CRT alone, the relative risk reduction in all-cause mortality of 24% only trended toward significance (p = 0.060). CRT with defibrillator backup provided 36% relative risk reduction in all-cause mortality compared with optimal drug therapy (p = 0.003). CARE-HF remains the single CRT pacing (without defibrillation) trial showing statistically significant reduction in mortality with CRT.

Number Needed to Treat

Meta-analyses by Bradley et al. [31] in 1,634 patients and McAllister et al. [32] in 3,216 patients demonstrated that CRT could potentially offer 23% and 20% relative reduction in all-cause mortality, respectively (largely driven by 51% and 40% reduction in deaths from progressive heart failure, respectively). The fairly wide confidence intervals reported in these meta-analyses suggest that the benefit from CRT may be offset by an increase in non–heart failure mortality. The number needed to treat for benefit (NNT) to prevent one death was estimated to be 24. Meta-analyses of time-to-death assessment suggest benefits of cardiac resynchronization therapy become apparent by about 3 months after implantation [32].

Complications

The average implant success rate for CRT devices is estimated to be $\geq 90\%$, and serious complications are uncommon. However, implantation of a biventricular pacemaker and, particularly, left ventricular lead implantation remain technically challenging and are not without risk. Systematic review estimates a 0.4% death rate during implantation [32]. This peri-implantation mortality is similar to the 0.7% reported in the Mode Selection in Sinus Node Dysfunction Trial in which conventional dual-chamber pacemakers were implanted in more than 2,000 patients [43]. Based on a systematic CRT review with a median 6-month follow-up [32], 9% of left ventricular leads became dislodged, and device malfunction occurred in 7% of CRT recipients [32]. Another review found rates of serious bleeding ranging from 1% to 6%, and pneumothorax in less than 1% of patients [44] and suggests that CRT patients might require more frequent monitoring. The electrophysiologic effects and the subsequent hemodynamic alterations of biventricular pacing in the setting of heart failure are complex; therefore careful programming may be important to accommodate each patient's physiology.

Cardiac Resynchronization Therapy: Areas for Future Investigation

Entry Criteria for Previous Randomized Clinical Trials

Knowledge of clinical trial inclusion and exclusion criteria remains critical in applying the evidence reported to clinical practice but also helps identify the limitations and uncertainties of therapy. Trials thus far reported show underrepresentation of NYHA class I, II and IV heart failure and atrial fibrillation as well as the absence of less severe left ventricular systolic dysfunction [i.e., left ventricular ejection fraction (LVEF) >35%)] and more narrow complex QRS (<120 ms). Consequently, CRT efficacy in these subpopulations is inconclusive. The vast majority of patients studied have been in sinus rhythm, with severe left ventricular systolic dysfunction (LVEF $\leq$35%), with symptomatic (predominately class III) heart failure with evidence of dyssynchrony as evidenced by prolonged QRS duration of 120 ms or longer in three trials [10,45,46]; 130 ms or longer in two trials [6,7]; longer than 140 ms in one trial [47]; longer than 150 ms in one trial [9]; longer than 180 ms in one trial [48]; and longer than 200 ms in one trial [49]. Although, recent data indicate that CRT may be efficacious in patients with mechanical dyssynchrony regardless of QRS duration [50], additional data are required before CRT can be recommended for these groups of patients excluded from previous trials.

Atrial Fibrillation and CRT

CRT has not been well studied in patients with atrial fibrillation (AF) despite the relatively large number of patients with concurrent heart failure (with other CRT indications) and AF. Most major clinical CRT trials, to date, have had inclusion or exclusion criteria that prohibited the enrollment of patients with AF. Small trials have attempted to assess the effect of CRT in AF. In MUSTIC-AF, a single-blind crossover study design was used to evaluate the efficacy of CRT versus conventional VVIR pacing in patients with a wide paced rhythm (the majority having received an AV nodal ablation). CRT was found to improve exercise tolerance and was preferred by patients [49]. In another trial, patients with a history of AV junction ablation for permanent AF who had received RV pacing for at least 6 months were upgraded to biventricular pacing. This resulted in improved NHYA functional class, decreased number of hospitalizations, increased mean left ventricular EF, and improved echocardiographically measured LV dimensions [51]. Finally, the PAVE study randomized AF patients, after AV nodal ablation, to receive CRT or a right ventricular pacing system [52]. CRT produced significant improvement in functional status and ejection fraction. While the benefit was greater in those patients with impaired systolic function ($\leq 45\%$), this was thought to be due to loss of function and lowered ejection fraction in the RV pacing group, suggesting not only that CRT can be successfully applied in patients with AF, but also that CRT may be superior regardless of QRS duration in patients in whom ventricular pacing is necessary.

Indirect assessment of CRT in atrial fibrillation can be taken from patients who were enrolled in the CARE-HF trial. Those who received CRT were no more likely to develop AF; but those who did develop AF still benefited from CRT with regard to all-cause mortality and other predefined end points [53]. These small studies are suggestive of benefit for patients in atrial fibrillation.

Future trials will evaluate AF and CRT. One such trial, MASCOT, will evaluate use of atrial tachyarrhythmia suppression algorithms in single-blind fashion, with the CRT-only group compared with the CRT with AF suppression group [54].

QRS Duration and Morphology in CRT

Right Bundle Branch Block

Most patients enrolled in major trials have had left bundle branch block. Little randomized trial data exist to evaluate the effect of CRT in patients with right bundle branch block (RBBB). Published data are conflicting in conclusions. For this subgroup of patients, the number included in trials has typically been ≤10% of the total. An initial analysis of MIRACLE data suggested that patients with RBBB or IVCD did benefit from CRT [55]. In COMPANION, patients classified as "BBB other than left" appear to have less benefit from CRT than those with LBBB. A pooled analysis of data from MIRACLE and CONTAK CD did not support the use of CRT in RBBB, likening the therapy to placebo in those patients [56]. Patients with such QRS morphology are currently eligible for CRT according to current criteria.

QRS Duration

Most trials have used QRS duration criteria for enrollment. For example, the COMPANION trial required a QRS of ≥120 ms. Most have excluded patients with QRS duration <120 to <130 ms. When COMPANION data was stratified by QRS duration, there were apparent differences in response to CRT using combined end points and death, which seem to favor a more significant response in those patients with a longer QRS (Fig. 8.3). CARE-HF showed a similar trend (Fig. 8.4). The CARE-HF trial inclusion criteria required not only the same QRS criteria (>120 ms) but also echocardiographically documented dyssynchrony if the QRS fell below 150 ms. Standard measures of dyssynchrony were used (aortic pre-ejection delay >140 ms, interventricular mechanical delay >40 ms, and posterolateral delay). This may account for some of the strength of the CARE-HF data.

Limited studies have demonstrated benefit of CRT to patients with narrow QRS. In the presence of documented interventricular and intraventricular dyssynchrony, the benefit is similar to that obtained in patients selected by standard criteria in a small study with 52 patients [57]. In patients with heart failure, intraventricular dyssynchrony can be documented in >40% of patients with QRS <120 ms and in three-quarters of patients with QRS >120 ms [58]. This leaves a rather large population of patients with normal to mildly prolonged QRS who might potentially benefit from CRT but in whom data are wanting.

Echocardiography in CRT

Echocardiography holds promise in determining, prior to implant, which patients may benefit the most from CRT. Novel modalities including tissue Doppler imaging (TDI), tissue tracking, strain rate analysis, and time to peak systolic velocity have been used to quantitate dyssynchrony, along with the previously mentioned M-mode parameters.

Studies have shown the promise of the use of echocardiographic techniques to prescribe CRT, possibly even favoring it over QRS duration. Using TDI, delayed longitudinal contraction (contraction during diastole indicating mechanical left ventricular dyssynchrony), but not QRS, has been shown to be predictive of response to CRT and improvement in standard outcome measures, both clinically and echocardiographically [39]. A tissue Doppler index of multiple measures accurately predicts response to CRT-induced left ventricular reverse remodeling, whereas baseline QRS did not (Fig. 8.5) [59]. These techniques may provide the ability to accurately delineate who might benefit from CRT prospectively.

Future trials will attempt prospective use of these parameters. The PROSPECT trial, which is currently in progress, is one such trial. It is

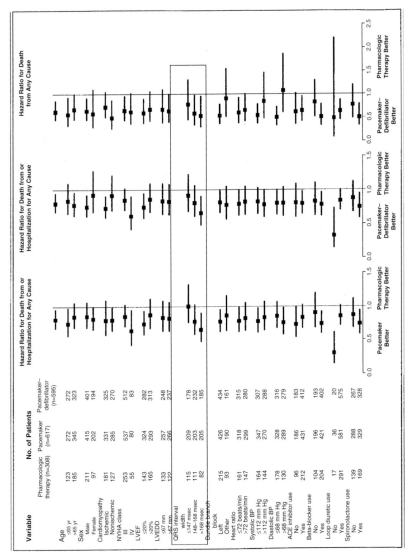

Fig. 8.3 Hazard ratios and 95% confidence intervals for the primary end point (death from or hospitalization for any cause) in COMPANION. The inserted box highlights the differences in response in patients with different QRS durations. (From Bristow MR, Saxon LA, Boehmer J, et al. Cardiac-resynchronization therapy with or without an implantable defibrillator in advanced chronic heart failure. N Engl J Med 2004:350:2140–50, permission and copyright 2004 Massachusetts Medical Society, all rights reserved).

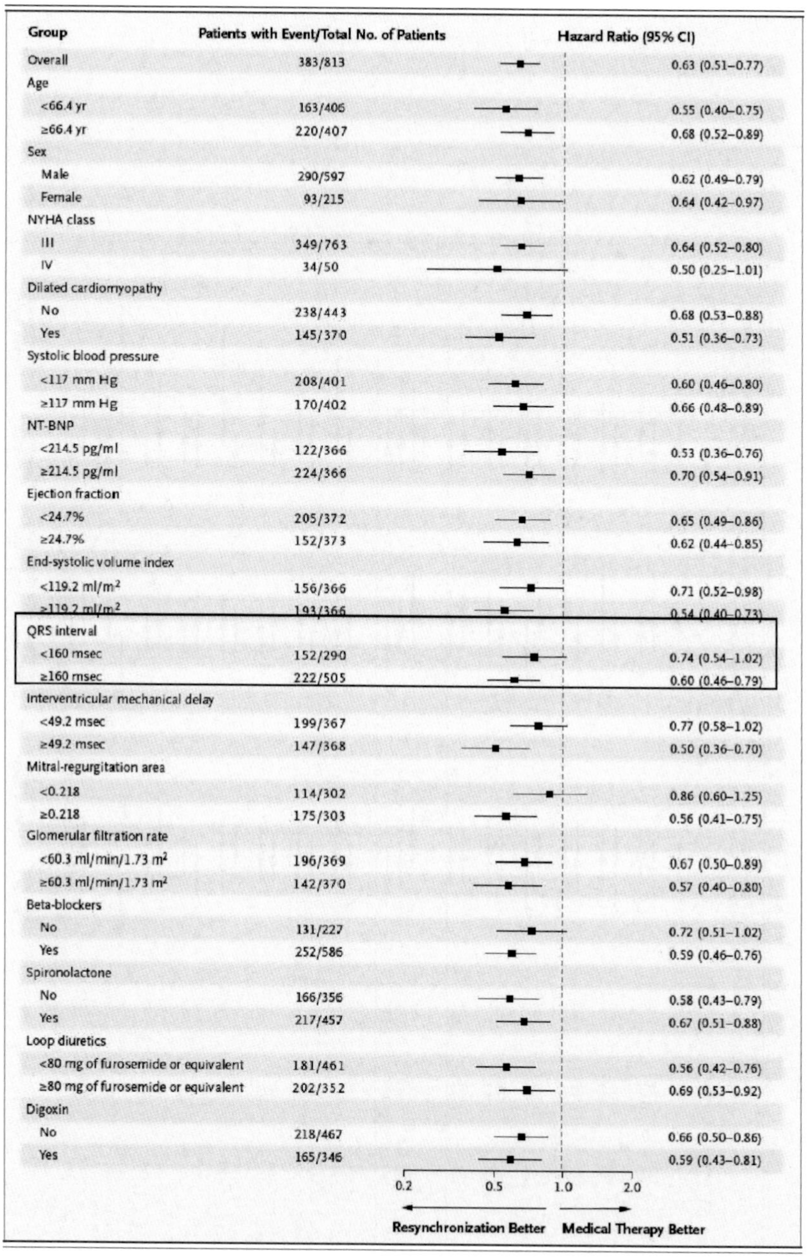

Fig. 8.4 Hazard ratios and 95% confidence intervals for the primary end point (death from any cause or hospitalization for major cardiovascular events) from CARE-HF. The inserted box highlights the differences in response in patients with different QRS durations, remembering that all patients with QRS duration ≤149 ms had to have echocardiographic dyssynchrony to be included in the study. (From Cleland JG, Daubert JC, Erdmann E, et al. Cardiac Resynchronization-Heart Failure (CARE-HF) Study Investigators. The effect of cardiac resynchronization on morbidity and mortality in heart failure. N Engl J Med 2005;352[15]:1539–49, permission and copyright 2005 Massachusetts Medical Society, all rights reserved).

a multicenter, nonrandomized prospective global trial to identify reliable echocardiographic predictors of positive response to CRT [60].

Echocardiographic use in postimplant optimization of CRT is an area that needs further clarification. Atrioventricular (A-V) optimization is performed with varying degrees of regularity, often dependent on center experience and in patients who are deemed to be "nonresponders" due to lack of clinical improvement. A recent retrospective analysis [61] showed that in patients who were assessed for the need for A-V optimization in the days after implant, 40% had significant changes made to their A-V interval in order to optimize diastolic filling but did not demonstrate differences in ejection fraction, NYHA class, or mortality. This report concluded that the importance of A-V optimization remains controversial and that inherent abnormalities of cardiac function (mitral regurgitation) may limit the application of A-V optimization, but that there was at least no harm demonstrated with changed settings.

Left Ventricular Pacing Site

The placement of the left ventricular lead in the CRT device is thought to have significant bearing on patient response to therapy. Early studies demonstrated poor hemodynamic response to pacing of the anterior wall (via the great cardiac vein) in comparison with pacing the LV free wall (lateral or posterior vein) [62]. A prospective study has concluded that reverse remodeling can be achieved by pacing at the site of maximum mechanical delay, more so than adjacent or remote areas [63].

Further questions remain regarding placement of the left ventricular lead including whether there are inherent differences in optimal pacing sites comparing patients with ischemic versus nonischemic cardiomyopathy.

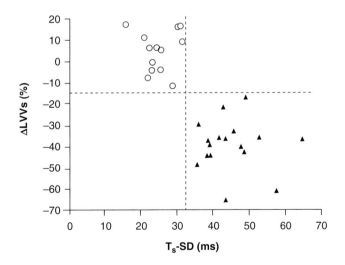

Fig. 8.5 An echocardiographic index of dyssynchrony can accurately delineate CRT responders from nonresponders (figure shows change in LV end systolic volume vs. severity of systolic dyssynchrony). (From Yu C, Fung W, Lin H, et al. Predictors of left ventricular reverse remodeling after cardiac resynchronization therapy for heart failure secondary to idiopathic dilated or ischemic cardiomyopathy. Am J Cardiol 2002;91:684–8).

16. Innes D, Keitch J, Fletcher P, et al. VDD pacing at short atrioventricular intervals does not improve cardiac output in patients with dilated heart failure [abstract]. PACE 1994;17:959.

17. Linde C, Gadler F, Edner M, et al. Results of atrioventricular synchronous pacing with optimized delay in patients with severe congestive heart failure [abstract]. Am J Cardiol 1995;75:919.

18. Brecker S, Gibson D. What is the role of pacing in dilated cardiomyopathy? Eur Heart J 1996;17:819.

19. Leclercq C, Cazeau S, Ritter P, et al. A pilot experience with permanent biventricular pacing to treat advanced heart failure. Am Heart J 2000;140(6):862–70.

20. Gras D, Leclercq C, Tang AS, et al. Cardiac resynchronization therapy in advanced heart failure the multicenter InSync clinical study. Eur J Heart Fail 2002;4(3): 311–20.

21. Kuhlkamp V, InSync 7272 ICD World Wide Investigators. Initial experience with an implantable cardioverter-defibrillator incorporating cardiac resynchronization therapy. J Am Coll Cardiol 2002;39(5):790–7.

22. Flather MD, Yusuf S, Kober L, et al. Long-term ACE-inhibitor therapy in patients with heart failure or left-ventricular dysfunction: A systematic overview of data from individual patients. ACE-Inhibitor Myocardial Infarction Collaborative Group. Lancet. 2000;355:1575–81.

23. Brophy JM, Joseph L, Rouleau JL. Beta-blockers in congestive heart failure. A Bayesian meta-analysis. Ann Intern Med 2001;134:550–60.

24. Pitt B, Zannad F, Remme WJ, et al. The effect of spironolactone on morbidity and mortality in patients with severe heart failure. Randomized Aldactone Evaluation Study Investigators. N Engl J Med 1999;341:709–17.

25. Pitt B, Remme W, Zannad F, et al. Eplerenone, a selective aldosterone blocker, in patients with left ventricular dysfunction after myocardial infarction. N Engl J Med 2003;348:1309–21.

26. Rector TS, Cohn JN. Assessment of patient outcome with the MinnesotaLiving with Heart Failure questionnaire: Reliability and validity during a randomized, double-blind, placebo-controlled trial of pimobendan. Pimobendan Multicenter Research Group. Am Heart J 1992;124:1017–25.

27. Rector TS, Kubo SH, Cohn JN. Validity of the Minnesota Living with Heart Failure questionnaire as a measure of therapeutic response to enalapril or placebo. Am J Cardiol 1993;71:1106–7.

28. Rector TS, Johnson G, Dunkman WB, et al. Evaluation by patients with heart failure of the effects of enalapril compared with hydralazine plus isosorbide dinitrate on quality of life. V-HeFT II. The V-HeFT VA Cooperative Studies Group. Circulation 1993;87:VI71–7.

29. Cohn JN, Tognoni G. A randomized trial of the angiotensin-receptor blocker valsartan in chronic heart failure. N Engl J Med 2001;345:1667–75.

30. Hjalmarson A, Goldstein S, Fagerberg B, et al. Effects of controlled-release metoprolol on total mortality, hospitalizations, and well-being in patients with heart failure: the Metoprolol CR/XL Randomized Intervention Trial in congestive heart failure (MERIT-HF). MERIT-HF Study Group. JAMA 2000;283:1295–302.

31. Bradley DJ, Bradley EA, Baughman KL, et al. Cardiac resynchronization and death from progressive heart failure: a meta-analysis of randomized controlled trials. JAMA 2003;289(6):730–40.

32. McAlister FA, Ezekowitz JA, Wiebe N, et al. Systematic review: Cardiac resynchronization in patients with symptomatic heart failure. Ann Intern Med 2004;141:381–90.

33. Davis DR, Krahn AD, Tang ASL, et al. Long-term outcome of cardiac resynchronization therapy in patients with severe congestive heart failure. Can J Cardiol 2005;21:413–7.

34. Bax JJ, Ansalone G, Breithardt OA, et al. Echocardiographic evaluation of cardiac resynchronization therapy: Ready for routine clinical use? A critical appraisal. J Am Coll Cardiol 2004;44:1–9.

35. Yu CM, Fung WH, Lin H, et al. Predictors of left ventricular reverse remodeling after cardiac resynchronization therapy for heart failure secondary to idiopathic dilated or ischemic cardiomyopathy. Am J Cardiol 2003;91:684–88.

36. Kim WY, Sogaard P, Mortensen PT, et al. Three dimensional echocardiography documents haemodynamic improvement by biventricular pacing in patients with severe heart failure. Heart 2001;85:514–20.

37. Pitzalis MV, Iacoviello M, Romito R, et al. Cardiac resynchronization therapy tailored by echocardiographic evaluation of ventricular asynchrony. J Am Coll Cardiol 2002;40:1615–22.

38. Reuter S, Garrigue S, Barold SS, et al. Comparison of characteristics in responders versus nonresponders with biventricular pacing for drug-resistant congestive heart failure. Am J Cardiol 2002;89:346–50.

39. Sogaard P, Egeblad H, Kim WY, et al. Tissue Doppler imaging predicts improved systolic performance and reversed left ventricular remodeling during long-term cardiac resynchronization therapy. J Am Coll Cardiol 2002;40:723–30.

40. Rossillo A, Verma A, Saad EB, et al. Impact of coronary sinus lead position on biventricular pacing: Mortality and echocardiographic evaluation during long-term follow-up. J Cardiovasc Electrophysiol 2004;15:1120–25.

41. Auricchio A, Fantoni C. Cardiac resynchronization therapy in heart failure. Ital Heart J 2005;6(3):256–60.

42. Bardy GH, Lee KL, Mark DB, et al, for the Sudden Cardiac Death in Heart Failure Trial (SCD-HeFT) Investigators. Amiodarone or an implantable cardioverter-defibrillator for congestive heart failure. N Engl J Med 2005;352:225–37.

43. Ellenbogen KA, Hellkamp AS, Wilkoff BL, et al. Complications arising after implantation of DDD pacemakers: the MOST experience. Am J Cardiol 2003;92:740–1.

44. Ezekowitz JA, Armstrong PW, McAlister FA. Implantable cardioverter defibrillators in primary and secondary prevention: A systematic review of randomized, controlled trials. Ann Intern Med 2003;138:445–52.

45. Higgins SL, Hummel JD, Niazi IK, et al. Cardiac resynchronization therapy for the treatment of heart failure in patients with intraventricular conduction delay and malignant ventricular tachyarrhythmias. J Am Coll Cardiol 2003;42:1454–59.

46. Auricchio A, Stellbrink C, Sack S, et al. Long-term clinical effect of hemodynamically optimized cardiac resynchronization therapy in patients with heart failure and ventricular conduction delay. J Am Coll Cardiol 2002;39:2026–33.

47. Garrigue S, Bordachar P, Reuter S, et al. Comparison of permanent left ventricular and biventricular pacing in patients with heart failure and chronic atrial fibrillation: prospective haemodynamic study. Heart 2002;87:529–34.

48. Leclercq C, Cazeau S, Lellouche D, et al. Upgrading from right ventricular pacing to biventricular pacing in previously paced patients with advanced heart failure: A randomized controlled study [the RD-CHF Trial] [abstract]. Presented at the European Society of Cardiology Congress, Vienna, Austria, 30 August–3 September 2003.

49. Leclercq C, Walker S, Linde C, et al. Comparative effects of permanent biventricular and right-univentricular pacing in heart failure patients with chronic atrial fibrillation. Eur Heart J 2002;23:1780–7.

50. Turner MS, Bleasdale RA, Vinereanu D, et al. Electrical and mechanical components of dyssynchrony in heart failure patients with normal QRS duration and left bundle-branch block: Impact of left and biventricular pacing. Circulation 2004;109:2544–9.

management with LVEF $\leq 35\%$, QRS ≤ 130 ms, and a class I indication for an implantable cardioverter defibrillator (ICD). The study randomized 186 patients who received a combined CRT-D (i.e., CRT and ICD) device to CRT-on (n = 85) or CRT-off (ICD only [n = 101] serving as the control group). A total of 98 control and 82 CRT patients completed the study through a 6-month follow-up. After 6 months, patients who received CRT demonstrated improvements over the control group in exercise time, 6-min walk distance, and peak VO_2 (the study's primary end point), although none of these parameters reached statistical significance. However, significant reverse LV remodeling was observed: The CRT group did show statistically significant differences compared with the control group in ventilatory response to exercise (VE/VCO_2; p = 0.01), NYHA class (p = 0.05), percentage of patients with improved overall clinical status (p = 0.01), and several echocardiographic functional parameters, including LV end diastolic volume (LVEDV) (p = 0.04), LV end systolic volume (LVESV) (p = 0.01), and LVEF (p = 0.02) (Fig. 9.1). According to the MIRACLE ICD II trial investigators, the fact that CRT did not significantly improve exercise capacity was not particularly surprising, because exercise capacity at baseline in class II patients is typically only mildly impaired. However, the workers noted that the patients in the study, despite having mild heart failure symptoms, already showed signs of extensive cardiac remodeling at baseline, comparable with that seen in class III/IV patients. The significant improvement of LVEDV, LVESV, and LVEF indicated that CRT promotes reverse remodeling even at an earlier stage in heart failure patients. The investigators also concluded that the improvement in the CRT group and the composite clinical response suggest that CRT acts to limit disease progression in patients with mild heart failure symptoms.

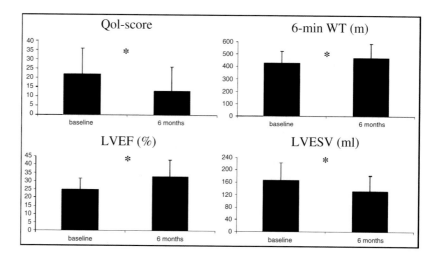

Fig. 9.1 Change in LV volumes and LVEF after 6 months of CRT or no pacing in NYHA class II patients. See text for details. (Reproduced with permission from Abraham WT, Young JB, Leon AR, et al. Multicenter InSync ICD II Study Group. Effects of cardiac resynchronization on disease progression in patients with left ventricular systolic dysfunction, an indication for an implantable cardioverter-defibrillator, and mildly symptomatic chronic heart failure. Circulation 2004;110:2864–2868).

CONTAK CD Trial: NYHA Class II Patients

The CONTAK CD trial [9] was another randomized, double-blind, parallel, controlled trial of CRT that included NYHA class II–IV heart failure patients; the trial's inclusion criteria were otherwise similar to those of the MIRACLE trials [6–8]. When the results were broken down by NYHA class III/IV and class II, the findings were very consistent with those seen in the aforementioned MIRACLE data. In addition to significant reductions in LV internal diameter in diastole and LV internal diameter in systole observed in class III/IV patients treated with CRT, significant reductions in both parameters were also noted with CRT (vs. control) in class II patients (p = 0.024 and p = 0.014, respectively).

Leiden Trial: NYHA Class II Patients

Fifty consecutive patients in NYHA class II heart failure and 50 consecutive patients in NYHA classes III to IV (control group) were prospectively evaluated for the impact of CRT [10]. All patients had LV ejection fraction ≤35% and QRS duration >120 ms. The effects of CRT in NYHA class II patients were compared with the results obtained in both groups. The severity of baseline LV dyssynchrony (assessed with color-coded tissue Doppler imaging) was comparable between patients in NYHA class II versus those in NYHA classes III to IV (83 ± 49 vs. 96 ± 51 ms, p = NS). Surprisingly, a modest but significant improvement in mean NYHA class was observed in the class II group from 2 ± 0 to 1.7 ± 0.6 (p < 0.01). The quality-of-life score improved from 22 ± 14 to 13 ± 13 (p < 0.001), and a small but significant improvement was observed in the 6-min walking distance (from 430 ± 94 to 469 ± 118 m, p < 0.01) (Figs. 9.2 and 9.3). In contrast with the minor improvements in clinical symptoms in class II patients, the improvements in LV function after 6 months of CRT were substantial, as evidenced by considerable LV reverse remodeling and markedly improved LVEF. NYHA class II patients showed a significant improvement in LVEF (from 25 ± 7% to 33 ± 10%, p < 0.001) and reduction in LVESV (from 168 ± 55 ml to 132 ± 51 ml, p < 0.001) after CRT, similar to patients in NYHA class III/IV. Only 8% of NYHA class II patients exhibited progression of heart failure symptoms. In line with previous studies, only the patients with substantial LV dyssynchrony demonstrated improved LV function and showed reduction in LV dyssynchrony. CRT had comparable effects in patients in NYHA class II and in NYHA classes III to IV heart failure in terms of LV resynchronization, improvement in LVEF, and LV reverse remodeling. The lack of a control group of NYHA class II patients without CRT represents a limitation of this study. However, the MIRACLE ICD study [7] had previously demonstrated less progression of heart failure in NYHA class II patients who underwent CRT than in a control group of NYHA class II patients treated medically.

HOBIPACE Trial: Moderate Impairment of Left Ventricular Function

The Homburg Biventricular Pacing Evaluation (HOBIPACE) was a randomized controlled study that compared the biventricular pacing approach with conventional right ventricular (RV) pacing in patients with LV

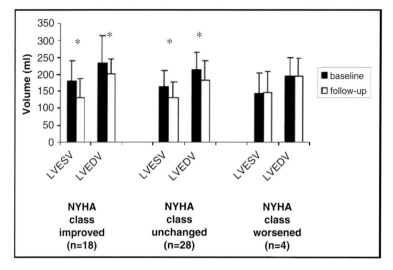

Fig. 9.2 Improvements in clinical and echocardiographic parameters at 6 months of CRT follow-up in patients in NYHA class II. *p < 0.05. 6-min WT, 6-min walking test; LVESV, left ventricular end-systolic volume; Qol, quality-of-life. See text for details. (Reproduced with permission from Bleeker GB, Schalij MJ, Holman ER, et al. Cardiac resynchronization therapy in patients with systolic left ventricular dysfunction and symptoms of mild heart failure secondary to ischemic or nonischemic cardiomyopathy. Am J Cardiol 2006;98:230–235).

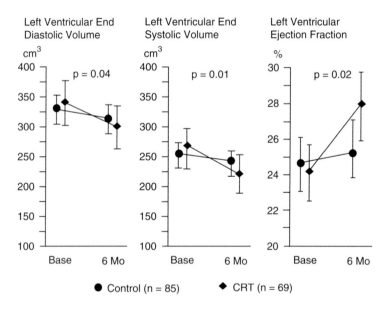

Fig. 9.3 Magnitude of LV reverse remodeling at 6 months of follow-up in CRT patients in NYHA class II with improvement in NYHA class (n = 18) versus those with unchanged NYHA class (n = 28) or with deterioration in NYHA class (n = 4). Black bars, baseline; white bars, follow-up. *p <0.05. LVEDV, left ventricular end-diastolic volume; other abbreviation as in Fig. 9.2. (Reproduced with permission from Bleeker GB, Schalij MJ, Holman ER, et al. Cardiac resynchronization therapy in patients with systolic left ventricular dysfunction and symptoms of mild heart failure secondary to ischemic or nonischemic cardiomyopathy. Am J Cardiol 2006;98:230–235).

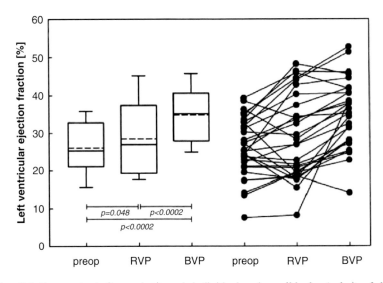

Fig. 9.4 Summarized (*box plots*) and individual values (*black circles*) of left ventricular ejection fraction before implantation of the study CRT device (*preop*) and after 3 months of right (*RVP*) and biventricular (*BVP*) pacing. In the box plot graph, the boundaries of the box indicate the 25th and 75th percentiles, the whiskers indicate the 10th and 90th percentiles, and the solid and dashed horizontal lines mark the median and mean value, respectively. (Reproduced with permission from Kindermann M, Hennen B, Jung J, et al. Biventricular versus conventional right ventricular stimulation for patients with standard pacing indication and left ventricular dysfunction: The Homburg Biventricular Pacing Evaluation (HOBIPACE). J Am Coll Cardiol 2006;47:1927–1937).

dysfunction and a standard indication for ventricular antibradycardia pacing [11]. Thirty patients with standard indication for permanent ventricular pacing and LV dysfunction defined by an LV end-diastolic diameter ≥60 mm, LVEF ≤40% and NYHA functional class II–IV were included. Using a prospective, randomized crossover design, 3 months of RV pacing were compared with 3 months of biventricular pacing with regard to LV function, N-terminal pro-B-type natriuretic peptide (NT-proBNP) serum concentration, exercise capacity, and quality of life. When compared with RV pacing, biventricular stimulation reduced LV end-diastolic (–9.0%, p = 0.022) and end-systolic volumes (–16.9%, p < 0.001), NT-proBNP level (–31.0%, p < 0.002), and the Minnesota Living with Heart Failure score (–18.9%, p = 0.01). LVEF (+22.1%), peak oxygen consumption (+12.0%), and oxygen uptake at the ventilatory threshold (+12.5%), were higher (p < 0.0002) with BV pacing (Fig. 9.4). The benefit of biventricular over RV pacing was similar for patients with (n = 9) and without (n = 21) atrial fibrillation. RV function was not affected by biventricular pacing.

NYHA Class III Patients with Moderate Depression of Left Ventricular Ejection Fraction

Fung et al. [12] conducted a prospective CRT study in 15 optimally treated patients (age: 66.1 ± 12.8 years; male = 13) with NYHA class III, LV ejection fraction >35% and <45% and QRS duration >120 ms. The magnitude of echocardiographic measurements was compared with 30 age, sex, NYHA class, and heart failure etiology matched patients with conventional CRT indication. After 3 months, there were significant reductions in LV end-systolic (86.2 ± 24.1 ml to 69.7 ± 22.2 ml, p < 0.01)/end-diastolic (135.5 ± 36.8 ml to 120.5 ± 34.6 ml, p < 0.01) volumes, improvement in LVEF (39.1 ± 2.2% to 44.2 ± 5.5%, p = 0.01), and NYHA class (3.0 ± 0.0 to 2.07 ± 0.46, p < 0.001). There was no difference in changes in LV volumes, LVEF, NYHA class, and exercise capacity before and after CRT between the study and conventional groups except for greater improvement in the quality of life score in the conventional group.

Overall Benefit of CRT in Patients with Less Advanced Heart Disease

It cannot be expected that patients with milder form of heart disease would show marked improvement compared with those with more severe forms of disease. However, in all the aforementioned studies, markers of deleterious ventricular remodeling were attenuated. LV function improved considerably with CRT (LV ejection fraction and reverse remodeling), and this improvement was comparable with that observed in those with more severe forms of a disease (NYHA class III/IV). Thus, it appears that CRT can provide significant benefit in terms of retardation or delay in heart failure progression for class II patients with LV ejection fraction ≤35% or class III patients with LV ejection fraction between 35% and 45% functional improvement as well as reverse LV remodeling.

Ongoing Trials in Patients with Less Advanced Heart Disease

Two large studies are under way to confirm these findings, which may result in future guidelines being expanded to include class II patients.

The REsynchronization reVErses Remodeling in Systolic left vEntricular dysfunction (REVERSE) study is a prospective, multicenter, randomized, double-blind, parallel, controlled clinical trial designed to establish whether CRT combined with optimal medical treatment can attenuate heart failure disease progression compared with optimal medical treatment alone in patients with either asymptomatic LV dysfunction (NYHA class I American College of Cardiology/American Heart Association stage C) or mild (NYHA functional class II) heart failure, QRS duration >120 ms, LVEF <40%, and LV end-diastolic diameter >55 mm [13]. The primary end point is the heart failure morbidity by clinical composite response, and reverse LV remodeling by LV end-systolic volume index is the first-order secondary end point. Approximately 600 patients from 100 centers in the United States, Canada, and Europe will be double-blinded randomized 2:1 to CRT versus no CRT. The follow-up is 5 years in total with the primary and first secondary end points reported at 12 months. Enrollment began in September 2004 and is expected to be completed in 2006.

The MADIT-CRT trial [14] aims at investigating whether prophylactic CRT inhibits or slows asymptomatic or mildly symptomatic heart failure. Patients with previous myocardial infarction and NYHA functional class I–II or patients with nonischemic cardiomyopathy in NYHA class II will be included if they have LVEF <30%, sinus rhythm, and QRS >130 ms. The primary end point is the time to first all-cause mortality or heart failure event analyzed from randomization. This study will include 1,820 subjects with an estimated follow-up time of 24 months.

CRT for Primary Implantation in Patients with a Conventional Indication for Antibradycardia Pacing

The widespread acceptance that long-term RV apical pacing can impair LV function and precipitate heart failure raises the question whether biventricular pacing should be considered for the "primary prevention" of LV remodeling and development of heart failure [15]. It would be useful to identify a subset of patients who are susceptible to the adverse effects of RV apex pacing before pacemaker implantation. Currently, only patients with preexisting LV dysfunction seem more likely to develop LV dyssynchrony after RV pacing. It can be hypothesized that patients requiring pacing for a conventional indication, NYHA class III/IV and LVEF $\leq$35% (regardless of the underlying configuration of the spontaneous QRS complex) might benefit from CRT at the time of the initial pacemaker implantation. The impressive 36% reduction in all-cause mortality (p = 0.002) produced by CRT (according to accepted indications) in the CARE-HF trial lends some validity to the idea of primary prevention [16]. The results of CRT in patients with less advanced heart disease (discussed above) could be logically extrapolated to selected patients requiring conventional RV antibradycardia pacing [17].

We believe that a CRT approach for initial pacemaker implantation might be worthwhile in selected patients with bradycardia. On the basis of little data [17, 18], a number of workers now believe that it is reasonable to consider biventricular pacing if frequent or continuous RV pacing (i.e., when a large cumulative percentage of RV pacing as in complete atrioventricular (AV) block) is expected in the setting of LVEF $\leq$35% (even without clinical heart failure) especially with associated mitral regurgitation. The cutoff point for LVEF is likely to change in the future with the emergence of more supportive data about the benefit of CRT in patients with less advanced forms of heart disease. At this juncture, all patients with sinus node dysfunction and especially with LVEF $\leq$35% should receive a conventional RV pacemaker with appropriate algorithms to minimize RV pacing if the clinical situation suggests that RV pacing is likely to be infrequent. The suggestion to consider biventricular pacing in selected patients requiring antibradycardia pacing is based on the concept derived from the Mode Selection Trial (MOST) that it is the cumulative percentage of RV pacing time that ultimately determines the incidence of hospitalizations for CHF, and the frequency of AF [19, 20].

Right Ventricular Pacing After AV Nodal Ablation for Atrial Fibrillation

PAVE Trial

The PAVE trial was the first randomized trial designed to evaluate prospectively the long-term effects of pacing in patients with chronic atrial fibrillation

Upgrading of Conventional Pacing Systems

Upgrading from RV to biventricular (BV) pacing now constitutes an important and rapidly growing segment of pacemaker practice involving NYHA class III–IV patients with heart failure and LVEF $\leq 35\%$ despite an optimal AV delay 11, 22–35]. About 20% of resynchronization devices are now implanted to upgrade a conventional RV pacemaker for the treatment of heart failure. The growing number of upgrading procedures from RV to biventricular pacing in regular pacemaker patients with heart failure should be interpreted as a wake-up call to seriously consider and investigate the role of primary prevention of heart failure in selected patients at the time of initial pacemaker implantation. In this setting, the potential advantages of CRT should be weighed against procedural difficulties and complications. The decision process would be facilitated with the future studies and development of faster and easier methods to achieve LV pacing.

In patients with systolic heart failure and an implanted RV pacemaker, upgrading to a biventricular system produces an immediate improvement in LV function and reduction of functional mitral regurgitation on the basis of a more coordinated LV contraction [22–35]. On a long-term basis, there is evidence that pacemaker patients with an upgraded system exhibit further improvement of LV function on the basis of reverse remodeling [22–35]. The acute and long-term responses to upgrading an RV pacing system appear similar to those seen in patients (without a pacemaker) undergoing cardiac resynchronization for standard indications (poor systolic LV function and LV dyssynchrony) [22–35]. The question of primary prevention of heart failure is becoming important in patients with conventional RV pacemakers. We believe that upgrading to a biventricular system should be considered earlier than waiting for the development of heart failure with an LVEF $\leq 35\%$. Hence the importance of careful follow-up to detect progressive deterioration of LV function.

Monitoring Left Ventricular Function in Pacemaker Patients

The impact of CRT therapy has increased the importance of monitoring LV function in patients attending a routine pacemaker follow-up service. In this respect, a study involving 307 pacemaker patients in a routine pacemaker follow-up service revealed an LVEF <40% in 31% of the patients [36]. These findings suggest that if "prevention is better than a cure," one should adopt a proactive approach and periodically evaluate the LVEF of pacemaker patients to determine whether upgrading to BV pacing might be beneficial before marked deterioration of LV function and the onset of heart failure, which carries a dismal prognosis in the elderly.

Deterioration of LV function over time was highlighted by the recent study [37] that evaluated the change of the nuclear determined LVEF (baseline 25–40%) over a period of approximately 18 months in 207 patients with a variety of conditions including some patients with RV pacemakers. The analysis was limited to patients with an increase of $\geq 10\%$ (148 patients) and those with a decrease of $\geq 7\%$ (59 patients) of the LVEF. Among pacemaker patients (mostly dual chamber rate responsive (DDDR)), 27% showed an increase in LVEF and 50% showed a decrease. The strongest independent predictor of LVEF decrease was the presence of a permanent RV pacemaker (odds ratio

6.6, p = 0.002). Although the presence of a pacemaker probably identified a sicker group of patients at the beginning of the study, the results do highlight the importance of carefully following LV function in pacemaker patients.

Thus, follow-up of LV function is an effective way to determine potential candidates for upgrading patients undergoing RV pacing. However, the main flaw of this approach, as well as usage of current indications for CRT, is absence of indices to prediction a positive response to upgrading.

The recently published report from the Ablate and Pace in Atrial Fibrillation (APAF) group [38] attempted to resolve this problem. This study evaluated how pacing from the RV apex affected LV electromechanical activation and assessed whether the extent of LV dyssynchrony during RV pacing can be predicted by clinical, ECG, or echocardiographic findings obtained during sinus rhythm. The authors evaluated 56 patients (all in sinus rhythm except for three in atrial fibrillation) with a normal QRS complex and preserved AV conduction who received permanent backup RV pacemakers. Intra-LV electromechanical activation was assessed during sinus rhythm and during RV pacing. An abnormal electromechanical LV delay was found in 27% of patients all during sinus rhythm and *only* in 50% of patients during RV pacing (p <0.001). This data is in full agreement with the results of the Leiden AF trial [21]. An abnormal baseline electromechanical LV delay (in sinus rhythm) and QRS >85 ms were independent predictors of an abnormal electromechanical LV delay during RV pacing. Thus, RV apical pacing induces mechanical LV dyssynchrony in a substantial percentage of pacemaker patients but not all. In some patients with complete AV block, RV pacing may even improve LV function [11, 37]. Although normal baseline electromechanical LV activation cannot exclude the development of significant dyssynchrony during RV pacing, the presence of preimplantation LV dyssynchrony predicts worsening of this detrimental problem. These observations should encourage the search of additional indices that predict a positive response to CRT in patients with conventional pacemakers (as well as in patients with accepted indications for CRT). These data can also begin to explain why not all the patients with RV pacing develop LV dysfunction and heart failure.

Enhanced Follow-up of Patients with Conventional Pacemakers and Preimplant Prediction of Deleterious Effect of RV Pacing

QRS Duration

Preimplantation and postimplantation paced QRS duration was recently shown to be a strong predictor of heart failure hospitalization (HFH) and death in pacemaker patients [20, 38–41]. According to Sweeney et al. [39], the risk of HFH increased incrementally with increasing QRS duration, independent of whether the prolonged QRS duration occurred spontaneously or was caused by RV apical pacing (Fig. 9.6). Importantly, the absolute risk of HFH was always twofold higher for a prolonged QRS duration that occurred spontaneously versus that due to RV apical pacing for any given value of QRS duration. This study also provided strong evidence that the increased relative risk of HFH associated with a more prolonged QRS duration is equivalent for prolongation that either occurs spontaneously or is due to RVA pacing. The increased risk of HFH associated with increasing QRS duration was slightly failure secondary to ischemic or nonischemic cardiomyopathy. Am J Cardiol 2006;98:230–235.

11. Kindermann M, Hennen B, Jung J, et al. Biventricular versus conventional right ventricular stimulation for patients with standard pacing indication and left ventricular dysfunction: The Homburg Biventricular Pacing Evaluation (HOBIPACE). J Am Coll Cardiol 2006;47:1927–1937.

12. Fung JW, Zhang Q, Yip GW, et al. Effect of cardiac resynchronization therapy in patients with moderate left ventricular systolic dysfunction and wide QRS Complex: A prospective study. J Cardiovasc Electrophysiol 2006; 17:1288–1292.

13. Linde C, Gold M, Abraham WT, Daubert J-C, for the REVERSE Study Group. Rationale and design of a randomized controlled trial to assess the safety and efficacy of cardiac resynchronization therapy in patients with asymptomatic left ventricular dysfunction with previous symptoms or mild heart failure—the REsynchronization reVErses Remodeling in Systolic left vEntricular dysfunction (REVERSE) study. Am Heart J 2006;151:288–294.

14. Moss AJ, Brown MW, Cannom DS, et al. Multicenter automatic defibrillator implantation trial-cardiac resynchronization therapy (MADIT-CRT): Design and clinical protocol. Ann Noninvasive Electrocardiol 2005;10(4 Suppl):34–43.

15. Barold SS, Lau CP. Primary prevention of heart failure in cardiac pacing. Pacing Clin Electrophysiol 2006; 29:271–219.

16. Cleland JGF, Daubert J-C, Erdmann E, et al, for the Cardiac Resynchronization—Heart Failure (CARE-HF) Study Investigators. The effect of cardiac resynchronization on morbidity and mortality in heart failure. N Engl J Med 2005;352:1539–1549.

17. Sweeney MO, Prinzen FW. A new paradigm for physiologic ventricular pacing. J Am Coll Cardiol 2006;47:282–288.

18. Doshi RN, Daoud EG, Fellows C, et al. Left ventricular- based cardiac stimulation post AV nodal ablation evaluation (The PAVE Study). J Cardiovasc Electrophysiol 2005;16:1160–1165.

19. Sweeney MO, Hellkamp AS, Ellenbogen KA, et al, for the MOST Investigators. Adverse effect of ventricular pacing on heart failure and atrial fibrillation among patients with normal baseline QRS duration in a clinical trial of pacemaker therapy for sinus node dysfunction. Circulation 2003;107:2932–2937.

20. Sweeney MO, Hellkamp AS. Heart failure during cardiac pacing. Circulation 2006;113:2082–2088.

21. Tops LF, Schalij MJ, Holman ER, et al. Right ventricular pacing can induce ventricular dyssynchrony in patients with atrial fibrillation after atrioventricular node ablation. J Am Coll Cardiol 2006;48:1642–1648.

22. Leon AR, Greenberg JM, Kanuru N, et al. Cardiac resynchronization in patients with congestive heart failure and chronic atrial fibrillation: Effect of upgrading to biventricular pacing after chronic right ventricular pacing. J Am Coll Cardiol 2002;39:1258–1263.

23. Horwich T, Foster E, DE Marco T, et al. Effects of resynchronization therapy on cardiac function in pacemaker patients "upgraded" to biventricular devices. J Cardiovasc Electrophysiol 2004;15:1284–1289.

24. Eldadah ZA, Rosen B, Hay I, et al. The benefit of upgrading chronically right ventricle-paced heart failure patients to resynchronization therapy demonstrated by strain rate imaging. Heart Rhythm 2006;3:435–442.

25. Marai I, Gurevitz O, Carasso S, et al. Improvement of congestive heart failure by upgrading of conventional to resynchronization pacemakers. Pacing Clin Electrophysiol 2006;29:880–884.

26. Linde C, Leclercq C, Rex S, et al. Long-term benefits of biventricular pacing in congestive heart failure: Results from the MUltisite STimulation in cardiomyopathy (MUSTIC) study. J Am Coll Cardiol 2002;40:111–118.

27. Baker CM, Christopher TJ, Smith PF, et al. Addition of a left ventricular lead to conventional pacing systems in patients with congestive heart failure: Feasibility, safety, and early results in 60 consecutive patients. PACE 2002;25:1166–1171.
28. Valls-Bertault V, Fatemi M, Gilard M, et al. Assessment of upgrading to biventricular pacing in patients with right ventricular pacing and congestive heart failure after atrioventricular junctional ablation for chronic atrial fibrillation. Europace 2004;6:438–443.
29. Rosen BD, Berger R. Resynchronization therapy upgrade. Turning coach into first class. J Cardiovasc Electrophysiol 2004;15:1290–1292.
30. Hoijer CJ, Meurling C, Brandt J. Upgrade to biventricular pacing in patients with conventional pacemakers and heart failure: A double-blind, randomized crossover study. Europace 2006;8:51–55.
31. Leclercq C, Cazeau S, Lellouche D, et al. Upgrading from right-ventricular pacing to biventricular pacing in previously paced patients with advanced heart failure: A randomized controlled study. Eur Heart J 2003;24(Suppl Aug/Sept):364A.
32. Bertault V, Fatemi M, Etienne Y, et al. Congestive heart failure in patients with right-ventricular pacing after atrioventricular node ablation. Is upgrading to biventricular pacing an effective treatment. Eur Heart J 2003;24(Suppl Aug/Sept24):521A.
33. Ritter O, Koller ML, Fey V, et al. Progression of heart failure in right univentricular pacing compared to biventricular pacing. Int J Cardiol 2006;110(3):359–365.
34. Rubaj A, Rucinski P, Rejdak K, et al. Biventricular versus right ventricular pacing decreases immune activation and augments nitric oxide production in patients with chronic heart failure. Eur J Heart Fail 2006; 8:615–620.
35. Leclercq C, Walker S, Linde C, et al. Comparative effects of permanent biventricular and right-univentricular pacing in heart failure patients with chronic atrial fibrillation. Eur Heart J 2002;23(22):1732–1736.
36. Thackray SD, Witte KK, Nikitin NP, et al. The prevalence of heart failure and asymptomatic left ventricular systolic dysfunction in a typical regional pacemaker population. Eur Heart J 2003;24:1143–1152.
37. O'Keefe JH Jr, Abuissa H, Jones PG, et al. Effect of chronic right ventricular apical pacing on left ventricular function. Am J Cardiol 2005;95:771–773.
38. Lupi G, Sassone B, Badano L, et al.; Ablate and Pace in Atrial Fibrillation (APAF) Pilot Echocardiographic Trial Investigators. Effects of right ventricular pacing on intra-left ventricular electromechanical activation in patients with native narrow QRS. Am J Cardiol 2006;98(2):219–222.
39. Sweeney MO, Hellkamp AS, Lee KL, Lamas GA; Mode Selection Trial (MOST) Investigators. Association of prolonged QRS duration with death in a clinical trial of pacemaker therapy for sinus node dysfunction. Circulation 2005;111: 2418–2423.
40. Miyoshi F, Kobayashi Y, Itou H, et al. Prolonged paced QRS duration as a predictor for congestive heart failure in patients with right ventricular apical pacing. Pacing Clin Electrophysiol 2005;28:1182–1188.
41. Hayes JJ, Sharma AD, Love JC, et al,; DAVID Investigators. Abnormal conduction increases risk of adverse outcomes from right ventricular pacing. J Am Coll Cardiol 2006;48:1628–1633.
42. Barold SS, Stroobandt RX. Harmful effects of long-term right ventricular pacing. Acta Cardiol 2006;61:103–110.
43. Manolis AS. The deleterious consequences of right ventricular apical pacing: Time to seek alternate site pacing. Pacing Clin Electrophysiol 2006;29:298–315.
44. Barold SS, Herweg B. Right ventricular outflow tract pacing: not ready for prime time. J Interv Card Electrophysiol 2005;13:39–46.

of 21% and 78 mm, respectively, and normal coronary angiography. Further, we carefully excluded those with a suspected known reversible causes of cardiomyopathy

Even if some cases of clear improvement of idiopathic DCM have been reported, "complete" recovery is rare, and when it did occur, the patients were usually young and had had a short duration of symptoms; neither of these characteristics apply to our study population. In our cases, the long-lasting (over several years) evolution of CHF symptoms essentially excludes the possibility of either "spontaneous" recovery or of the DCM being of acute myocarditis origin. Consequently, it could be reasonably assumed that our patients indeed had exhibited a severe idiopathic DCM upon entry into this study.

Was the Reversal of LV Dysfunction Real?

Our findings indicate that the reversal of LV dysfunction encompassed not only LVEF but also end diastolic diameter and mitral regurgitation. A remaining important question to consider is whether this reversal is complete or not. It seems complete, comparing baseline values of radionuclide angiography and echocardiography with those at the 12-month follow-up, supporting the view that the cardiac status of the group 1 patients could be considered "normal."

Mechanism of LV Dysfunction

It has long been known that LBBB induces an abnormal LV contraction pattern resulting in LV dysfunction with a decrease in EF. Whether this abnormal contraction pattern could provoke over time a DCM remains unknown, but the possibility is supported by Framingham data in which LBBB was reported to precede appearance of CHF in a subset of individuals.

Exclusion of LBBB induced by LV-based cardiac pacing may substantially diminish the mechanically deleterious effects of the intraventricular dyssynchrony. The outcome is progressive improvement in LV function. Further, the observation that after cessation of pacing the QRS duration tended to decrease in group 1 patients supports the notion that LBBB-induced dyssynchrony leads to a form of LV dysfunction that aggravates intraventricular conduction disturbances. Presumably, LV-based pacing interrupts this vicious circle and thereby tends to improve intraventricular contractions synchrony over time.

Predictive Factors of LV Dysfunction Reversal

The small number of patients who normalized their LV function limits identification of predictors of reverse remodeling. It should be stressed that many potential discriminating factors have not been analyzed either because they were not included in the database or because they are still undetermined.

How Many Patients with DCM Could Be Cured?

In series evaluating patients with DCM, a wide QRS complex was found in approximately 25% to 30% of the population. Considering the 17% reversal rate observed in our study, it seems that 5% of all the patients with DCM could have a complete reversal to normal of their left ventricular function.

Unresolved Issues

There remain many unresolved issues with respect to the LBBB-induced DCM issue. Why some patients with long-term evolution of well-defined DCM and LBBB had, after LV pacing, normalization of their LV function whereas others did not is unclear. Had the left ventricular lead pacing site some influence? Are some environmental or genetically transmitted factors responsible for different outcomes?

Conclusion

Among patients with DCM and LBBB, there is a significant subset of patients (17%) that can be cured by left ventricular–based pacing. This observation gives rise to the new concept of LBBB-induced DCM or more extensively to the concept of dyssynchrony or mechanical-induced DCM.

References

1. Maron BJ, Towbin JA, Thiene G, et al.; American Heart Association; Council on Clinical Cardiology, Heart Failure and Transplantation Committee; Quality of Care and Outcomes Research and Functional Genomics and Translational Biology Interdisciplinary Working Groups; Council on Epidemiology and Prevention. Contemporary definitions and classification of the cardiomyopathies: An American Heart Association Scientific Statement from the Council on Clinical Cardiology, Heart Failure and Transplantation Committee; Quality of Care and Outcomes Research and Functional Genomics and Translational Biology Interdisciplinary Working Groups; and Council on Epidemiology and Prevention. Circulation 2006;113: 1807–16.
2. Blanc JJ, Fatemi M, Bertault V, et al. Evaluation of left bundle branch block as a reversible cause of non-ischaemic dilated cardiomyopathy with severe heart failure. A new concept of left ventricular dyssynchrony-induced cardiomyopathy. Europace 2005;7:604–10.

(A)

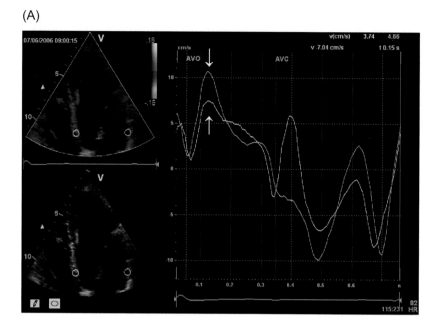

(B)

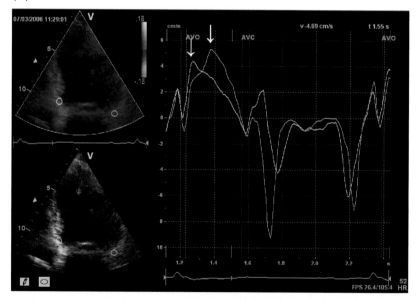

Fig. 11.5 (**A**) Color-coded tissue Doppler image of a normal individual without LV dyssynchrony. The sample volumes are placed in the basal part of the septum and lateral wall, and tracings are derived (*yellow curve*, septum; *green curve*, lateral wall; *arrows* indicate peak systolic velocities). (**B**) Color-coded tissue Doppler image of a patient with severe heart failure and substantial LV dyssynchrony (*yellow curve*, septum; *green curve*, lateral wall; *arrows* indicate peak systolic velocity).

velocities were measured in the six basal LV segments (septal, lateral, inferior, anterior, anteroseptal, and posterior). Calculating the difference between the longest and shortest time to peak systolic velocity across the six regions yielded the peak systolic difference. Again, the TDI-derived parameter of LV dyssynchrony was the only baseline parameter that predicted (echocardiographic) response to CRT. A predefined cutoff value of 110 ms in peak systolic difference had a sensitivity of 97% with a specificity of 55% to predict LV reverse remodeling at 3 months follow-up [9].

Yu et al. have published extensively on the use of color-coded TDI to predict response to CRT. The authors developed a 12-segment model of LV dyssynchrony by measuring the peak systolic velocities from six basal and six mid-LV segments on the three apical views. The dyssynchrony index was calculated as the standard deviation of the time to peak systolic velocity from all 12 segments [7, 15–17]. Preliminary data showed that the dyssynchrony index improved significantly in 25 patients undergoing CRT (from 37.7 ± 10.9 to 29.3 ± 8.3, $p < 0.05$), and it was concluded that improvement of LV dyssynchrony seemed to be the predominant mechanism of response to CRT [7]. In subsequent studies, the dyssynchrony index proved highly predictive of response [15]. Sophisticated analysis revealed that the optimal cutoff value of 31.4 ms yielded a sensitivity of 96% with a specificity of 78% to predict LV reverse remodeling at 3 months follow-up [16].

Pulsed-Wave TDI

Pulsed-wave TDI can be used for the on-line recording of myocardial velocity curves by placing the pulsed-wave Doppler sample in the region of interest. This approach does not allow simultaneous calculations of multiple segments in one view, and changes in cardiac frequency should be avoided in different recordings in order to obtain an accurate comparison of the timing of systolic events among different LV segments.

Studies using pulsed-wave TDI usually calculate the time from beginning of the QRS complex to the *onset of systolic velocity*, because the peak systolic velocity is often less clearly defined compared with color-coded TDI (Figs. 11.3 and 11.4).

Ansalone et al. used a six-segment model in 21 nonischemic heart failure patients and demonstrated that CRT significantly reduced desynchronized contractions in at least one third of the LV basal segments [19].

Bordachar et al. studied 41 patients by measuring both the largest delay in peak and the onset of systolic velocity and the standard deviation of peak to systolic velocity in six basal and six mid-LV segments from the apical views. The authors concluded that the improvement in cardiac output and the reduction in mitral regurgitation were significantly correlated with the degree of preimplantation LV dyssynchrony. In addition, the authors conclude that the degree in interventricular dyssynchrony was not related to hemodynamic improvements following CRT [20]. The work by Penicka et al. defined LV dyssynchrony as the maximal electromechanical delay among the three basal LV segments (septal, lateral, and posterior wall) and interventricular dyssynchrony as the maximal delay between the basal right ventricular segment and the three LV sites [22]. The authors suggested that summation of the LV and interventricular dyssynchrony had a high predictive

routine echocardiography LV dyssynchrony was calculated as the standard deviation of times to minimal regional volume for each of the 16 segments, referred to as the systolic dyssynchrony index. The authors concluded that RT3DE is highly reproducible and able to quantify global LV dyssynchrony. In addition, preliminary results in 26 patients undergoing CRT showed that the baseline systolic dyssynchrony index was significantly different between responders and nonresponders [31]. To date, no study has provided an optimal cutoff value for the systolic dyssynchrony index assessed by RT3DE to predict response to CRT.

Besides its use for the detection and quantification of LV dyssynchrony, RT3DE can potentially play an important role in identifying the most suitable location for the LV pacing lead. Recent studies have indicated that the LV pacing lead should ideally be positioned in the area of latest LV activation [22, 29]. Because of its ability to quantify regional LV dyssynchrony in a large number of LV segments, in a 3D fashion, RT3DE may prove to be an ideal tool to guide LV lead placement.

Another method to obtain 3D information on LV dyssynchrony is now available in the form of triplane TSI (Fig. 11.9). This technique allows simultaneous recording and analysis of peak systolic velocity in the four-, two-, and three-chamber views in one single heartbeat. Off-line analysis

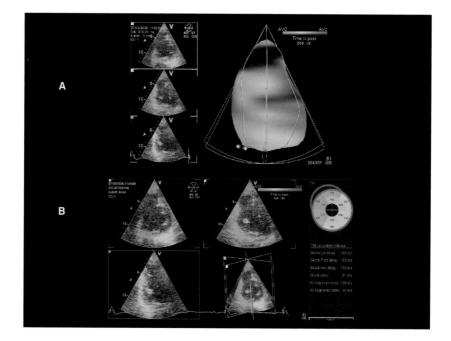

Fig. 11.9 Triplane tissue synchronization imaging (TSI) allows automatic analysis of time to peak systolic velocities in various LV segments during the same heartbeat. Panel *A* illustrates TSI combined with surface mapping. The 3D reconstructed image of the left ventricle shows a delayed activation of the anterolateral wall represented by the yellow color. Panel *B* shows that by placing markers in 12 left ventricular segments, TSI automatically generates the time to peak systolic velocity of these segments. The results are presented in a polar plot confirming delayed activation of the anterolateral segments. Septal to lateral delay and standard deviation of the six basal or all 12 left ventricular segments are calculated automatically.

with a dedicated software program (Echopac, General Electric-Vingmed, Milwaukee, Wis., USA) allows parametric imaging with a 3D color-coded volume based on the triplane data set allowing a visual representation of the area of latest mechanical activation. The software program also automatically calculates the time to peak systolic velocity in 12 segments of the left ventricle and summarizes these quantitative data in a polar plot. Various indices of dyssynchrony such as septal to lateral delay and standard deviations are calculated automatically. Future studies are needed to show the value of this technique for assessment of the area of latest LV activation.

Other Factors Related to Response

Although a large number of studies has demonstrated the value of substantial LV dyssynchrony to predict response to CRT [8,9,15,16], other factors may also influence the response to CRT. In particular, the location of the LV pacing lead and the presence of (posterolateral) scar tissue (in patients with ischemic cardiomyopathy) may be important factors influencing response to CRT.

Currently, the LV pacing lead is preferably positioned in the lateral or the posterolateral LV region. Several studies have indeed indicated that positioning the LV lead in this region resulted in the largest improvement in hemodynamics. For example, Rossillo et al. retrospectively evaluated 233 patients showing who underwent successful CRT implantation and noted that patients with an anterior or anterolateral lead position (n = 66) did not improve in LV ejection fraction, whereas patients with a lateral or posterolateral lead position showed a significant increase in LV ejection fraction (from 19% to 27%, p < 0.01) [46].

More recent studies emphasized the importance of positioning the LV lead in the area of latest LV activation, which is usually the posterior/lateral region. Murphy et al. [22] used TSI to study the effects of LV lead positioning in relation to the area of latest LV activation. The authors demonstrated a larger reduction in end-systolic volume (indicating reverse LV remodeling) in patients with the LV lead positioned in the area of latest activation (23% reduction in LV end-systolic volume) compared with patients with the lead positioned in an adjacent (15% reduction) or a remote (9% increase) region. Similar results were reported by Suffoletto et al. showing that LV pacing in the area of latest activation increased LV ejection fraction by 10 ± 5% compared with 6 ± 5% (p < 0.05) when a remote area was paced [29].

LV lead placement in the area of latest LV activation will require a patient-tailored approach, and 3D TSI or RT3DE may be the preferred techniques to provide this information.

A second factor that influences the response to CRT and may have potential implications for patient selection is the presence and localization of myocardial scar tissue; this is an issue only in patients with ischemic cardiomyopathy and previous infarction. Bleeker et al. recently addressed this issue in an elegant study using contrast-enhanced magnetic resonance imaging (MRI) to assess scar tissue [47]. Contrast-enhanced MRI is an excellent technique for this purpose, because the high spatial resolution permits precise delineation of scar tissue and even permits distinction between subendocardial

The role of the echocardiography, then, consists in optimizing the end of the filling phase by adapting the AV delay according to Ritter's formula or any other method, with a view to program the shortest delay that allows the longest filling without encroaching on the A-wave by premature closure of the mitral valve. This maneuver is performed during VDD (on sensed waves) pacing, with P wave sensing, and during atrial (DDD (on paced atria)) pacing, in order to correct for electromechanical delays during atrial stimulation.

Ritter's formula uses transmitral inflow Doppler measurements made with two different AV delays. Both AV delays must be applied under the same condition of either atrial sensing or atrial pacing. It is recommended to begin with sensed P-waves, that is, atrial contraction must be spontaneous (not paced), and ventricular contraction must be stimulated. The same measurements are repeated during atrial pacing. The paced AV delay must be longer than the sensed AV delay.

Instructions:

1. Program a long AVD (e.g., 150 ms) and record the transmitral inflow Doppler from the apical view and measure the QA interval from ventricular pacing spike to end of the A-wave of the transmitral Doppler signal (Fig. 12.6).
2. Program a short AV delay (e.g., 50 ms) and record the transmitral inflow Doppler from the apical view and measure the QA interval from ventricular pacing spike to end of the A-wave of the transmitral Doppler signal (Fig. 12.7).
3. Calculate the optimal AV delay.

The difference between the long and short AV delays, minus the difference between the short and long QA, is the excess shortening of the AV delay. This value should be added to the short AV delay to obtain the optimal AV delay for

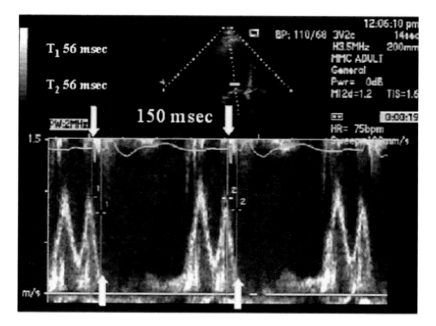

Fig. 12.6 Measurement of the QA interval. In this example, a long AV delay of 150 ms results in a QA interval of 56 ms.

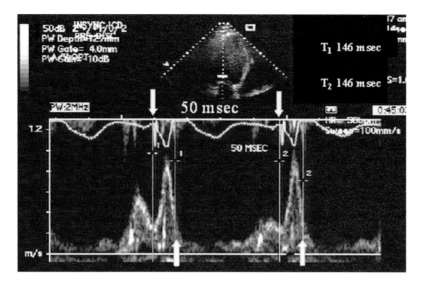

Fig. 12.7 Measurement of the QA interval for the short AV Delay. In this example, a short AV delay of 50 ms results in a QA interval of 146 ms.

ventricular filling. It represents the shortest AV delay that allows the longest filling period without interrupting the end of the A-wave by premature mitral valve closure. In this particular example, the value is $[(150 \text{ ms} - 50 \text{ ms}) - (146 \text{ ms} - 56 \text{ ms})] = 10$ ms. This is the value that is added to the short AV delay (i.e., 50 ms). According to Ritter's formula, the optimal AV delay is 60 ms.

However, when AV conduction is partially preserved, this standard approach might not be the best, because a prolongation of the AV delay might, paradoxically, lengthen the period of ventricular filling. Indeed, lengthening of the AV delay can result in fusion between activation originating from the stimulating leads and activation via the Purkinje system. This causes shortening of systole by the earlier activation of a greater number of sites and, therefore, a considerable increase in the time occupied by diastole and ventricular filling. This action affects the beginning of the filling phase only and is possible for a short range of values of the AV delay. To maintain the same fusion between spontaneous activation and stimulated activation, the AV delay value should closely follow the variations in spontaneous PR interval, modulated by the autonomic nervous system. This, however, is not systematically the case, and a flawless optimization at rest is often accompanied by loss of capture during activity.

Interventricular Resynchronization and Interventricular Delay

At the interventricular level, the preoperative mechanical interventricular delay, considered abnormal beyond 40 ms, must be shortened. This is the duty of biventricular stimulation, which hinges more on a proper lead placement than on postoperative reprogramming of the device. There are, nevertheless, two means of shortening of the interventricular interval: (1) by shortening the abnormally long left pre-ejection interval or (2) by shortening the right pre-ejection interval, which is often within normal limits. The improvement of interventricular synchrony between the left ventricle and right ventricle (RV) by CRT is far less important clinically than the reduction or elimination of intraventricular LV dyssynchrony.

It remains to be determined whether the interventricular interval is a marker or a cause of dyssynchrony, though it is clear that its shortening after implantation of the CRT system has an impact on the optimal AV delay. The persistence of a long interval implies that an AV delay that is optimal for the filling of the left cardiac chambers is not optimal for RV filling. Indeed, in the presence of a persistently long interventricular delay, the AV delay associated with the longest filling period in the left cardiac chambers will certainly be too short for the RV and is likely to encroach on the end of the right-sided A-wave. The equalization of the left and right pre-ejection intervals allows the programming of the same optimal AV delay for the left and right cardiac chambers (Fig. 12.8).

The V-V interval can be used to shorten the interventricular delay by "advancing" the delayed ventricle [7]. Although it shortens the interventricular delay by shortening the pre-ejection interval of that ventricle, this programming step is also likely to have an opposite effect on the pre-ejection interval of the other ventricle. While the interventricular delay has been shortened, the overall duration of systole is sometimes ultimately lengthened. The clinical value of V-V programming and its precise indications have not been fully established at the present time.

Intraventricular Resynchronization

The assessment of intraventricular resynchronization is a critical step in the echocardiographic evaluation after CRT implantation. Intraventricular dyssynchronization can be detected (a) in the spatial dimension, by comparing the contraction delays among the various myocardial segments, or (b) in the time dimension, by the detection of one or several segments that end their contraction after the aortic valve closure or even during the next cardiac filling cycle.

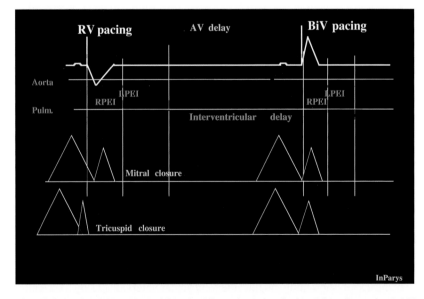

Fig. 12.8 During RV pacing with a significant interventricular delay, the optimal AV delay for LV filling is too short for optimal RV filling. During biventricular pacing, equalization of left and right pre-ejection intervals enhances the programming of an AV delay "optimal" for both the right and left ventricles. *LPEI* and *RPEI* are the respective left and right pre-ejection intervals.

Spatial intraventricular dyssynchrony can be corrected by either delaying the contraction of the earliest segments or by advancing the most delayed ones. Whereas the latter choice seems intuitively the most judicious, its merit has never been confirmed. Spatial dyssynchronization is, in fact, a heterogeneous temporal dyssynchronization among the various myocardial segments. Reducing temporal dyssynchronization invariably reduces spatial dyssynchronization. Reducing temporal dyssynchronization also shortens the duration of systole, hence it lengthens diastole.

Echocardiography performed immediately after CRT implantation is complex with conflicting issues as attempts are being made to optimize resynchronization. Its value, however, has been abundantly demonstrated in CRT patients undergoing a first implantation, as well as in patients whose standard DDD pacing systems have been upgraded.

The acute effect of CRT occurs within one heartbeat and is manifested by an increase in the aortic systolic pressure, stroke volume, and the maximum rate of rise of LV pressure (dP/dt) as well as a reduction in functional mitral regurgitation.

At the end of the echocardiographic procedure, one should not forget to program basic rate, upper rate limit, refractory periods, safety algorithms, and Holter function of the device. One should be cognizant of the fact that AV delay is a somewhat "tricky" parameter not only linked to AV synchronization but also to atrial refractory periods, 2 to 1 upper rate point, and a timing cycle with the potential of interfering with safety algorithms such as mode switching or anti-pacemaker-mediated tachycardia functions. The automatic shortening of the AV delay on exercise may be programmed if it can be demonstrated that this function is beneficial on exercise.

Long-term Considerations

Postimplantation echocardiography is indispensable for the long-term follow-up of the underlying heart disease, for the standard measurements of chamber diameters and volumes, ventricular ejection fractions, pressures, for the estimation of AV valve regurgitation, and for the regulation of medical therapy with a view to decreasing the dose of diuretics and increasing the administration of beta-adrenergic blockade and angiotensin-converting enzyme inhibitors. There is no consensus on whether LV reverse remodeling or clinical status should be employed as end points for assessing response to CRT.

Several studies have shown the beneficial time-dependent effects of CRT on ventricular geometry (less spherical LV shape) and function consistent with reverse LV remodeling of the heart, judged by a decrease in end-systolic LV volume, end-diastolic LV volume (8–15%), and increase in LV ejection fraction (4–7%) [8–17]. There is also further reduction of mitral regurgitation related to distortion of mitral apparatus by LV dyssynchrony (compared with the immediate reduction at the start of CRT) as a result of improved myocardial contractility, reduction of ventricular size, and improved coordinated timing of mechanical activation of papillary muscle insertion sites, left atrial size, and attenuation of the interventricular electromechanical delay [8] (Table 12.1). Reverse remodeling (greater in patients with nonischemic

Table 12.1 Effects of CRT on LV function and dimensions in patients with moderate to severe heart failure (NYHA class III–IV).

Study	Baseline	CRT FU	Control FU	p
MUSTIC [18, 19] (n = 34)		9 months		
LVED (mm)	73 ± 8	64 ± 7		<0.001
LVESD (mm)	62 ± 8	53 ± 8		<0.001
Aortic ITV (cm)	14.9 ± 5.6	17.9 ± 6.6		<0.001
PATH-CHF [20] (n = 25)		6 months		
LVESD (mm)	63 ± 11	58 ± 11		0.007
FS (%)	12 ± 6	15 ± 7		NS
CONTAK-CD [21] (n = 227)		6 months	6 months	
LVEDD (mm)	71.5 ± 10.5	−4.9 ± 1	−0.2 ± 1.1	0.001
LVESD	59.5 ± 11	−5.4 ± 1.1	−0.6 ± 1.1	0.002
LVEF (%)	21 ± 6	6 ± 1.1	2.3 ± 1.2	0.029
MIRACLE [22] (n = 172)		6 months	6 months	
LVED volume (ml)	295.6 ± 102.6	−27.2	+4.7	<0.05
LVES volume (ml)	227.7 ± 93.7	−25.6	+0.3	<0.05
LVEF (%)	24.5 ± 6.8	+3.6	−0.4	<0.05
CARE-HF [8] (n = 409)		18 months	18 months	
LVESVI (ml/m^2)	121 (92–151)	−84.4	−26.4	<0.0001
LVEF (%)	25 (21–29)	+6.9	+2.1	<0.0001

LVESD, left ventricular end-systolic diameter; LVED volume, left ventricular end-diastolic volume; LVES volume, left ventricular end-systolic volume; LVESVI, left ventricular end-systolic volume index; FS, fractional shortening ; FS, TVI, total isovolumic time; LVEDD, Left ventriculae end-diastolic diameter; FU, followup. In parentheses are figured the changes observed in the control group of each randomized study in opposition to changes observed in the CRT group. MUSTIC and PATH-CHF were crossover studies without any control group.
Source: Reproduced with permission from Donal E, Leclercq C, Linde C, Daubert JC. Effects of cardiac resynchronization therapy on disease progression in chronic heart failure. Eur Heart J 2006;27:1018–25.

cardiomyopathy) is correlated with the presence of mechanical LV dyssynchrony before device implantation and appears as early as 1 month after implantation and can be documented at 3 months after which it is mostly sustained on a long-term basis with data available as long as 2–3 years after the onset of CRT. Improvement may take as long as 6 months. A reduction in LV end-systolic volume of 10% signifies clinically relevant reverse remodeling, which is a strong predictor of lower long-term mortality and heart failure events [15]. Reverse remodeling provides a stimulus for regression of LV mass and improved contractile function. Regression of LV mass occurs more slowly than the reduction of LV volumes. Patients who do not improve clinically generally show little or no evidence of reverse remodeling and no change in LV ejection fraction.

In a study where pacing was transiently discontinued after 3 months of CRT, the LV volumes did not change despite an acute reversal of dP/dt max, a response consistent with a true remodeling effect. When pacing was kept off for the next month, further reversal of the systolic benefit was observed together with reappearance of LV dilatation [4].

Refractory Heart Failure After Initial Improvement with CRT

Postoperative echocardiography is also useful on a long-term basis for the detection of the late development of recurrent dyssynchronization despite satisfactory initial resynchronization and considerable early hemodynamic improvement. In patients who present with recurrent, refractory congestive heart failure (CHF), the addition of a third ventricular lead may be helpful in the presence of LV dyssynchrony. We investigated the addition of a third lead in the RV in such patients (two RV leads and one LV lead) [23]. These three-ventricular lead systems were evaluated clinically and echocardiographically before versus during biventricular stimulation, and before versus after the addition of the third ventricular lead, in five men and two women (mean age = 74 ± 9 years) with idiopathic (n = 5) or ischemic (n = 2) cardiomyopathy. All patients initially had undergone implantation of a CRT system for the management of New York Heart Association (NYHA) functional class III (n = 3) or IV (n = 4) for CHF despite optimal drug therapy. Chronic atrial fibrillation was present in three patients at the time of implantation. A significant improvement was observed in six patients after implantation of the biventricular stimulation system. However, after a mean of 40 ± 26 months (range, 2 to 75), refractory CHF reappeared. The LV lead had originally been placed in a lateral vein in five and in a posterolateral vein in two patients. The original RV lead was apical in six and septal in one patient. The additional third ventricular lead was affixed to the right interventricular septum in six and to the RV outflow tract in one patient. Late, recurrent inter- and intraventricular dyssynchrony was corrected by the third ventricular lead, and an increase in mean LV ejection fraction and decrease in mean NYHA functional class were observed. These pilot observations warrant pursuit in controlled trials.

References

1. Cazeau S, Gras D, Lazarus A, Ritter P, Mugica J. Multisite stimulation for correction of cardiac asynchrony. Heart 2000;84:579–81.
2. Kindermann M, Fröhlig G, Doerr T, Schieffer H. Optimizing the AV delay in DDD pacemaker patients with high degree AV block : mitral valve Doppler versus impedance cardiography. Pacing Clin Electrophysiol 1997;20:2453–62.
3. Bax JJ, Marwick TH, Molhoek SG, et al. Left ventricular dyssynchrony predicts benefit of cardiac resynchronization therapy in patients with end-stage heart failure before pacemaker implantation. Am J Cardiol 2003;92:1238–40.
4. Yu CM, Chau E, Sanderson JE, et al. Tissue Doppler echocardiographic evidence of reverse remodeling and improved synchronicity by simultaneously delaying regional contraction after biventricular pacing therapy in heart failure. Circulation 2002;105:438–45.
5. Pitzalis MV, Iacoviello M, Romito R, et al. Cardiac resynchronization therapy tailored by echocardiographic evaluation of ventricular asynchrony. J Am Coll Cardiol. 2002;40:1615–22.
6. Cazeau S, Bordachar P, Jauvert G, et al. Echocardiographic modeling of cardiac dyssynchrony before and during multisite stimulation: a prospective study. Pacing Clin Electrophysiol 2003;26:137–43.
7. Sogaard P, Egeblad H, Pedersen AK, et al. Sequential versus simultaneous biventricular resynchronization for severe heart failure: evaluation by tissue Doppler imaging. Circulation. 2002;106:2078–84.

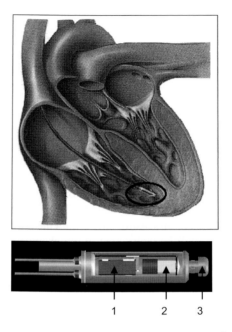

Fig. 13.10 Measurement of the peak endocardial acceleration (PEA) for automatic optimization of the AV and VV delay. Located in the lead tip, a piezoelectric crystal measures myocardial contractility. Automatic AV optimization based on this measurement correlates with echocardiographic optimization to an extent of 93%. *1*, electronic converter; *2*, piezo crystal; *3*, electrode tip.

be programmed just above the threshold value, reducing battery current drain, improving resynchronization success, and decreasing phrenic nerve stimulation.

Atrial Tachyarrhythmia Therapies

Atrial tachyarrhythmias, particularly atrial fibrillation, are a frequent problem in CRT patients. They may cause CRT interruption, loss of atrial systole, and high ventricular rates that frequently cause clinical deterioration (see Fig. 13.4). New CRT devices provide a wide range of therapies for the prevention and termination of atrial tachyarrhythmias (Table 13.4):

1. *Atrial preventive pacing.* These algorithms are designed to permanently overdrive intrinsic atrial rhythms (suppression of ectopic activity), prevent post-extrasystolic pauses (reduction of dispersion of atrial refractoriness), and provide temporary high-rate overdrive pacing after arrhythmia termination (prevention of immediate reinitiation of atrial tachyarrhythmia).
2. *Atrial antitachycardia pacing (ATP).* Several burst, ramp, scan, and high-rate burst (e.g., 50 Hz) therapies are programmable; these may start immediately after tachyarrhythmia detection, after a delay of 1 or several minutes (to verify persistence of atrial tachyarrhythmia), or later when the device automatically detects transition of the arrhythmia to a higher degree of organization ("reactive ATP") rendering pace-termination more likely. Typically, these therapies should not be applied if the arrhythmia persists for more than 48 h to prevent embolic complications in patients without anticoagulation.

Table 13.4 CRT devices with atrial therapies.

	APP	Post-APB	Post-MS	Burst/ Ramp/Scan	20–50 Hz	Automatic shocks	Patient-triggered shocks
Biotronik Tupos LV/ATx	–	–	–	+	+	+	–
Ela Talent MSP AF	+	+	–	–	–	–	–
Guidant Renewal 4	+	+	+	+	+	+	+
Medtronic Concerto	+	+	+	+	+	+	+
St. Jude Medical Frontier II	+	–	–	–	–	–	–
St. Jude Medical Atlas II HF/Epic II HF	+	–	–	–	–	–	–

APP, atrial preventive pacing (continuous sinus rhythm overdrive pacing); post-APB, pacing after atrial premature beats; post-MS, pacing after mode switching back to tracking mode.

3. *Atrial shocks.* Modern CRT devices offer R-wave–synchronized atrial shocks with an output programmable from 0.1 J to 41 J. These can be applied via conventional defibrillation electrodes (best via dual-coil shock electrodes) in mono- or biphasic shape and with reverse polarity. Of note, shocks can be applied immediately after detection of atrial fibrillation or with a delay programmable to a maximum of several hours. This delay can refer to an automatic or patient-activated ICD discharge. In the latter mode, the patient applies a special activator triggering device-confirmation of atrial tachyarrhythmia. Upon this, the device can apply an R-wave–synchronized shock immediately or after a delay of 20 s to 6 h (e.g., if the patient prefers to take a sedative before ICD discharge). As a safety feature, the maximum number of atrial shocks in a programmable time interval (e.g., 24 h) can be limited to 1–5.

Results on pacing for prevention of atrial tachyarrhythmias have been less promising than expected, therefore it is not considered as a "stand-alone" indication [18]. However, if patients receive a device for an indication other than atrial tachyarrhythmia, these algorithms may prove highly successful and beneficial in individual patients. This may particularly apply to patients with CRT devices because one of the shortcomings of atrial preventive pacing therapy was the increase in right ventricular pacing in dual-chamber devices [19], which may cancel all positive effects of atrial preventive pacing. Similarly, atrial antitachycardia pacing has been successful in some studies [20, 21] while unsuccessful in others [22–24] in reducing the cumulative arrhythmia burden, mainly due to methodological shortcomings in these studies (arrhythmia burden too low in the control groups). A significant effect of atrial antitachycardia pacing can only be expected if it exceeds a success rate of approximately 60%, leading to reverse electrical atrial remodeling [25]. Interestingly, antitachycardia pacing is much more successful than it could be expected in patients with atrial fibrillation because most patients with atrial fibrillation also have intermittent periods of highly organized atrial tachyarrhythmia, which may represent forms of atrial flutter (Figs. 13.11 and 13.12) [26]. Such arrhythmias precede the development of atrial fibrillation

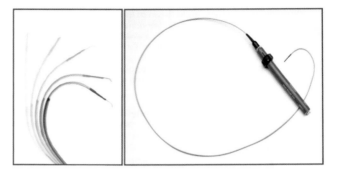

Fig. 14.6 Steerable inner catheter.

Left Ventricular Leads

The integrated system of steerable and fixed-shape catheters and over-the-wire leads have increased implantation success rate, lowered dislodgment rates, and improved electrical performance. The currently available over-the-wire leads have different diameters and lengths, straight and preshaped tip unipolar leads, straight and preshaped tip bipolar leads, allowing advancement and fixation of the lead into small and large branch veins, at the desired pacing site.

The straight lead must be wedged deep in the vein for stability, but in the bipolar configuration the ring may be floating in the vein, without electric contact. (Fig 14.7). Preshaped end leads allow navigation of acute angles and can be positioned at a stable site in a wide range of vein sizes and tortuousities. Different tip shapes have been introduced: angled, S-shaped,

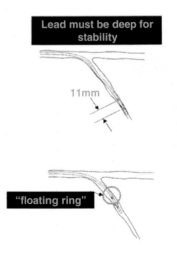

Fig. 14.7 Floating ring of a bipolar straight lead.

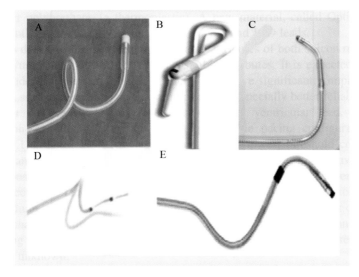

Fig. 14.8 Different tip shapes available: *A*, Helix tip; *B*, double leftward curve tip; *C*, angled tip; *D*, spiral tip; *E*, S-shaped tip.

helix, spiral, double-leftward curvature (Fig 14.8). Steroid elution ensures low acute and chronic thresholds. The proximal body may be coated by polyurethane for better pushing and handling, while the flexible distal body is coated by silicone for tracking. The leads may also be equipped with a stylet, whose stop is located near the tip, which allows full straightening of and maximal load transmission to the distal end of the lead. Some manufacturers provide an integrated distal tip seal, which prevents or reduces blood intrusion into the lead lumen during the implantation procedure and once implanted (Fig. 14.9). A fluoroscopic marker, when present, is a further assist in correct placement. Preshaped and bipolar leads allowing a more basal stimulation are the best way to avoid phrenic nerve stimulation and to obtain acceptable thresholds. Moreover, thresholds tend to become lower when anodal surface area is significantly larger than the cathodal surface area.

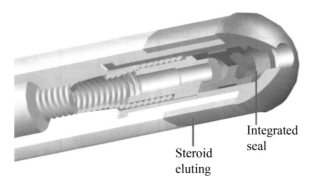

Integrated
seal

Steroid
eluting

Fig. 14.9 Section of the tip of bipolar lead.

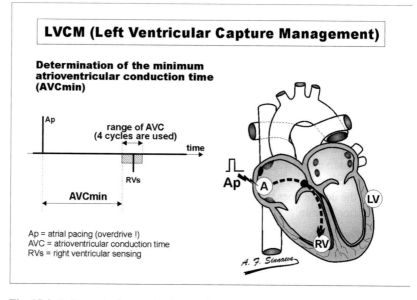

Fig. 15.4 Atrioventricular conduction test (see text for explanation). *AV min*, minimum AV interval

extrasystoles), the measurement is delayed by 30 min. The threshold search starts at a setting below the last measured threshold and decrements until a subthreshold setting is discovered (Fig. 15.6). The output is then incremented until a suprathreshold impulse is confirmed. The nominal voltage safety margin is 1.5 V greater than the LV threshold. The clinician can choose to limit the output to maximum-adapted amplitude to avoid phrenic

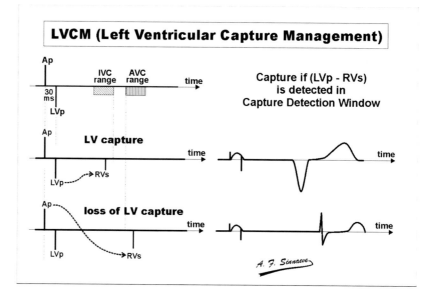

Fig. 15.5 LV capture (see text for explanation). *Ap*, atrial pacing; *LVp*, left ventricular pacing; *IVC*, interventricular conduction time; *AVC*, atrioventricular conduction time; *RVs*, sensed RV event.

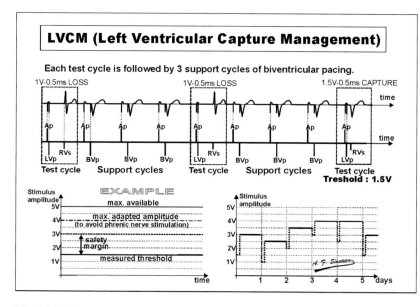

Fig. 15.6 LV threshold measurement *Upper panel*: During a test cycle, the threshold search starts at a setting below the last measured threshold and decrements the output until a subthreshold setting is discovered (loss of capture). Each test cycle is followed by a support cycle. The output is then incremented until a suprathreshold impulse is confirmed (capture). *Left lower panel*: After determining the LV threshold, the output will be set at a safety margin of 1.5 V above threshold. To avoid phrenic nerve stimulation, a maximum LV amplitude can be programmed. *Right lower panel*: Example of daily LV threshold measurements. *Ap*, atrial pacing; *LVp*, left ventricular pacing; *RVs*, sensed RV event; *BVp*, biventricular pacing; *V*, volt.

nerve stimulation. The LV amplitude value will not be increased above this setting, even if the voltage margin cannot be maintained. The maximum programmable output in the Concerto-D, Medtronic is up to 8 V.

LVCM in Non-Tracking Modes

LVCM also operates in nontracking modes (VVIR or DDIR). In this situation, the test paced event is delivered early enough to differentiate interventricular conduction (LV–RV) from the underlying rhythm. With a *subthreshold LVp*, the time measured to the RVs event reflects the underlying ventricular rhythm, while with a *suprathreshold LVp event,* the time measured to the RVs event constitutes the LV–RV interval.

Automatic Optimization of AV Delay and VV Timing

Maximum hemodynamic benefit requires optimization of atrioventricular (AV) and interventricular (VV) intervals [8]. These procedures not only need a lot of expertise but they are also time-consuming and costly.

AV Optimization

A number of *Doppler echocardiographic indices* has been investigated and correlated with invasive hemodynamic measurements to determine the optimal AV delay in CRT patients [5] (Fig. 15.7).

10. Vanderheyden M, De Backer T, Rivero-Ayerza M, et al. Tailored echocardiographic interventricular delay programming further optimizes left ventricular performance after cardiac resynchronization therapy. Heart Rhythm 2005;2: 1066–1072.

11. Meine M, Min X, Paris M, et al. An intracardiac EGM method for VV optimization during cardiac resynchronization therapy. Heart Rhythm 2006;3 [abstract AB 30-5].

16

Significance of Latency During Left Ventricular Pacing for Cardiac Resynchronization Therapy

Bengt Herweg, Arzu Ilercil, Chris Madramootoo, Nadim G. Khan, and S. Serge Barold

Simultaneous biventricular pacing is unsuccessful in approximately 30% of patients [1–6]. In some patients, lack of hemodynamic improvement with cardiac resynchronization therapy (CRT) may be due to regional variations in electrical excitability and impulse propagation such as electrical latency, slow impulse propagation in proximity of the lead, or more globally delayed intra– and interventricular conduction [7–10]. All of these conditions may affect the balance between right ventricular (RV) and left ventricular (LV) activation during biventricular stimulation and affect LV contractility. This discussion reviews the significance of electrical latency during LV stimulation from the coronary venous system and describes the electrocardiographic and hemodynamic findings encountered in patients with LV latency complicating CRT.

Definition and Pathophysiology of Latency

The interval from the pacemaker stimulus to the onset of the earliest paced QRS complex on the 12-lead ECG is called *latency*, and during RV pacing this interval normally measures <40 ms. Pronounced latency is uncommon during RV pacing at physiologic rates [11]. A prolonged latency interval represents first-degree pacemaker exit block [12]. The latter may progress to type I second-degree Wenckebach exit block characterized by gradual prolongation of the spike to QRS interval eventually resulting in an ineffectual stimulus (Fig. 16.1) [7, 12, 13]. Further progression leads to 2:1 or more severe forms of exit block and eventually to complete loss of capture. Latency must be differentiated from so-called exit block, which is a physiologic phenomenon related to complete or occasional failure of ventricular depolarization at the pacing threshold in the absence of a prolonged stimulus–QRS interval.

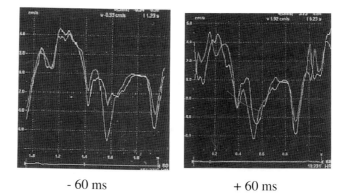

- 60 ms   + 60 ms

Fig. 17.3 Tissue Doppler imaging evaluation of V-V programming. In this patient, a V-V interval of –60 ms (left ventricle before right ventricle) resulted in the highest aortic velocity time integral (VTI) and perfect left ventricular synchronicity indicated by the superposition of the peak myocardial systolic velocities sampled from the septal and lateral segments. In contrast, the lowest aortic VTI and the highest degree of dyssynchrony was found at a V-V interval of 60 ms (right ventricle before left ventricle). (Reproduced with permission from Schalij MJ, van Erven L, Bleeker GB, Bax JJ. Device-specific features in cardiac resynchronization therapy. In: Yu CM,. Hayes DL, Auricchio A, eds. Cardiac Resynchronization Therapy. Malden, MA: Blackwell Futura; 2006:141–51).

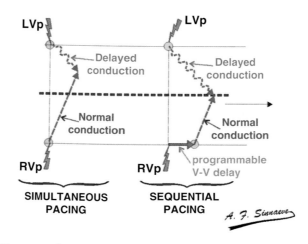

Fig. 17.4 Diagrammatic representation of left ventricular (*LV*) conduction delay interfering with synchronous activation of the two ventricles at the broken horizontal line. Programmability of the interventricular (*V-V*) interval permits preactivation of the LV to compensate for the LV conduction delay. In this way, both ventricles are activated synchronously at the broken horizontal line. *LVp*, left ventricular pacing event; *RVp*, right ventricular pacing event.

Clinical Considerations

On the basis of the above arguments, it is therefore not surprising that V-V programmability has shown a heterogeneous response with great variability of the optimal V-V delay from patient to patient. V-V programmability may partially compensate for less than optimal LV lead position by tailoring ventricular timing and may also correct for individual heterogeneous ventricular activation patterns commonly found in patients with LV dysfunction and HF. The benefit of V-V programming is additive to AV delay optimization. The optimal V-V delay cannot be identified clinically in the majority of patients (Table 17.1) [3, 12–15, 29–36]. Consequently adjustment of the V-V delay like the AV delay must be individualized (Table 17.1; Fig. 17.1). In addition, assessment of the role of V-V programmability reported in the literature is difficult to evaluate because of the varied cutoff of the spontaneous QRS duration for inclusion in the various studies, the different testing procedures to determine the optimum V-V delay, and the timing and methodology of AV delay optimization performed in the setting of V-V programming.

Although V-V programmability produces a rather limited improvement in LV function or stroke volume, the response is important in patients with a less than desirable response to CRT (Fig. 17.5). It is currently unknown whether AV and/or V-V interval optimization can actually decrease the percentage of nonresponders to CRT. The optimal V-V delay should decrease LV dyssynchrony and provide a more homogeneous LV activation with faster LV emptying and improved and longer diastolic filling. V-V programmability may increase LV ejection fraction and other indices of LV function and may also reduce mitral regurgitation in some patients [37], but overall improvement is only moderate (Fig. 17.6).

The range of optimal V-V delays is relatively narrow and most commonly involves LV preexcitation by 20 ms. LV preexcitation is required in most patients.

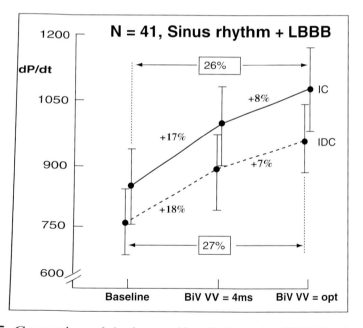

Fig. 17.5 Comparison of simultaneous biventricular pacing (*BiV V-V* = 4 ms), and optimized biventricular pacing (*BiV V-V opt*) on left ventricular dP/dt max in patients with sinus rhythm and ischemic cardiomyopathy (*IC*) and idiopathic dilated cardiomyopathy (*IDC*). *LBBB*, left bundle branch block. p < 0.05 for differences between baseline and simultaneous biventricular pacing and between simultaneous biventricular pacing and optimized pacing. (Reproduced with permission from van Gelder BM, Bracke FA, Meijer A, Lakerveld LJ, Pijls NH. Effect of optimizing the VV interval on left ventricular contractility in cardiac resynchronization therapy. Am J Cardiol 2004;93:1500–1503).

respectively, along with an increase in velocity integral by 21% and 37%, respectively. The ability to use this sensor to monitor and optimize AV and VV interval is under study.

Other Sensors

Other sensors have been proposed to monitor heart failure. Minute ventilation and respiratory rate have already been used as sensors for rate adaptation, and these parameters may be useful as an adjunct to monitor respiratory changes during heart failure. A dilated LV is associated with a decrease in evoked response and can be detected with a LV lead in a CRT device. It

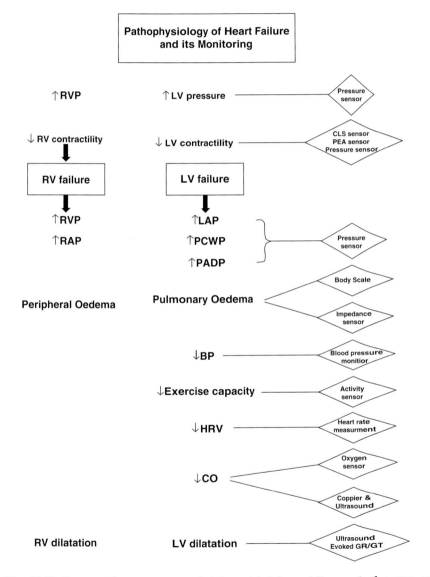

Fig. 18.10 Causes and consequences of right and left heart failure and the use of sensors for their detection. RVP = Right Ventricular Pressure, LV = Left Ventricle, RV = Right Ventricle, LAP- Left Atrial Pressure, RAP = Right Atrial Pressure, PCWP = Pulmonary Capillary Wedge Pressure, PADP = Pulmonary Arterial Diastolic Pressure, BP = Blood Pressure, HRV = Heart rate variability, CO = cardiac output.

Table 18.4 Current feasibility of implantable sensors for heart failure

Type	Activity	HRV	CVo2	RVP	PEA	Pulmonary impedance
Special lead	–	–	+	+	+	–
Energy consumption	Low	Low	Moderate	Moderate	Moderate	Moderate
Changes precedes HF	–	16 days	–	4–5 days	–	18 days
Web-based data availability	Yes	–	–	Yes	–	Pending
False-positive	N/A	2.4/year	N/A	N/A	N/A	1.5/year
Clinical proof in randomized trials	–	–	–	+	–	–

HRV, heart rate variability; CVO_2, central venous oxygen saturation; RVP, right ventricular pressures; PEA, peak endocardial acceleration.

may be able to track the extent of LV reverse remodeling over time after CRT. Likewise, QT interval may change with the onset of heart failure or ischemia and may be a useful detection method for heart failure. It is possible to combine data from an implanted system with clinical measures that can be taken by patients themselves such as their own body weight and blood pressure. All this information can be incorporated in a Web-based system for fine-tuning heart failure monitoring and treatment. Figure 18.10 shows the pathophysiologic consequences of right and left heart failure that can be monitored by sensors to guide heart failure therapy.

Conclusion

The current possibility of sensors to monitor heart failure is detailed in Table 18.4. Impedance and RV pressure sensing are now in clinical use. It is expected that advances will be made such that a sensor will be used in all heart failure devices for monitoring, rate adaptation, and to assist programming. It is expected that multiple sensors will be available to look at different pathophysiologic consequences of heart failure.

References

1. Lau CP. The range of sensors and algorithms used in rate adaptive cardiac pacing. Pacing Clin Electrophysiol 1992;15:1177–211.
2. Karlof I. Haemodynamic effect of atrial triggered versus fixed rate pacing at rest and during exercise in complete heart block. Acta Med Scand 1975;197:195–206.
3. Greenberg B, Chatterjee K, Parmley WW, et al. The influence of left ventricular filling pressure on atrial contribution to cardiac output. Am Heart J 1979;98:742–51.
4. Vollmann D, Luthje L, Schott P, et al. Biventricular pacing improves the blunted force-frequency relation present during univentricular pacing in patients with heart failure and conduction delay. Circulation 2006;113:953–9.

A step-up DFT is used more commonly for atrial defibrillation testing, where the duration of the arrhythmia is not of concern. Surprisingly, a comparison of step-up and binary search protocols has also shown no difference in DFT, with the average total time in VF actually less for the step-up method, even though longer single episodes of VF may occur [15].

Other methods of ensuring an adequate defibrillation safety margin have been developed. Swerdlow reported that inductionless implantations could be performed using a vulnerability safety margin based on a T-wave scan at 15 J. Instead of the traditional induction of VF at implant, the minimal shock energy required to induce VF (upper limit of vulnerability) plus a safety margin could be reliably used to define defibrillation threshold. They estimate that >80% of ICD implants could be implanted using this method, avoiding VF induction [16]. Critics of this method note this technique may require a greater number of shocks, as well as the failure to document adequate sensing of VF during testing.

Defibrillation Efficacy Testing

Though important for defibrillation research, a true DFT is measured in <10% of ICD implants at present. Rather, shocks are most often given at a single energy level to assess the defibrillation safety margin. This is based on empiric observations of patients with epicardial patch electrodes and monophasic waveform ICDs; the presence of at least a 10-J safety margin was predictive of a high success rates for terminating spontaneous ventricular arrhythmias [17]. Defibrillation testing of modern-day implants is still most often performed by observing success using two inductions with termination by shocks at 10 J below the maximum output of the ICD (i.e., 10-J safety margin). Although these strategies are supported by long-standing clinical practice, statistical models provide evidence that the sensitivity and specificity of implant test protocols are significantly less than perceived, bringing into question the value of basing implant decisions on such limited testing [20, 21].

It is common for patients with limited defibrillation success at implant and apparently high DFTs to exhibit adequate defibrillation efficacy during testing on another day. It is not clear if this was merely a probabilistic phenomenon (e.g., regression to the mean) or a transient period when the patient has higher defibrillation energy requirements. In either case, these observations imply that extensive lead revision or subcutaneous array placement should not be performed at initial ICD implant. Rather, retesting several days later or adding a class III antiarrhythmic drug, such as dofetilide or sotalol, may be a simpler strategy [20, 21].

As noted above, another important reason for defibrillation testing is to demonstrate adequate sensing capabilities at implantation. Without proper R-wave sensing, ventricular fibrillation may go undetected, so shocks are never delivered. R-waves of at least 5 mV in sinus rhythm usually ensure adequate sensing of VF [22], but the most reliable and direct assessment of sensing is to observe the ICD response to induced VF in a controlled environment during DFT evaluation. This also allows the evaluation of oversensing due to T-waves or diaphragmatic myopotentials.

The Low Energy Safety Study (LESS) was designed to test the hypothesis that a 5-J safety margin may be adequate if three successive terminations of

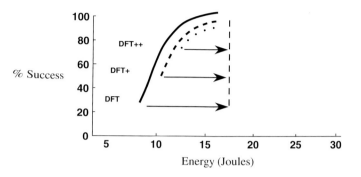

Fig. 19.3 The effect of enhanced DFT step-down testing on the probability of defibrillation success. Confirmation testing to establish two (DFT+) or three (DFT++) consecutive successful defibrillations at the DFT energy results in progressive reductions of the probability distribution of defibrillation success. This allows for programming with a smaller safety margin, as the DFT is ensured to be closer to the maximum or top of the defibrillation efficacy distribution.

VF are demonstrated [23]. This is because the more successive successful shocks for VF termination that are obtained, the more likely that this energy is at the higher part of the DFT probability curve. This is shown graphically in Figure 19.3. Although a step-down DFT may most commonly predict the DFT_{70} point on the defibrillation efficacy curve, there is a wide range of error in this point estimate. As the number of successive shocks at DFT increases (e.g., DFT+ and DFT++), the distribution on the defibrillation efficacy curve decreases with higher probabilities of being at the upper end and thus requiring lower safety margins.

In LESS, 720 patients were enrolled of whom 636 had full testing in the protocol. The first trial of DFT testing was at 14 J stored energy. If successful, the energy was decreased in small steps of about 2–3 J on successive trials. After a failed first shock to establish the DFT, subsequent inductions were performed at the next highest energy to establish the energy that was successful two consecutive times (DFT+) and three consecutive times (DFT++). The DFT was 7.9 ± 3.7 J for this cohort, whereas the DFT++ was 9.1 ± 3.8 J. The DFT++ energy is used for subsequent induced VF testing and for a randomized comparison of low energy safety margin versus full output shocks for spontaneous episodes of ventricular tachyarrhythmias [24]. In this study, programming the first two shocks at two steps (4–6 J) above the DFT++ resulted in comparable defibrillation efficacy as full output shocks, both for induced episodes of VF and spontaneous episodes of rapid ventricular tachyarrhythmias.

One-Shock DFT Testing

The long-term safety and efficacy of single-shock defibrillation testing has not been evaluated prospectively. LESS was not designed specifically to evaluate one-shock DFT testing. Rather, it was intended to evaluate more extensive testing to allow for downsized lower output pulse generators. With improvements in capacitor technology and ICD design, low-output devices are no

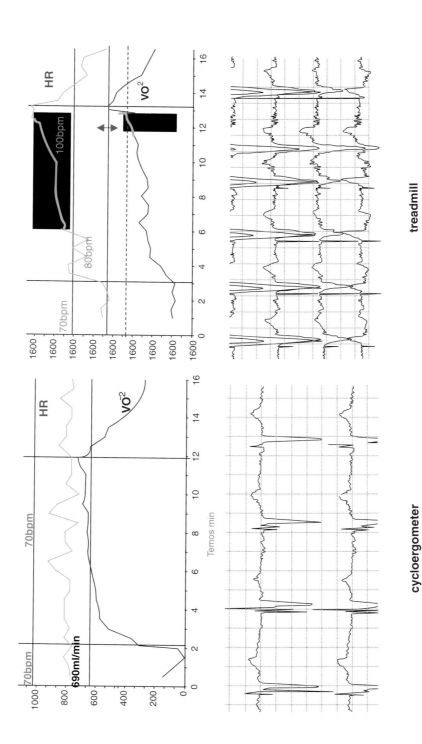

Fig. 20.13 Importance of the type of exercise test in patients with sensor-driven pacemakers. In the *left panel* with an exercise test performed on a cyclo-ergometer, the programmed sensor was not activated and the heart rate (*HR*) remained below 70 bpm. By contrast, in the *right panel*, when the exercise test was performed on a treadmill, the sensor with the same settings was activated with a significant increase in heart rate.

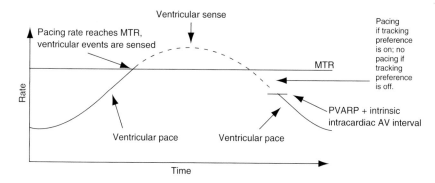

Fig. 20.14 Tracking preference is designed to maintain atrial-tracked ventricular pacing in DDD(R) and VDD modes by identifying atrial events that should be tracked but are hidden in the PVARP. Hidden atrial events can occur when a patient has a combination of long intrinsic intracardiac AV interval and a long PVARP. This algorithm allows the delivery of cardiac resynchronization therapy for atrial rates below but near the maximal tracking rate (Courtesy of Guidant Corporation, St Paul, MN, USA).

of the upper rate interval. It is therefore sensed by the device, and ventricular pacing is preempted. This form of upper rate response is more likely observed with relatively normal AV conduction, a short programmed AV delay, a relatively slow programmed upper rate (driven by the atria), and a sinus rate greater than the programmed upper rate. Moreover, this phenomenon may occur on exercise or in circumstances with a high adrenergic tone.

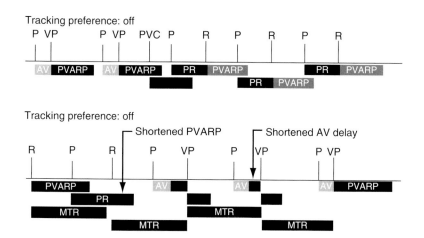

Fig. 20.15 Atrial tracking preference function of the Guidant Renewal ICD. If two successive cycles occur in which a sensed RV event is preceded by an atrial event that occurs in the PVARP, the PVARP shortens until normal atrial tracking is established. By programming "Tracking Preference On," continuous cardiac resynchronization therapy is delivered at rates below maximal tracking rate, rates that otherwise might be inhibited when the sum of PVARP and intrinsic intracardiac atrioventricular interval is longer than the prevailing maximal tracking rate interval. At rates above maximal rate tracking (MRT), atrial tracking preference is disabled. (Courtesy of Guidant Corporation, St Paul, MN, USA).

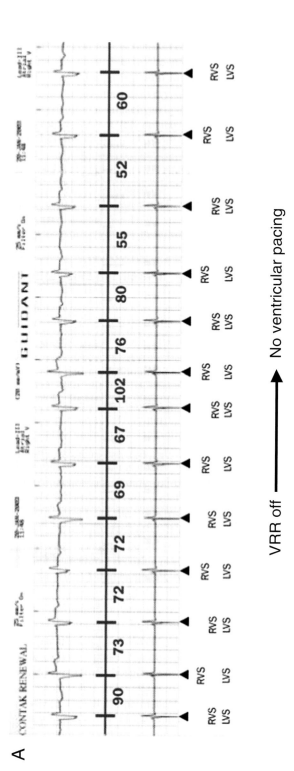

Fig. 20.21 Ventricular rate regularization. (**A**) Recording from a patient with a CRT device and permanent atrial fibrillation with a spontaneous ventricular rate ranging from 55 to 102 bpm. The ventricular rate regularization algorithm is not activated and the RV and LV are not paced. (**B**) In the same patient after switching on the ventricular rate regularization (VRR) feature, there is biventricular pacing in 84% of the cardiac cycles with a more regular heart rate. (Courtesy of Guidant Corporation. St Paul, MN, USA).

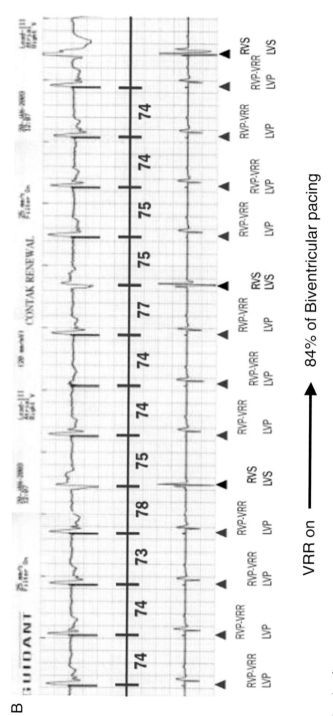

B

VRR on 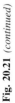 84% of Biventricular pacing

Fig. 20.21 *(continued)*

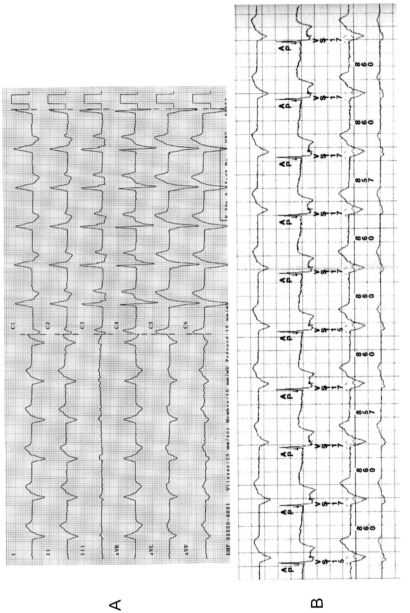
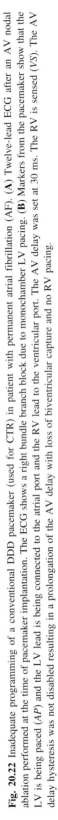

Fig. 20.22 Inadequate programming of a conventional DDD pacemaker (used for CTR) in patient with permanent atrial fibrillation (AF). (**A**) Twelve-lead ECG after an AV nodal ablation performed at the time of pacemaker implantation. The ECG shows a right bundle branch block due to monochamber LV pacing. (**B**) Markers from the pacemaker show that the LV is being paced (*AP*) and the LV lead is being connected to the atrial port and the RV lead to the ventricular port. The AV delay was set at 30 ms. The RV is sensed (*VS*). The AV delay hysteresis was not disabled resulting in a prolongation of the AV delay with loss of biventricular capture and no RV pacing.

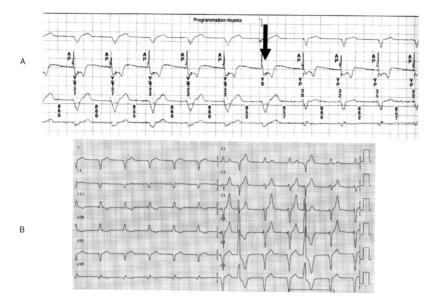

Fig. 20.23 Correction of the inappropriate programming shown in Figure 20.22. (**A**) By switching off the AV delay hysteresis (*arrow*), RV and LV were paced (AP and VP). (**B**) The 12-lead ECG displays biventricular paced complexes.

use of routine AV ablation at the time of CRT implantation or 1 month later after verification of proper device function. Gasparini et al. did show that the efficacy of CRT on exercise tolerance and disease progression in patients with AF and AV node ablation was similar than those observed in sinus rhythm patients. By contrast, AF patients without AV node ablation did not improve with CRT, underlying the importance of AV node ablation [32].

Classically, to provide CRT in patients with permanent AF, a conventional dual-chamber pacemaker can be implanted with the LV lead connected to the atrial port and the RV lead to the ventricular port. The pacemaker is programmed to the DDDR or best to the DVIR mode with the shortest available AV delay to achieve near-simultaneous biventricular pacing. Figures 20.22 and 20.23 illustrate loss of biventricular capture due to inadequate device programming. The pacemaker was programmed to the DDDR mode with an AV delay of 30 ms. However, AV hysteresis was programmed resulting in a prolongation of the AV delay of 52 ms, the RV was sensed, and the patient was paced only in the LV. This case illustrates the limitation of conventional dual-chamber pacemakers for CRT and suggests the superiority of a dedicated triple-chamber device (plugging the atrial port) for patients with permanent AF. Furthermore, triple-chamber devices allow V-V interval optimization if necessary.

Programming and Premature Ventricular Complexes

The presence of frequent premature ventricular complexes (PVCs) represents another potential cause of CRT loss or reduction of CRT "dosage."

A device generally defines a PVC as a sensed ventricular event following a ventricular event without an intervening detected atrial event. In a common

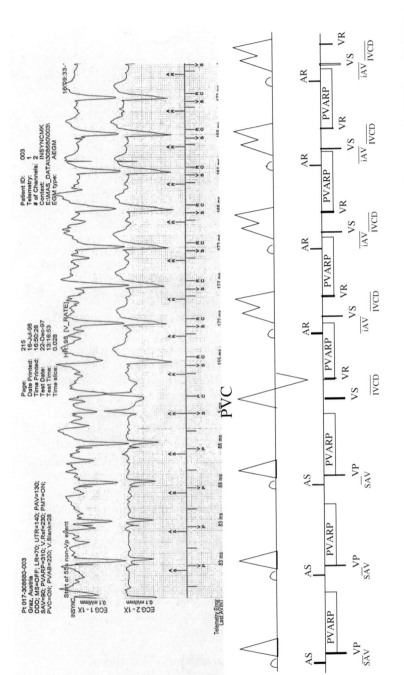

Fig. 20.24 Loss of biventricular capture in a CRT device with a common ventricular sensing channel. induced by a premature ventricular complex (*PVC*) associated with double counting of the ventricular electrogram. A new PVARP is initiated by the second sensed ventricular signal. This shifts the timing of the PVARP so that the following atrial event falls within the reset PVARP where it cannot be tracked. This results in inhibition of biventricular capture and emergence of the intrinsic rhythm. (Courtesy of Medtronic Inc., Minneapolis, MN, USA).

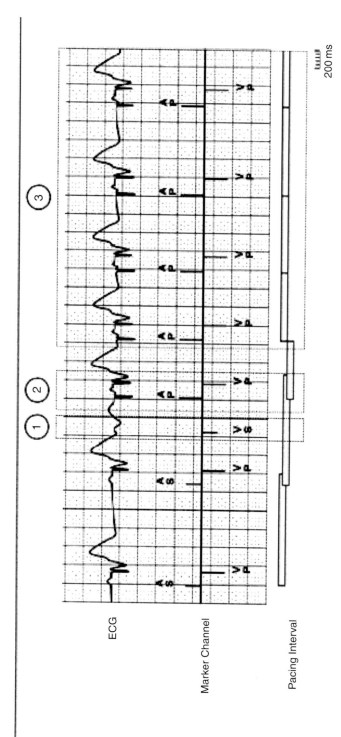

Fig. 20.25 Ventricular rate stabilization of the Medtronic InSync Sentry. *1*, A PVC occurs, causing a short *V-V* interval. *2*, VRS paces the ventricle at the previous *V-V* interval plus the programmed "Interval Increment" (and schedules the atrial pace early to maintain AV synchrony). *3*, With each successive VRS pace, the pacing interval increases by the programmed "Interval Increment." *PVC*, premature ventricular contraction; *VRS*, ventricular rate stabilization.

special pacemaker function, the detection of a PVC generates a PVARP extension (e.g., 400 ms) to prevent pacemaker-mediated tachycardia. This feature need not be programmed routinely. It should be used cautiously in CRT devices. With extension of the PVARP or a relatively long PVARP, a P-wave may occur during the atrial refractory period where it cannot trigger a ventricular stimulus. This situation favors the occurrence of a conducted spontaneous QRS complex as most CRT patients do not have AV block [21]. Intrinsic AV conduction then begets intrinsic AV conduction resulting in permanent loss of biventricular capture. In order to restore atrial tracking and CRT delivery, atrial events have to fall outside the intrinsic total atrial refractory period (equal to intrinsic PR interval plus PVARP). Some algorithms by temporally shortening the PVARP and so reducing the total atrial refractory period may restore atrial tracking and CRT delivery (Fig. 20.24). In some devices, a ventricular event detected during the AV interval may trigger an immediate ventricular pacing stimulus with a 2.5 ms V-V pace delay.

Premature ventricular contractions are generally followed by a long pause. These short–long interval sequences may generate in some cases spontaneous ventricular arrhythmias. To eliminate these short–long sequences, some algorithms have been developed to stabilize the ventricular rate (Fig. 20.25).

Programming and Slow Ventricular Tachycardia

In CRT patients, slow ventricular tachycardia (VT) may cause loss of biventricular capture. Moreover, there is an interaction between CRT and ICD tachycardia detection zones without the possibility of antitachycardia pacing to address slow VT. For CRT ICDs, the lowest programmable VT detection zone is 5 bpm above the maximal tracking rate. This may result in trade-offs between the rates of CRT delivery and the slowest detected VT rate. For example, a patient with a monomorphic VT at 130 bpm will require programming of the VT detection rate to 120 bpm. With this VT detection rate, CRT will be limited to tracking of atrial rates <115 bpm. With an increase in the maximal tracking rate, for example up to 140 bpm, the slow VT at 130 bpm will not be detected. Some devices now offer the capability to treat slow VT with antitachycardia pacing within a zone below the upper tracking limit. Thus, in patients with slow VT, alternative VT therapies such as antiarrhythmic drugs or radiofrequency ablation should be explored to ensure effective CRT at physiologic rates.

Interventricular Refractory Period

The interventricular refractory period prevents restarting the ventricular refractory period, postventricular atrial blanking and refractory periods, and upper rate timers when a second sensed depolarization is seen after a paced or sensed event (Fig. 20.26). This function is not required during monochamber sensing but may be useful with biventricular sensing (from RV tip to LV tip; the interventricular refractory period should be programmed to the patient's intraventricular conduction delay + 30 ms).

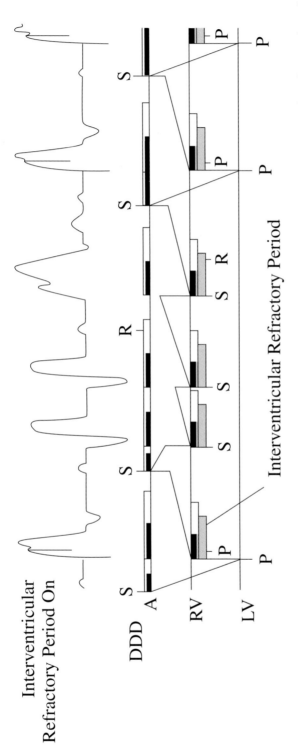

Fig. 20.26 Diagrammatic representation of the interventricular refractory period (IRP) in the Medtronic InSync III pacemaker. The IRP prevents sensing of a second ventricular depolarization when the RV and LV do not depolarize simultaneously. Thus, a sensed event in the IRP (either after a ventricular paced event or a nonrefractory sensed event) does not initiate new timing cycles. A, atrium; RV, right ventricle; LV, left ventricle; S, nonrefractory sensed event; P, paced event; R, refractory sensed event. Note the short P-P intervals representing the V-V delay or the timing difference between LV and RV stimulation. (Courtesy of Medtronic Inc., Minneapolis, MN, USA).

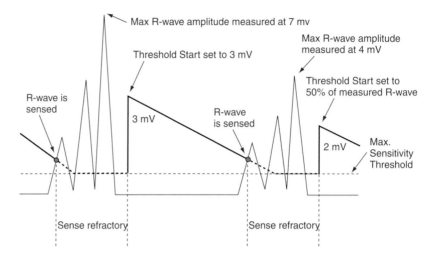

Fig. 20.27 "Automatic Sensitivity Control." This feature allows accurate sensing in both the atrium and the right ventricle over a wide range of signal amplitudes. "Threshold Start" begins at 50% of the measured R-wave (if the R-wave is between 2 and 6 mV) and decays linearly until the next sensed beat or until it reaches the "Maximum Sensitivity Threshold." If the maximum R-wave amplitude is greater than 6 mV or less than 2 mV, "Threshold Start" is set to 3 mV or 1 mV, respectively. Sensing in the atrium is identical, with the "Threshold Start" being 50% of the measured P-waveif the P-wave is between 0.6 and 3 mV. After a paced event, the "Threshold Start" is nominally set to 0.8 mV in the atrium and to adjust automatically based on the pacing rate in the right ventricle. (Courtesy of St. Jude Medical, Sylmar, CA).

Automatic Sensitivity Control

Automatic sensitivity controls allow accurate sensing in both the atrium and the ventricle over a wide range of signal amplitudes. As shown in Figure 20.27, threshold starts at 50% of the measured R-wave (if the R-wave is between 2 and 6 mV) and decays linearly until the next sensed beat or until it reaches the maximum sensitivity threshold. If the maximum R-wave amplitude is greater than 6 mV or less than 2 mV, "Threshold Start" is set to 3 mV or 1 mV, respectively. To prevent oversensing, a *decay delay* can be programmed: decay delay is the amount of time after the sensed or paced refractory period

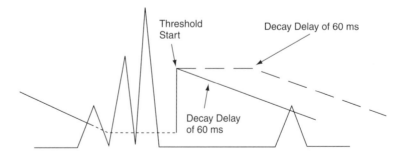

Fig. 20.28 St. Jude Medical algorithm to prevent oversensing from the decay delay in the St. Jude Atlas + HF. Decay delay is the amount of time after the sensed or paced refractory period that the threshold remains at the "Threshold Start" value before beginning its decay. If necessary, increasing the decay delay can prevent oversensing of P-waves in the atrium and T-waves in the ventricle. (Courtesy of St. Jude Medical, Sylmar, CA).

that the threshold remains at the "Threshold Start" value before beginning its decay (Fig. 20.28). If necessary, increasing the decay delay can prevent oversensing of P-waves in the atrium and T-waves in the ventricle.

Diaphragmatic Stimulation

Diaphragmatic stimulation is a complication related to LV lead implantation. In CRT patients, permanent or paroxysmal diaphragmatic stimulation may occur in up to 5% to 10% of patients, resulting in major discomfort [11–14]. This complication is related to the anatomic vicinity of the left phrenic nerve to the LV pacing site, especially when the LV lead is implanted into a posterior or posterolateral vein of the coronary sinus. It may also be caused by LV lead dislodgment. With the recent development of thinner LV leads, and using the over-the-wire technology, this complication seems to occur more frequently, perhaps due to the more distal position of the LV lead in the coronary vein. During the LV lead implantation, phrenic nerve stimulation is assessed by using a high-voltage output at 10 V and deep breathing maneuvers. In case of phrenic nerve stimulation during LV lead implantation, it is recommended to consider another LV pacing site. However, despite various precautions, permanent or paroxysmal diaphragmatic stimulation (during upright posture or physical activity) may occur, requiring active therapy. An alternative strategy involves keeping the same pacing site only if the LV pacing threshold is low and the phrenic nerve stimulation threshold is high, but the absence of recurrent phrenic nerve stimulation with this approach cannot be guaranteed.

The occurrence of phrenic nerve stimulation early after LV lead implantation may signal LV lead migration, sometimes without significant changes

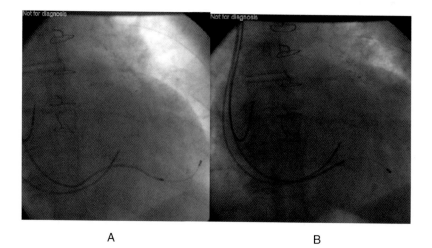

A   B

Fig. 20.29 Phrenic nerve stimulation. (**A**) Intraoperative chest x-ray film showing an atrial lead placed in the right appendage, an RV lead screwed in the mid interventricular septum, and an LV lead inserted into a posterolateral vein of the coronary sinus. Diaphragmatic stimulation occurred even with a low LV output (1 V). The LV pacing threshold was measured at 0.75 V with a pulse width of 0.5 ms. (**B**) With a more proximal position of the LV lead in the posterolateral vein, diaphragmatic stimulation disappeared even at a high output (10 V) in the setting of an acceptable LV pacing threshold at 1.25 V.

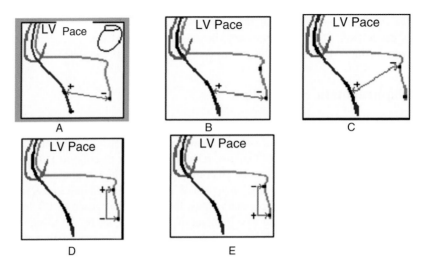

Fig. 20.30 Programmability of pacing configurations of the Guidant Renewal. (**A**) When the "Single" (extended bipolar) configuration is programmed, the pacing stimulus is applied between the LV coronary venous lead tip and the RV distal coil electrode (Tip≫Coil). (**B**) When "Tip≫Coil" (extended bipolar) is selected for dual configuration, the pacing stimulus is applied between the LV coronary venous lead tip and the RV distal coil electrode. (**C**) When "Ring≫Coil" (extended bipolar) is selected for "Dual" configuration, the pacing stimulus is applied between the left ventricular coronary venous (proximal) lead ring and the right ventricular distal coil electrode. (**D**) When "Tip≫Ring" (standard bipolar) is selected for "Dual" configuration, the pacing stimulus is applied between the LV coronary venous lead tip and the LV coronary venous (proximal) lead ring electrode. (**E**) When "Ring≫Tip" (standard bipolar) is selected for "Dual" configuration, the pacing stimulus is applied between the LV coronary venous (proximal) lead ring electrode and the LV coronary venous lead tip electrode. (Courtesy of Guidant Corporation, St Paul, MN, USA).

in the chest x-ray. The LV capture threshold and that of phrenic nerve stimulation thresholds should be assessed. If the LV capture threshold falls far from below the phrenic nerve stimulation threshold, a reduction of LV pacing amplitude below the phrenic nerve stimulation threshold may simply solve the problem. However, overlapping or minimally different thresholds that preclude a programmable solution mandate repositioning of the LV lead as illustrated in Figure 20.29. Programming the LV amplitude at or barely above the LV capture may result in the loss of CRT. One alternative solution in some cases is to decrease the LV ventricular output and to increase the pulse width. With this compromise, LV capture may be achieved without the discomfort of phrenic nerve stimulation. Recently, bipolar pacing LV leads and devices allowing reprogramming of the LV lead pacing configuration may be useful to decrease phrenic nerve stimulation without the need of invasive LV lead manipulation or replacement (Fig. 20.30).

Conclusion

The clinical follow-up of CRT patients requires a multidisciplinary approach. Programming of CRT devices has to be carefully evaluated to ensure continual biventricular capture at rest and during exercise. This requires aggressive therapy of atrial and/or ventricular tachyarrhythmias. With the technical improvement of recent CRT devices and appropriate fine-tuning of devices with specific algorithms designed to improve CRT delivery, we can reasonably expect that the relatively high number of partial or complete nonresponders will decrease. However, programming of a CRT device remains complex and has to be tailored for the individual patient.

References

1. Swedberg K, Cleland J, Dargie H, et al. Task Force for the Diagnosis and Treatment of Chronic Heart Failure of the European Society of Cardiology. Guidelines for the diagnosis and treatment of chronic heart failure: executive summary (update 2005): The Task Force for the Diagnosis and Treatment of Chronic Heart Failure of the European Society of Cardiology. Eur Heart J 2005;26:1115–40.
2. Hunt S, Abraham W, Chin M, et al. ACC/AHA 2005 guideline update for the diagnosis and management of chronic heart failure in the adult. J Am Coll Cardiol 2005;46:1116–43.
3. Cazeau S, Leclercq C, Lavergne T, et al. Effects of multisite biventricular pacing in patients with heart failure and intraventricular conduction delay. N Eng J Med 2001;344:873–80.
4. Auricchio A, Stellbrink C, Sack S, et al. Long-term clinical effect of hemodynamically optimized cardiac resynchronization therapy in patients with heart failure and ventricular conduction delay. J Am Coll Cardiol 2002;39:2026–33.
5. Abraham Wt, Fisher GW, Smith A, et al. Cardiac resynchronization in heart failure. N Engl J Med 2002;40:111–8.
6. Bristow M, Saxon L, Boehmer J, et al. Cardiac-resynchronization therapy with or without an implantable defibrillator in advanced chronic heart failure. N Engl J Med 2004;350:2140–50.
7. Cleland JGF, Daubert JC, Erdmann E, et al. Cardiac Resynchronization-Heart Failure (CARE-HF) Study Investigators. The effect of cardiac resynchronization therapy on morbidity and mortality in heart failure (the CArdiac REsynchronization-Heart Failure [CARE-HF] Trial). N Eng J Med 2005;352:1539–49.
8. Cleland J, Tavazzi L, Freemantle N. CARE-HF: Long-term effects of cardiac resynchronization therapy on mortality in the CARE-HF extension study. Paper presented at Clinical Trial Update II. European Society of Cardiology meeting, Stockholm, 3 September 2005.
9. Feldmann A, de Lissovoy G, Bristow M, et al. Cost-effectiveness of cardiac resynchronization therapy with and without a defibrillator in COMPANION heart failure patients. J Am Coll Cardiol 2005;45:160A.
10. Bernheim A, Ammann P, Bernheim P, et al. Right atrial pacing impairs cardiac function during resynchronization therapy: Acute effects of DDD pacing compared to VDD pacing. J Am Coll Cardiol 2005;45:1482–5.
11. Gassis S, Leon A. Cardiac resynchronization therapy: strategies for device programming, troubleshooting and follow-up. J Interv Card Electrophysiol 2005;13:209–22.
12. Vardas P. Pacing follow up techniques and trouble shooting during biventricular pacing. J Interv Card Electrophysiol 2003;9:183–7.
13. Ellery S, Paul V. Complications of biventricular pacing. Eur Heart J 2004;6(Suppl D):D117–D121.
14. Bhatta L, Luck J, Wolbrette D, et al. Complications of biventricular pacing. Curr Opin Cardiol 2004;19(1):31–5.
15. Linde C, Leclercq C, Rex S, et al. Long-terms benefits of biventricular pacing in congestive heart failure: results from the MUSTIC study. J Am Coll Cardiol 2002;40:111–8.

16. Barold S. Herweg B, Giudici M. Electrocardiographic follow-up of biventricular pacemakers. Ann Noninvasive Electrocardiol 2005;10:231–55.
17. Asirvatham S. Electrocardiogram interpretation with biventricular pacing devices. In: Hayes DL, Wang PJ, Sackner-Bernstein J, Asirvatham S, eds. Resynchronization and Defibrillation for Heart Failure: A Practical Approach. Elmsford, NY: Blackwell-Futura; 2004:73–98.
18. Garrigue S, Barold SS, Clementy J. Electrocardiography of multisite ventricular pacing. In: Barold SS, Mugica J, eds. The Fifth Decade of Cardiac Pacing. Elmsford, NY: Blackwell-Futura; 2004:84–100.
19. Steinberg J, Maniar P, Higgins S, et al. Noninvasive assessment of the biventricular pacing system. Ann Noninvasive Electrocardiol 2004;9:58–70.
20. Lau C, Barold S, Tse H, et al. Advances in devices for cardiac resynchronization in herat failure. J Interv Card Electrophysiol 2003;9:167–81.
21. Barold SS, Garrigue S, Israel CW, Gallardo I, Clementy J. Arrhythmias of biventricular pacemakers and implantable cardioverter defibrillators. In Barold SS, Mugica J, eds. The Fifth Decade of Cardiac Pacing. Elmsford, NY: Blackwell-Futura; 2004:100–117.
22. Barold S, Herweg B. Upper rate response of biventricular pacing devices. J Interv Card Electrophysiol 2005;12:129–36.
23. Wang P, Kramer A, Estes N III, et al. Timing cycles for biventricular pacing. Pacing Clin Electrophysiol 2002;25(1):62–75.
24. Leclercq C, Kass DA. Retiming the failing heart: principles and current clinical status of cardiac resynchronization. J Am Coll Cardiol 2002;39:194–201.
25. Leclercq C, Hare J. Ventricular resynchronization. Current state of the art. Circulation 2004;10:296–99.
26. CIBIS II Investigators and Committees. The Cardiac Insufficiency Bisoprolol Study II (CIBIS II): A randomized trial. Lancet 1999;353:9–13.
27. MERIT-HF Study Group. Effect of Metoprolol CR/XL in chronic heart failure: Metroprolol CR/XL Randomized Intervention in Congestive Heart Failure (MERIT-HF). Lancet 1999;353:2001–2007.
28. Middelkauf HR, Stevenson WG, Stevenson LW. Prognostic significance of atrial fibrillation in advanced heart failure. A study of 390 patients. Circulation 1991;84:40–48.
29. Knight B, Desai A, Coman J, et al. Long-term retention of cardiac resynchronization therapy. J Am Coll Cardiol 2004;44:72–7.
30. Leclercq C, Walker S, Linde C, et al. Comparative effects of permanent biventricular and right-univentricular pacing in heart failure patients with chronic atrial fibrillation. Eur Heart J 2002;23:1780–7.
31. Brignole M, Gammage M, Puggioni E, et al. Comparative assessment of right, left, and biventricular pacing in patients with permanent atrial fibrillation. Eur Heart J 2005 ;26(7):712–22.
32. Gasparini M, Auricchio A, Regoli F, et al. Four-year efficacy of cardiac resynchronization therapy on exercise tolerance and disease progression. J Am Coll Cardiol 2006;48:734–43.

21

Programming and Follow-up of CRT and CRTD Devices

Michael O. Sweeney

Introduction

Optimal programming of implanted electrical devices for cardiac resynchronization therapy (CRT) requires a sophisticated understanding of the pathophysiologic electrical and mechanical substrates that occur in some patients with symptomatic heart failure due to dilated cardiomyopathy (DCM). Furthermore, it cannot be overemphasized that optimal CRT programming is an active process that requires sustained vigilance for the remainder of the patient's life and must anticipate the potential for dynamic and related changes in patient condition or device system operation. This is a critically important distinction to conventional pacemakers, which reliably provide bradycardia support with minimal need for periodic programming intervention, particularly with recent enhancements to automaticity. Similarly, though conventional implantable cardioverter-defibrillators (ICDs) require a slightly higher level of surveillance than pacemakers due to the possibility of clinically silent but important ventricular detections and therapies and several other considerations, they reside primarily in a passive state for the duration of the patient's life. The hybridization of CRT with defibrillation systems (CRTD) therefore invokes all of the complex considerations of optimal CRT and ICD programming. This introduces particularly unique challenges because the device must simultaneously exist in two fundamentally opposed states of operation: continuous delivery of ventricular pacing and continuous surveillance for ventricular arrhythmia.

Abnormal Electrical Timing in Heart Failure Associated with Dilated Cardiomyopathy

Disordered electrical timing frequently accompanies heart failure associated with DCM. Abnormal electrical timing alters critical mechanical relationships that further impair left ventricular (LV) performance. It is now recognized that there are four levels of electromechanical abnormalities associated with heart failure associated with DCM [1,2]. These must be understood and applied to optimal CRT programming and troubleshooting.

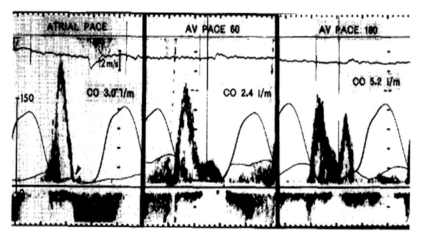

Fig. 21.2 Doppler mitral inflow patterns at various AV delays. *Left:* Atrial pacing with long PR interval. Arrow indicates increase in left ventricular end-diastolic pressure above left atrial pressure during atrial relaxation in mid-diastole, resulting in shortening of diastolic filling time and diastolic mitral regurgitation. *Middle:* AV pacing at short AV delay. Diastolic filling occurs throughout diastole but cardiac output declines due to ineffectual atrial contraction, which occurs synchronously with ventricular contraction. Note significantly elevated atrial pressure throughout. *Right:* AV pacing at optimal AV delay. Diastolic filling occurs throughout diastole and the relation of atrial to ventricular contraction is now optimal, just before ventricular contraction. Mean left atrial pressure is low and cardiac output is higher. (From Nishimura RA, Hayes DL, Holmes DR, Tajik AJ. Mechanism of hemodynamic improvement by dual-chamber pacing for severe left ventricular dysfunction: An acute Doppler and catheterization study. J Am Coll Cardiol 1995;25:281–288.)

in mechanical activation of each ventricle, most commonly LBBB where the right ventricle begins its contraction before the left ventricle. The delay in onset of left ventricular activation results in reversal of the normal sequence between right and left ventricular mechanical events that persists throughout the cardiac cycle [5]. Asynchronous ventricular contraction and relaxation results in dynamic changes in ventricular pressures and volumes throughout the cardiac cycle. This results in abnormal septal deflections that alter the regional contribution to global ejection fraction. Earliest ventricular depolarization is recorded over the anterior surface of the right ventricle and latest at the basal-lateral left ventricle [6]. In canine models with induced LBBB, increasing the delay between right ventricular (RV) and LV contraction increases the delay between the upslope of LV and RV systolic pressure. The increase in interventricular delay was associated with decreased LV +dP/dt and decreased stroke work, presumptively the result of ventricular interdependence and impairment of the septal contribution to LV ejection due to displacement after onset of RV ejection [7].

Intraventricular Delay
The third level of synchrony exists within each ventricle, most importantly the left ventricle. Rapid spread of contraction from the LV septum endocardially to the base of the heart creates coordinated, efficient contraction. Synchrony of contraction is important because it results in a more effective and energetically efficient ejection [8]. Asynchronous electrical activation reduces LV

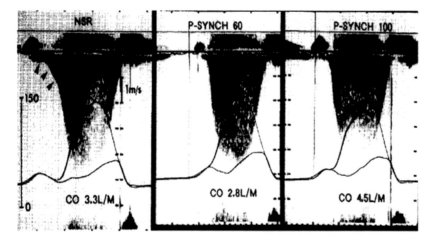

Fig. 21.3 Effect of various AV delays on mitral regurgitation, left atrial pressure, and cardiac output. *Left:* Sinus rhythm with long PR interval. Diastolic mitral regurgitation is due to an increase in left ventricular end-diastolic pressure above left atrial pressure before ventricular contraction. *Middle:* During atrial synchronous pacing at AV delay 60 ms, diastolic mitral regurgitation is eliminated, but there is a decrease in cardiac output due to atrial contraction that is ineffective because it occurs coincident with ventricular contraction. *Right:* Atrial synchronous ventricular pacing at optimal AV delay 100 ms; diastolic mitral regurgitation is no longer present. Left ventricular end-diastolic pressure increases appropriate at onset of ventricular contraction. (From Nishimura RA, Hayes DL, Holmes DR, Tajik AJ. Mechanism of hemodynamic improvement by dual-chamber pacing for severe left ventricular dysfunction: An acute Doppler and catheterization study. J Am Coll Cardiol 1995;25:281–288.)

pump function [9]. The mechanical effect of asynchronous electrical activation is quite dramatic, because the various regions not only differ in the time of onset of contraction but also in the pattern of contraction. Early contraction of regions close to the pacing site cause stretching of not yet activated remote regions. This stretching further delays shortening of these late-activation regions and increases their force of local contraction by virtue of the (local) Frank–Starling mechanism. Due to their vigorous contraction, the late-activated regions imposed loading on the earlier-activated territories, which now undergo systolic paradoxical stretch. This reciprocated stretching of regions within the LV wall causes a less effective and energetically efficient contraction [8].

The hemodynamic consequences of the discoordinate LV contraction are reduction in contractility and relaxation. The poorer contractility is reflected by decreases in stroke work and rate of rise of LV pressure, and a rightward shift of the LV end-systolic pressure–volume relationship [9]. The latter indicates that the left ventricle operates at a consistently larger volume [10,11]. The combination of these effects leads to a decrease in LV ejection time and ejection fraction (EF).

Premature relaxation in early-activated regions and delayed contraction in others also causes abnormal relaxation [9]. This is expressed as decrease in –dP/dt (maximal rate of fall of LV pressure), increase in the relaxation time constant tau, and decrease of E-wave velocity amplitude on Doppler echocardiograms. Moreover, the longer contraction and relaxation times lead to a reduction in diastolic filling time, leading to reduced preload.

has been elegantly described by Breithardt et al. [16]. This is strongly dependent on alterations in ventricular shape as the tethering forces that act on the mitral leaflets are higher in dilated, more spherical ventricles. These geometric changes alter the balance between tethering and closing forces and impede effective mitral closure. Ventricular dilatation and increased chamber sphericity increase the distance between the papillary muscles to the enlarged mitral annulus as well as to each other, restricting leaflet motion and increasing the force needed for effective mitral valve closure. This mitral valve closing force is determined by the systolic left ventricular pressure–left atrial pressure difference, which is called the transmitral pressure gradient. Under these conditions, the mitral regurgitant orifice area will be largely determined by the phasic changes in transmitral pressure. Increasing the transmitral pressure can reduce the effective regurgitant orifice area. CRT acutely reduces the severity of functional MR, and this reduction is quantitatively related to an increase in LV $+dP/dt_{max}$ and transmitral pressure [16] (Figs. 21.9 and 21.10). This is distinct from the reduction in MR due to reduced LV dimensions from remodeling associated with chronic CRT.

Delayed sequential activation of the papillary muscles due to intraventricular delay also contributes to functional mitral regurgitation. Kanzaki et al. used longitudinal strain to produce mechanical activation maps of the left ventricle immediately before and after CRT. Patients with intraventricular

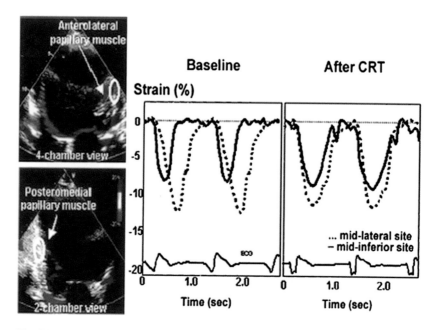

Fig. 21.11 Reduced interpapillary muscle delay during CRT. Echocardiographic strain images from the four-chamber view and two-chamber view, with corresponding time–strain plots from sites adjacent to papillary muscles before and after CRT. Baseline plots demonstrate delayed peak strain occurring in the anterolateral papillary muscle site compared with the posteromedial papillary muscle site. CRT results in time alignment of peak strain at papillary muscles. (From Kanzaki H, Bazaz R, Schwartzman D, Dohi K, Sade LE, Gorscan J 3rd. A mechanism for immediate reduction in mitral regurgitation after cardiac resynchronization therapy: Insights from mechanical activation strain mapping. J Am Coll Cardiol 2004;44(8):1619–1625.)

conduction delay had significantly increased times to peak strain between papillary muscle insertion sites compared with normal controls (Figs. 21.11 and 21.12). This interpapillary muscle delay shortened from 106 ± 74 ms to 39 ± 43 ms immediately after institution of CRT and was correlated with significant reduction in mitral regurgitant fraction [33]. This suggests that the acute reduction in MR associated with CRT is likely due to a complexity of factors, including increased +dP/dt as well as more coordinate papillary muscle activation.

Alterations in regional distribution of mechanical strain probably account for the development of severe MR reported in some patients after institution of RV apical pacing that mimics the activation sequence of LBBB and causes

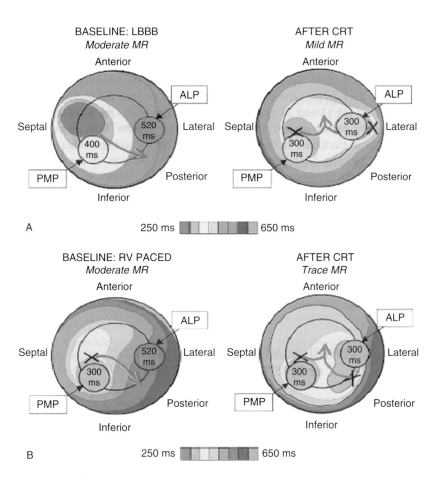

Fig. 21.12 Effect of CRT on interpapillary muscle time delay during LBBB (**A**) and RV apical pacing (**B**). Time to peak systolic strain is color-coded with lines representing isochromes of mechanical activation times at 50-ms intervals. The X indicates sites of lead placement, and the arrow indicates the direction of the propagating mechanical activation. Time to peak strain of sites adjacent to anterolateral (ALP) and posteromedial (PMP) papillary muscles are shown. A decrease in interpapillary muscle time delay was associated with decreased mitral regurgitation (MR). (From Kanzaki H, Bazaz R, Schwartzman D, Dohi K, Sade LE, Gorscan J 3rd. A mechanism for immediate reduction in mitral regurgitation after cardiac resynchronization therapy: Insights from mechanical activation strain mapping. J Am Coll Cardiol 2004;44(8):1619–1625.)

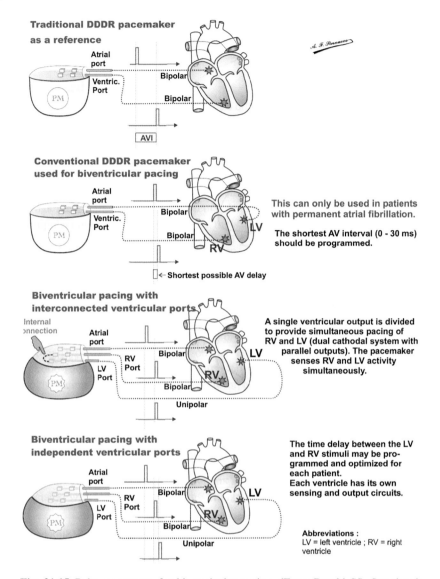

Fig. 21.15 Pulse generators for biventricular pacing. (From Barold SS, Stroobandt RX, Sinnaeve AF. Cardiac Pacemakers Step by Step: An Illustrated Guide. Malden, MA: Blackwell; 2004.)

or pacemaker inhibition in the case of LV lead dislodgment into the coronary sinus with sensing of atrial activity [42].

First-generation multisite pacing pulse generators similarly provide a single ventricular output for simultaneous RV and LV stimulation, however, two separate ventricular channels internally connect in parallel. This connection is made for both the lead tip and ring connections and eliminates the need for a Y-adaptor. However, this configuration still provides simultaneous RV and LV sensing with associated limitations.

Second-generation multisite pacing pulse generators have independent ventricular ports. Each ventricular lead therefore has separate sensing and output circuits. This arrangement permits optimal programming of outputs and time delay between RV and LV stimulation for each patient. It also eliminates the potential complications of biventricular sensing.

Programming Considerations for CRT

Pacing Modes

It is axiomatic that for maximal delivery of CRT, ventricular pacing must be continuous. DDD mode (atrial and ventricular pacing/sensing) guarantees AV synchrony by synchronizing ventricular pacing to all atrial events except during episodes of atrial tachycardia or atrial fibrillation. However, DDD mode increases the probability of atrial pacing (depending upon programmed lower rate limit) that may alter the left-sided AV timing relationship due to interatrial conduction time and atrial pacing latency.

VDD mode (atrial sensing only, ventricular pacing and sensing) guarantees the absence of atrial pacing and synchronizes all atrial events to ventricular pacing at the programmed AV delay. However, if the sinus rate is below the lower programmed rate limit, AV synchrony is lost because the VDD mode is operationally VVI (ventricular-only sensing and pacing).

Although conventional dual-chamber pacing systems are not designed for biventricular pacing and generally do not allow programming of an AV delay of zero, or near zero, they are being increasingly used with their shortest AV delay (0–30 ms) for CRT in patients with permanent AF. The advantages include programming flexibility, elimination of the Y-adaptor (required for conventional VVIR devices), protection against far-field sensing of atrial activity (an inherent risk of dual cathodal devices with simultaneous sensing from both ventricles), and cost. When a conventional dual-chamber pacemaker is used for CRT, the LV lead is usually connected to the atrial port and the RV lead to the ventricular port. This provides for (1) LV stimulation before RV activation (LV preexcitation); (2) protection against ventricular asystole related to oversensing of far-field atrial activity when the LV lead is dislodged toward the AV groove. The DVIR mode is ideally suited for this application. The DVIR mode (committed atrial pacing, ventricular pacing and sensing) behaves like the VVIR mode except that there are always two closely coupled independent ventricular stimuli thereby facilitating comprehensive evaluation of RV and LV pacing and sensing performance. The DVIR mode also provides absolute protection against far-field sensing of atrial activity in case of LV lead dislodgment, as no sensing occurs on the "atrial" (LV) lead in the DVIR mode.

Determining LV and RV Capture: Importance of Electrocardiography

The 12-lead ECG is essential to ascertain RV and LV capture during follow-up of CRT systems without separately programmable ventricular outputs. It is recognized that 6 distinct 12-lead ventricular activation patterns may be seen during threshold determination. These are (1) intrinsic rhythm during loss of RV and LV capture or pacing inhibition (native QRS), (2) isolated RV stimulation, (3) isolated LV stimulation, (4) biventricular stimulation with complete capture, (5) biventricular pacing with fusion between native activation and pacing capture, (6) biventricular stimulation with anodal capture.

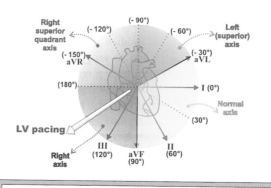

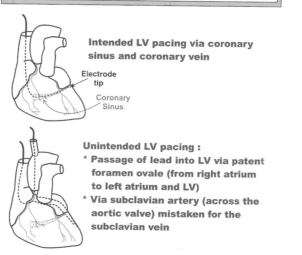

Fig. 21.18 ECG QRS patterns during LV free wall pacing. (From Barold SS, Stroobandt RX, Sinnaeve AF. Cardiac Pacemakers Step by Step: An Illustrated Guide. Malden, MA: Blackwell; 2004.)

Anodal capture refers to the situation when myocardial capture occurs at the RV anode. This could theoretically occur in isolation with the LV cathode but most commonly occurs with both RV and LV cathodes and is referred to as *triple site* pacing. Anodal capture is more common at high voltage output and with true bipolar RV leads due to the small surface area and higher current density of the ring electrode, as opposed to the larger surface area and lower current density of the coil electrode in integrated bipolar leads.

Anodal capture results in a distinct change in activation pattern compared with biventricular pacing that can only be appreciated on the 12-lead ECG (Fig. 21.21). The electrical axis is shifted leftwards and the QRS duration may be shorter as a consequence of increased ventricular fusion. The change in QRS morphology related to loss of anodal capture as voltage output is

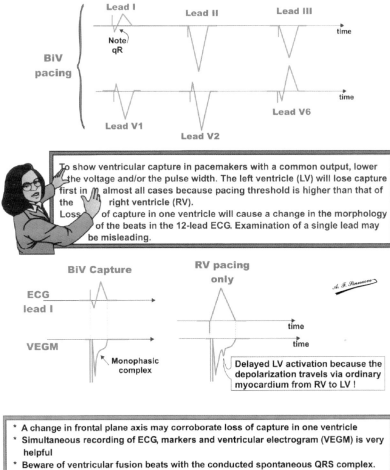

Fig. 21.19 Analysis of ECG QRS patterns to ascertain RV and LV capture in CRT systems without separately programmable ventricular outputs. (From Barold SS, Stroobandt RX, Sinnaeve AF. Cardiac Pacemakers Step by Step: An Illustrated Guide. Malden, MA: Blackwell; 2004.)

decremented during a temporary threshold test using a single ECG lead may be misinterpreted as loss of LV capture and result in erroneous overestimation of the LV threshold.

The physiologic consequences of anodal capture are uncertain. One study demonstrated that anodal capture might be advantageous during CRT by counteracting the regional activation delay located at the inferior wall of the left ventricle and improving regional measures of intraventricular dyssynchrony [43].

Programming Pacing Outputs

It is critically important that voltage output be adjusted to exceed ventricular capture threshold for left ventricle and right ventricle in common cathodal

AV Optimization

AV optimization is important for maximal hemodynamic response to CRT but not essential, as ventricular pumping function can be improved by CRT even in the presence of permanent AF. Nonetheless, acute hemodynamic studies have consistently demonstrated that AV optimization "re-times" the left atrial–left ventricular relationship and can result in 15–40% improvement in indices of left ventricular systolic performance acutely. Furthermore, small changes in AV delay may nullify hemodynamic benefit of CRT.

AV Optimization Using Invasive Hemodynamic Monitoring (Fig. 21.22)

Techniques for AV optimization using invasive left ventricular pressure monitoring have been described [20–22]. The optimal AV delay is assumed to be the value that yields at least a 5% increase in aortic pulse pressure or LV $+dP/dt_{max}$ compared with baseline. These indices are useful because they correlate with stroke volume and global contractile function. However, pulse pressure and LV $+dP/dt$ can be confounded by changes in preload and arterial impedance (afterload). Though this technique is useful for assessing the effects of acute manipulations of AV delay, ventricular stimulation sites, and ventricular sequencing on LV pumping function, this is an impractical approach for routine clinical care. Furthermore, there is some evidence that

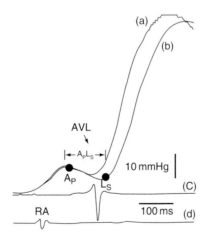

Fig. 21.22 AV optimization using invasive hemodynamic monitoring. Example of systolic left ventricular (LV) pressure during pacing (**a**) and intrinsic condition (**b**), intrinsic LV electrogram (**c**) and intrinsic right atrial (RA) electrogram (**d**) recorded from one patient. Also shown here is the presystolic peak (AP) due to atrial contraction and the start of pressure development in the LV (LS), the latter obtained as the point that first attained a slope >10% of maximum rate of increase of LV pressure. The interval (APLS) between AP and LS is defined as atrioventricular mechanical latency (AVL). When the ventricle is preexcited with pacing, the LS point moves to the left, as shown here in curve **a**. To obtain the LS point in paced condition, the pressure curves in pacing and intrinsic condition are aligned at the right atrium electrical activation (RA). Thereafter, the difference between the two curves is obtained. The LS is the first point on the difference curve at which the slope is 10% of the maximum slope. (From Auricchio A, Stellbrink C, Sack S, et al., Pacing Therapies in Congestive Heart Failure (PATH-CHF) Study Group. Long-term clinical effect of hemodynamically optimized cardiac resynchronization therapy in patients with heart failure and ventricular conduction delay. J Am Coll Cardiol 2002;39(12):2026–2033.)

acute hemodynamic response is not highly correlated with long-term clinical response including reverse ventricular remodeling.

AV Optimization Using Conventional Echocardiography

Several methods of AV optimization using echo-guided pulsed Doppler analysis of transmitral blood flow velocities to approximate an optimal timing relationship between atrial systole and ventricular filling have been described. The goal is manipulation of the AV delay until the end of the untruncated A-wave occurs coincident with mitral valve closure, which represents the onset of ventricular contraction. The common assumption of these methods is that this optimized AV delay will yield the longest diastolic filling time and best acute LV pumping function.

According to the method of Ritter et al. [44,45], optimal sensed AV (SAV) delay can be stated algebraically as $SAV_{optimal} = SAV_{short} + d$, where $d = (SAV_{long} + QA_{long}) - (SAV_{short} + QA_{short})$, Q = ventricular pacing stimulus, and A = termination of A-wave. This process is performed in three steps. First, the SAV_{long} and QA_{long} are determined by programming a "long" sensed AV delay (SAV_{long}). The AV delay should be long enough to maintain full ventricular capture but allow spontaneous closure of the mitral valve prior to aortic outflow (Fig. 21.23). QA_{long} is then measured as the time from the ventricular pacing stimulus to the end of the A-wave. Second, the SAV_{short} and QA_{short} are determined by programming a "short" sensed AV delay (SAV_{short}) that results in forced closure of the mitral valve (Fig. 21.24). QA_{short} is then measured as the time from the ventricular pacing stimulus to the end of the A-wave. Caution must be applied to not extrapolate to the end of the A-wave but to use the observed end of the A-wave. Third, AV optimization is confirmed by noting the return of normal E- and A-wave separation indicating improved diastolic filling time and optimized AV timing relationship (Fig. 21.25).

This is a rather tedious process and highly operator dependent, as visualization of the terminal portion of the A-wave is often difficult and subjective. A potentially more critical limitation is that the basis for the technique was

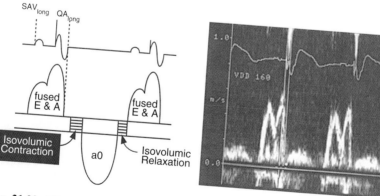
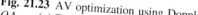

Fig. 21.23 AV optimization using Doppler mitral inflow. Determining SAV_{long} and QA_{long}. (**a**) To determine SAV_{long}, a long sensed AV delay that maintains ventricular preexcitation, yet allows spontaneous closure of the mitral valve prior to aortic ejection (e.g., 150 ms), is programmed. Next, the time from V-pace to the end of the A-wave is measured. This is QA_{long}, which refers to the QA distance measured when a "long" SAV is programmed. (**b**) Doppler echo of transmitral blood flow with a long AV delay.

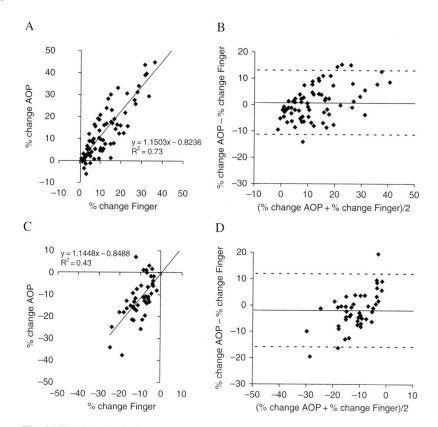

Fig. 21.27 AV optimization using finger plethysmography. Correlation of aortic pulse pressure change versus finger pulse change and the corresponding Bland–Altmann plots. (**A**) Correlation for significantly positive finger responses. (**B**) Bland–Altmann plot for significantly positive finger responses. (**C**) Correlation for significantly negative finger responses. (**D**) Bland–Altmann plot for significantly negative finger responses. (From Butter C, Stellbrink C, Belalcazar A, et al. Cardiac resynchronization therapy optimization by finger plethysmography. Heart Rhythm 2005;1:568–578.)

changes was well correlated with positive aortic pulse pressure changes ($R^2 = 0.73$). However, the correlation with negative aortic pressure changes was poor ($R^2 = 0.43$). FPPG identified 78% of the patients having positive aortic pulse pressure changes to CRT and identified the AV delay giving maximum aortic pulse pressure change in all selected patients. This approach has not been clinically validated but offers the appeal of a quick, noninvasive measure for correlating changes in AV delay with some meaningful measure of cardiac output.

Clinical Experience with AV Optimization

Previous studies have emphasized the importance of a short AV delay during standard dual-chamber pacing in patients with HF to optimize the acute hemodynamic response when native AV conduction is prolonged [50, 51]. However, in another study, the same benefit could not be documented [52]. It is now recognized that the acute hemodynamic benefit of AV optimization in conventional dual-chamber pacing is negated by the chronic adverse effects of ventricular desynchronization on LV pump function due to RV apical pacing, particularly among patients with systolic heart failure.

However, because biventricular pacing overcomes the problem of ventricular desynchronization caused by RV only pacing, AV optimization has been incorporated into RCTs of CRT. Using variations on the method of Ritter et al. [44] or invasive hemodynamic monitoring, the optimized AV delay in studies of CRT is almost invariably in the range 80–110 ms regardless of other considerations [20,21,48,53,54]. Because of this, some have argued empiric programming of the AV delay at ~100 ms. It is almost certainly true that the optimal AV delay will likely differ as heart rate and cardiac loading conditions change, such that the optimal AV delay at one point in time may not be optimal under other conditions. Furthermore, the importance of AV delay optimization at rest for chronic clinical and hemodynamic effect remains to be shown. It has also become clear that optimal ventricular synchronization is far more important than AV optimization. The atrial contribution to ventricular filling is probably minimal when the left ventricle is operating at persistently elevated diastolic pressures and atrial mechanical transport is diminished due to myopathic processes.

Recently, Sawhney et al. [55] reported a randomized, prospective, single-blind trial of echo-guided AV optimization using the aortic velocity–time integral (VTI) versus an empiric AV delay at 120 ms in 40 CRT patients. Optimal AV delay was defined as the AV delay that yielded the largest mean aortic VTI at one of eight tested AV intervals (between 60 and 200 ms). A small improvement in ejection fraction was demonstrated in the VTI-optimized group compared with the empiric AV delay group immediately after implementation of CRT. After 3 months, modest improvements in New York Heart Association (NYHA) functional class and standardized quality of life scores were observed in the VTI-optimized group. Not unexpectedly, the mean optimized AV delay program and empiric AV delay were almost identical (119 vs. 120 ms, respectively). The authors speculated that individual patient variation accounted for the slight differences in outcomes between groups. However, due to the large range of optimal AV delays observed (60–200 ms), many patients in the empiric AV delay group had an AV delay that was significantly different than their optimized AV delay. This data, though of interest, is insufficient to recommend AV optimization in all patients who receive CRT.

Interventricular Timing Considerations

First- and second-generation CRTP and CRTD systems delivered simultaneous biventricular stimulation, even when RV and LV stimulation outputs were separately programmable. Simultaneous biventricular stimulation has reproducibly been shown to be effective in the majority of patients in RCTs of CRT. However, despite similar prolongation of the QRS duration and morphology of LBBB, considerable heterogeneity in the location of regional mechanical dyssynchrony has been revealed by sophisticated echocardiographic techniques [27,56,57]. For example, the posterobasal left ventricle most commonly shows the greatest electromechanical delay in LBBB associated with nonischemic DCM (NDCM). However, the greatest electromechanical delay occurs in the interventricular septum (paradoxical septal contraction) in some patients with LBBB and NDCM. The situation is even more complex in ischemic cardiomyopathy where regional electrome-chanical delays are influenced by infarct location. It is therefore reasonable to hypothesize that timed stimulation of different left regions might be necessary for optimal resynchronization therapy. In practical application, RV stimu-lation serves as a surrogate for septal stimulation, but this may be influenced by RV lead position (RV apex [RVA] vs. septum).

Logically, enhancements to biventricular pacing systems might permit tailoring of ventricular stimulation by site and timing to optimally address the diversity of electromechanical phenomenon observed between individual patients. In third-generation systems, the relative timing of RV and LV stimulation can be varied. This requires separately programmable RV and LV stimulation outputs and circuitry to permit timing delay between outputs by stimulation site (V-V timing). The goal of V-V timing is site-selective, sequential ventricular stimulation. Theoretically, V-V timing could be achieved with unipolar or dual cathodal electrode configurations. From a practical perspective, unipolar pacing is inapplicable in CRTD, and anodal capture at high outputs with dual cathodal electrode configurations results in unintended biventricular stimulation and could disrupt V-V timing. This is probably only relevant when RV stimulation precedes LV stimulation, as RV capture will render the local myocardium refractory and anodal capture during high-output LV stimulation will not occur. Accordingly, the use of V-V timing where RV precedes LV stimulation with dual cathodal electrode configurations mandates exclusion of anodal capture by 12-lead electrocar-diography at programmed outputs (see above). Therefore, V-V timing is optimally delivered with true bipolar (RV and LV) electrode configurations.

Interventricular Timing Operation

Interventricular timing operation in the Medtronic InSync III CRTP system is shown in Figure 21.28. Nominally, selection of biventricular (RV + LV) pacing results in delivery of a pacing stimulus to the other chamber after a 4-ms delay. However, the first chamber paced and delay interval of a paced stimulus to the first and second chamber are separately programmable. The V-V Pace Delay parameter sets the amount of time that elapses between delivery of a stimulus to the first ventricle paced and delivery of a stimulus to the other ventricle. This can be varied between 4 and 80 ms. The V-V Pace Delay parameter necessitates timing interactions to guarantee proper operation of Ventricular Safety Pacing and Ventricular Sense Response. When these are enabled, paces generated in response to a ventricular sense will be delivered at the minimum (4 ms) V-V delay.

Clinical Experience with Sequential Versus Biventricular Stimulation

The long-term clinical experience with sequential biventricular stimulation is limited, and no RCTs have reported on outcomes based on the use of this potential enhancement to CRT. Sogaard et al. [27] used tissue tracking to quantify regions of delayed longitudinal contraction and three-dimensional echocardiography to measure the effects of sequential ventricular stimu-lation in 21 patients with systolic heart failure and LBBB and QRSd <130 ms. After AV optimization using the Ritter method [44] and simultaneous

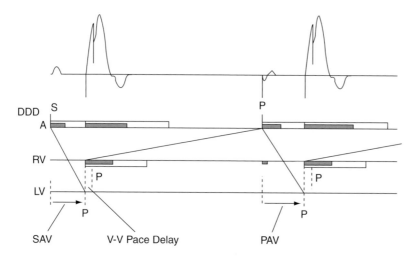

Fig. 21.28 Interventricular timing operation (Medtronic).

biventricular pacing, the number of regions displaying delayed longitudinal contraction was reduced and ejection fraction increased in all patients. These measurements were then repeated at five different interventricular delay intervals(12,20,40,60,and 80ms) with either LV or RV preactivation. Optimized sequential ventricular stimulation caused further reductions in regions displaying delayed longitudinal contraction and increases in ejection fraction, which were sustained for at least 3 months. Additionally, sequential ventricular stimulation increased diastolic filling time by about 7% even after AV optimization.

An interesting observation was that the location of myocardial regions displaying delayed longitudinal contraction varied between patients despite similar patterns of LBBB on the surface ECG. Although not uniformly observed, in most patients with nonischemic DCM (NDCM), the delayed regions were located in the posterobasal LV (Fig. 21.29), whereas in ischemic DCM the delayed regions were more frequently in the interventricular septum and inferior wall (Fig. 21.30). Correspondingly, optimal sequential ventricular stimulation was achieved with LV preexcitation when the posterobasal region was delayed and with RV preexcitation when the inferoseptal region was delayed. These beneficial effects were observed over a short range of ventricular timing intervals (±20 ms) and further increases in interventricular delay, or preexcitation of already early activated regions, resulted in worsened mechanical dyssynchrony and reduced pumping function.

Similar benefits of optimized sequential biventricular stimulation were observed by Bordachar [57]. Using combined measures of LV diastolic filling time, cardiac output, mitral regurgitant volume, and effective regurgitant orifice surface area (Fig. 21.31), systolic dyssynchrony index using tissue Doppler imaging, and extent of myocardium displaying delayed longitudinal contraction (tissue tracking), simultaneous biventricular pacing was the optimal stimulation configuration in only 15% of patients. LV preexcitation was optimal for 61% of patients with V-V interval ranging between 12 and 40 ms, whereas RV preexcitation was optimal in 24% patients with V-V interval ranging between 12 and 20 ms. All patients demonstrated clinical

A   Non- IHD systolic performance at baseline

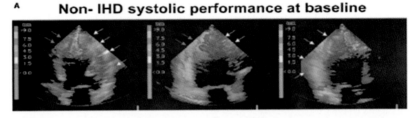

Non- IHD baseline delayed longitudinal contraction

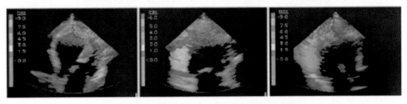

B   Non- IHD systolic performance during CRT (simultaneous)

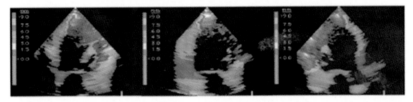

Non- IHD systolic performance during CRT (LV preactivated by 20 ms)

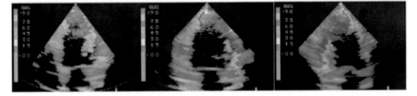

Fig. 21.29 Effect of sequential ventricular stimulation on LV systolic shortening. Color-coded scaling at left side of each image indicates regional motion amplitude. (**A**) *Top:* Baseline tissue tracking images in apical four-chamber, two-chamber, and long-axis views during systole in a patient with idiopathic dilated cardiomyopathy. Note lack of systolic motion in lateral wall, posterior wall, and distal parts of anterior wall, denoted by gray color and white arrows. Mechanical function of interventricular septum and inferior walls is abnormal, with greater motion amplitude in segments adjacent to apex (green arrows). *Bottom:* Extent of myocardium (colored segments) with delayed longitudinal contraction in diastole (mitral valve open). DLC is present in lateral, posterior, and inferior walls. Note that remaining part of LV is gray, indicating either no motion or motion toward base of heart (relaxation). (**B**) Same patient and views as in (**A**) (systole). *Top:* Simultaneous CRT resulting in contraction of larger proportion of lateral wall and posterior wall. In addition, each segment shows improved systolic shortening as seen from color coding. Abnormal distribution of myocardial motion in interventricular septum has been normalized. *Bottom:* Impact of sequential CRT with LV activated by 20 ms before RV. Compared with simultaneous CRT, sequential CRT yields further improvement in overall proportion of contracting myocardium in lateral and posterior walls. In addition, each segment shows further improvement in systolic shortening amplitude. (From Sogaard P, Egeblad H, Pedersen AK, et al. Sequential versus simultaneous biventricular resynchronization for severe heart failure: Evaluation by tissue Doppler imaging. Circulation 2002;106:2078–2084.)

A **IHD systolic performance at baseline**

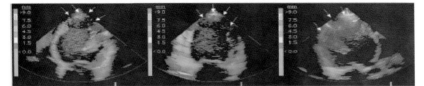

IHD delayed longitudinal contraction at baseline

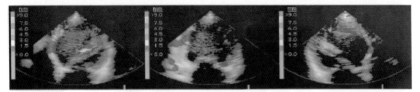

B **IHD systolic performance during CRT (simultaneous)**

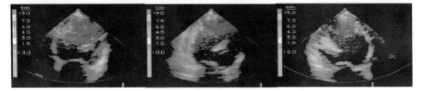

IHD systolic performance during CRT (RV preactivated by 12 ms)

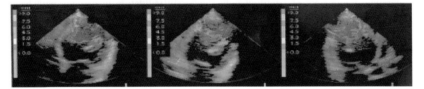

Fig. 21.30 Effect of V-V sequential ventricular stimulation on LV systolic shortening. (**A**) *Top:* Baseline tissue tracking images in apical four-chamber, two-chamber, and long-axis views during systole in a patient with idiopathic ischemic cardiomyopathy. Tissue tracking and strain rate analysis indicated apical infarct (*arrows*). *Bottom:* Extent of myocardium (colored segments) with delayed longitudinal contraction in interventricular septum and anterior and inferior walls (diastole). Extent of myocardium displaying delayed longitudinal contraction is less than that in patient with idiopathic dilated cardiomyopathy. (**B**) *Top:* Same patient as in (**A**) during simultaneous CRT, resulting in overall improvement in regional systolic shortening. *Bottom:* Impact of sequential CRT with RV lead activated 12 ms before LV lead. Compared with simultaneous CRT, sequential CRT yields further improvement in systolic contraction amplitude. (From Sogaard P, Egeblad H, Pedersen AK, et al. Sequential versus simultaneous biventricular resynchronization for severe heart failure: Evaluation by tissue Doppler imaging. Circulation 2002;106:2078–2084.)

responsiveness (improved NYHA class, quality of life, and 6-min hall walk) and evidence of reverse remodeling (improved ejection fraction, decreased LV end systolic and end diastolic volumes) at 3 months.

It is currently unclear what chronic benefit on a population scale, if any, manipulation of interventricular timing would provide during biventricular pacing. This is highlighted by the emerging evidence that univentricular left ventricular pacing is probably either equivalent or superior to biventricular pacing acutely and chronically (see below).

Ventricular Therapies in Primary Versus Secondary Prevention Patients

In general, secondary prevention patients have a greater frequency of spontaneous ventricular arrhythmia than primary prevention patients. Several retrospective analyses have preliminarily addressed these issues. It is important to note there have been no prospective, randomized clinical trials of specific empiric programming of ventricular therapies by ICD indication or substrate.

Wilkoff et al. [75] analyzed the frequency and characteristics of spontaneous VT and VF between patients with a primary versus secondary prevention indication for ICD therapy in the MIRACLE ICD study of CRTD. Primary prevention patients had a lower frequency of appropriate VT and VF episodes (0.12 vs. 0.53 episodes/month) at significantly faster CLs (303 ± 53 ms vs. 367 ± 54 ms, $p < 0.0001$). Primary prevention patients also had a significantly higher percentage of device-classified VF (40% vs. 14%, $p < 0.0001$). The absolute rate of inappropriate detections in the primary prevention group was lower but constituted a much higher portion of all episodes for that group (32% vs. 14% for the secondary prevention group). Most inappropriate detections in the primary prevention group were due to rapidly conducted SVT with 1:1 AV relationship (sinus tachycardia or atrial tachycardia) and were treated as VT.

Russo et al. [76] examined spontaneous therapies in primary prevention patients. Over 21 ± 18 months, 23% patients had appropriate therapies and 14% had inappropriate therapies for SVT. Clinical VT rates were higher than SVT rates (211 ± 38 bpm vs. 179 ± 14 bpm). Only 10% of the patients with appropriate therapies had VT rates <190 bpm. The authors concluded that although there was some overlap in VT and SVT rates, VT rates less than 190 bpm were uncommon and avoidance of programming to nominal VF detection rates may reduce inappropriate shocks for SVT.

These preliminary observations provoke examination of tachyarrhythmia detection and therapy programming based on indication for ICD therapy. "Overtreatment" in primary prevention patients is an important concern, potentially at the cost of spurious therapies for inappropriate ventricular detections due to SVT. A more detailed analysis of the incidence of appropriate therapies for specific ventricular rhythms, inappropriate ventricular therapies, quality of life, and mortality was recently performed in the PainFREE RX II Trial study population [77]. Appropriate therapies for specific ventricular rhythms and inappropriate therapies for SVT, quality of life, and mortality were compared in 582 patients (primary prevention = 248; second prevention= 334). ICDs were identically programmed with three zones (VT <188 bpm; FVT = 188–250 bpm; VF >250 bpm) but randomized to ATP or shock as initial therapy for FVT. All treated episodes with electrograms were adjudicated. Primary prevention patients had lower ejection fractions and were more likely to have ischemic cardiomyopathy, however, beta-blockers, antiarrhythmic drugs, and follow-up duration were similar. Over 11 ± 3 months, 1563 treated episodes were classified as 740 VT, 350 FVT, 77 VF, and 396 SVT. The distribution of VT, FVT, and VF was not different between primary and secondary prevention (VT 52% vs. 54%; FVT 35% vs. 35%; VF 14% vs. 10%). More secondary prevention patients had appropriate therapies (26% vs. 18%, $p = 0.02$), but among these patients, median episodes/patient was similar. Inappropriate therapies occurred in 15% of both groups and accounted for similar proportions of all detected and treated episodes. Quality of life improved modestly in both groups, and mortality was similar.

Because the relative frequency of specific ventricular rhythms is similar between primary and secondary prevention patients, an equivalent efficacy of ATP could be anticipated assuming similar arrhythmia substrate (i.e., reentrant VT). Therefore, it is reasonable to conclude that if any VT therapy is to be prescribed in either group, it should include ATP with the expectation that 70–90% of episodes will be painlessly terminated. The more difficult issue is whether *any* slow VT therapy should be prescribed in primary prevention patients, particularly those in who programmed stimulation has not been performed. Elimination of slow VT detection might reduce spurious therapies for some specific SVTs (such as sinus tachycardia) but might not be as effective for others, such as atrial fibrillation with a rapid ventricular response. The zeal for reducing the probability of spurious therapies by eliminating a slow VT detection zone must be balanced against the risk of failing to treat unanticipated VT. This issue was indirectly addressed by a retrospective study by Bansch et al. [78]. The risk of VT above the VT detection interval ranged between 2.7% and 3.5% per year during the first 4 years after ICD implantation. Fifty-four (88.5%) of the VT episodes above the VT detection interval were associated with significant symptoms, and 10% of patients had to be resuscitated. Risk factors for VT above the initial VT detection interval were heart failure, lower EF, spontaneous or inducible monomorphic VT, and use of class III antiarrhythmic drugs. The risk of recurrent VT above the VT detection interval was 11.8%, 12.5%, and 26.6% during the first, second, and third year after the first occurrence above the VT detection interval. This suggests that elimination of a slow VT zone in some patients will result in clinically consequential undertreatment of slow VT.

RV only, LV only, or Biventricular ATP in CRTD

An interesting recent development in the clinical application of ATP is stimulation site of origin. It is important to note that the pathophysiologic mechanism of reentrant VT is not dependent on, or influenced by, site of origin of the VT circuit. From a practical perspective, site of origin might be very important because the majority of VT circuits arise in the left ventricle, and pacing stimuli are conventionally delivered from the right ventricular apex. Because distance and conduction time between stimulation site and site of origin affect the ability of pacing stimuli to interact with the reentrant circuit, ATP delivered from the left ventricular pacing lead or biventricular pacing leads in CRTD might improve efficacy compared with right ventricular ATP.

Scientific evidence regarding the relative differences between RV, LV, or biventricular ATP for terminating monomorphic VT is limited. In the Ventak CHF/CONTAK CD study [79], all ATP among patients randomized to CRT was delivered simultaneously from right ventricle and left ventricle (biventricular ATP). Monomorphic VT was successfully terminated in 927 of 1053 (88%) episodes. Though this is in alignment with success rates for ATP delivered from the RV apex in other studies [60, 80–87], no comparison was made between biventricular ATP and RV only ATP (i.e., patients randomized to no CRT).

The relative efficacy of right ventricular versus biventricular ATP was evaluated in the InSync ICD OUS (Outside United States) Study [88]. ATP termination success was 2.4 times greater with biventricular versus right ventricular ATP and appeared to be associated with fewer accelerations for both slow VT and fast VT. A similar result was observed in the MIRACLE ICD study that randomized RV versus biventricular ATP for monomorphic VT induced during implantation. Biventricular ATP had a higher efficacy than RV ATP (622/658 [95%] versus 297/336 [88%] episodes, respectively, p < 0.001). A preliminary report from the VENTAK CHF/CONTAK CD study also showed that biventricular ATP was more successful in patients randomized to CRT pacing therapy [89]. This effect was influenced by left ventricular pacing lead location (improving in lateral locations, worsening in anterior locations) and improved over time in the patients who were receiving CRT.

These data are insufficient to support definitive conclusions regarding the role of alternate site ATP for terminating VT. Due to technical limitations, the CRTD ICDs in both studies were only capable of right ventricular or biventricular stimulation and therefore provide no insights on a possible role for isolated left ventricular stimulation. From a theoretical perspective, it is not immediately obvious that left ventricular stimulation should improve ATP success in coronary artery disease, as many reentrant VT circuits arise in the interventricular septum, closer to a RV stimulation site than a left ventricular free wall stimulation site. Conduction delay out of left ventricular stimulation sites due to interposed infarction and fibrosis might modify any advantage related to proximity to site of VT origin, and this effect may be different in the right ventricle. How these and other factors might influence the relative efficacy of left ventricular ATP is unknown.

Summary of Ventricular Therapy Programming in CRTD

Antitachycardia pacing reliably terminates ~85–90% of slow VT (cycle lengths [CL] <300–320 ms) with a low risk of acceleration (1–5%). Similar high success and low acceleration rates for fast VT (CL 320–240 ms) have recently been demonstrated. These results are probably consistent across different substrates (ischemic versus nonischemic DCM) when the common mechanism of VT is reentry. Therefore, ATP should be routinely applied in CRTD regardless of substrate.

Some general recommendations on programming ATP schemes are possible. For VT CL >300–330 ms, burst and ramp pacing are equivalently effective for terminating VT and equivalently low risk for causing acceleration. For VT CL <300–330 ms, burst pacing is more effective and less likely to result in acceleration than ramp pacing. In either case, the risk of acceleration is inversely related to the VT CL. "Less aggressive" burst stimulation (e.g., 91% of VT CL vs. 81% of VT CL) is more effective and causes less acceleration, especially for fast VT (CL <320 ms) [90]. "Tailoring" of ATP to specific induced VTs is not necessary in most situations.

Loss of CRT: Causes and Corrective Actions

Optimal CRT operation requires continuous delivery of ventricular pacing. In practical experience, 100% ventricular pacing is difficult to achieve. A reasonable goal is 90–95% cumulative ventricular pacing with verified left ventricular capture. A retrospective analysis of the VENTAK CHF/CONTAK CD Biventricular Pacing Study revealed that CRT is interrupted transiently in 36% if patients and permanently in 5% within 2 years of follow-up and the causes are diverse [91]. Restoration of CRT can usually be accomplished noninvasively and less commonly requires surgical intervention.

Loss of CRT Related to Pacing Operation

Obviously, programming parameters during CRT operation should reflect the goal of continuous ventricular pacing. Therefore, any parameter choice that might reduce the frequency of ventricular pacing should be avoided. The consequence of programmed parameters on continuous delivery of CRT is influenced by the patient's AV conduction status. The majority of patients who receive CRT have reliable AV conduction, and therefore any programming choice that permits the emergence of native ventricular activation will reduce delivery of CRT. In dual-chamber CRT systems, examples include pacing modes that do not synchronize ventricular pacing to atrial activity (such as DDI or VVI), inappropriately long AV delays or use of automatic AV interval extension, or any parameter that compromises continuous atrial tracking (true undersensing or pseudo-undersensing due to a long postventricular atrial refractory period [PVARP], automatic PVARP extensions, or a low upper tracking rate). In single-chamber CRT systems among patients with permanent AF, the lower rate should be programmed to continuously exceed the spontaneous ventricular rate. The absence of AV conduction renders loss of CRT due to poor programming choices unlikely because ventricular pacing cannot be inadvertently minimized by competition with native ventricular activation; however, considerations regarding optimal AV delay still apply. Even when these recommendations are implemented, loss of CRT can occur due to the complex interplay between spontaneous electrical activity and inviolable elements of timing cycle operation.

Pseudo-atrial Undersensing

A reduction in ventricular pacing due to loss of atrial tracking at high sinus rates (*pseudo-atrial undersensing*) is common. In this circumstance, high sinus rates and first-degree AV block (AVB), which are common in heart failure patients, displace the P-wave into the PVARP resulting in simultaneous loss of atrial tracking and synchronous ventricular pacing. This situation is commonly triggered by automatic PVARP extensions after a premature ventricular contraction (PVC) or other circumstances intended to prevent pacemaker-mediated tachycardia [92]. Spontaneous AV conduction occurs in the form of a preempted upper rate Wenckebach response (Fig. 21.32).

Though not required for pseudo-atrial undersensing, double counting (see below) of the native ventricular electrogram often participates in the initiation and maintenance of the phenomenon in nondedicated (Y-adaptors) or first-generation dual cathodal CRTP/CRTD systems where pacing and sensing from the right ventricle and left ventricle occurs simultaneously (Fig. 21.33). When spontaneous conduction with LBBB (or any form of ventricular conduction delay) emerges, the LV EGM may be sensed sometime after detection of the RV EGM if the LV signal extends beyond the relatively short ventricular blanking period initiated by RV sensing. The LV signal

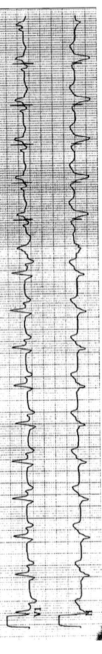

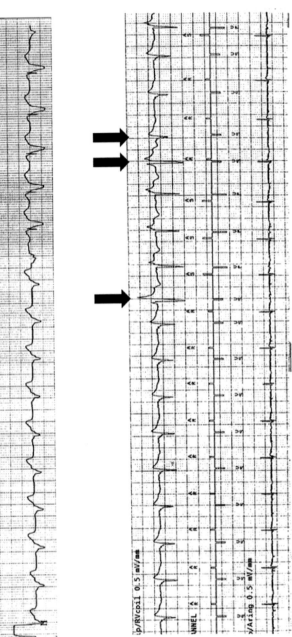

Fig. 21.32 Loss of CRT due to pseudo-atrial undersensing. *Top:* Telemetry strip. Note sinus tachycardia with marked first degree AV block (PR 400 ms) and loss of atrial synchronous biventricular pacing on left. Note restoration of atrial synchronous biventricular pacing after PVC (*arrow*) on right. *Bottom:* Same patient. Sinus rate exceeds the programmed upper rate limit, displacing P-waves into the PVARP (marked as AR). Spontaneous AV conduction occurs in the form of a preempted Wenckebach upper rate response. First PVC resets PVARP and restores atrial tracking. Second PVC (*arrow*) occurs coincident with sinus event, which falls into the post-ventricular atrial blanking period (PVAB). Third PVC (*arrow*) resets PVARP and reinitiates pseudo-atrial undersensing. Atrial tracking is restored when sinus rate slows slightly at the end of the strip.

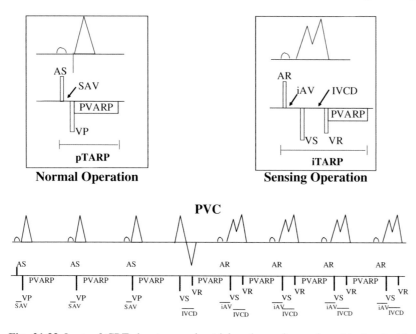

Fig. 21.33 Loss of CRT due to pseudo-atrial undersensing and ventricular double counting with implied total atrial refractory period. Premature ventricular contraction (PVC) is double counted; second component resets the PVARP, which initiates pseudo-atrial sensing. Loss of CRT results in emergence of spontaneous AV conduction. Double counting of the native ventricular electrogram continuously resets the PVARP, perpetuating pseudo-atrial sensing. Implied total atrial refractory period = SAV + PVARP + interventricular conduction delay.

continuously resets the PVARP resulting in an "implied total atrial refractory period (iTARP)" conflict and maintenance of pseudo-atrial undersensing.

Failure to deliver CRT at high sinus rates can be minimized by shortening the PVARP, increasing the upper tracking limit, and deactivating the PVC response in the DDD mode. Newer CRT systems minimize ventricular double counting by employing an interventricular ventricular refractory period (IVRP). Ventricular sensed events (i.e., LV sensing) during the IVRP do not reset the PVARP and eliminates the "implied TARP" conflict (Fig. 21.34). Another method for dealing with disruptions to CRT delivery when PVCs cause the following atrial events to fall into the PVARP is Atrial Tracking Recovery (Medtronic, Inc., Minneapolis, MN, USA) (Figs. 21.35–21.37). Atrial Tracking Recovery operates in the DDD/R mode when a mode switch episode is not in effect. Under certain conditions, Atrial Tracking Recovery temporarily shortens PVARP to reduce the intrinsic TARP. The device monitors for eight consecutive pacing cycles where all the following occur: (1) the current ventricular event is sensed, not paced, (2) the last ventricular interval contains exactly one refractory atrial event, (3) the last two atrial intervals vary from each other by less than 50 ms, (4) the last atrial interval is longer than the upper tracking rate (UTR) interval by at least 50 ms, (5) the last atrial interval is greater than current SAV plus current PVARP, (6) the last VS-AR interval (from the previous ventricular event to the atrial refractory event) is greater than Post Ventricular Atrial Blanking (PVAB).

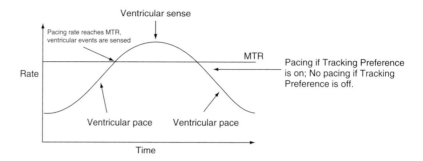

Fig. 21.38 Atrial Tracking Preference (Guidant).

alternating pattern of atrial cycle lengths with one signal timed close to the ventricular EGM. Less common causes of spurious mode switching include "near-field" or "early" R-wave oversensing (atrial R-wave sensing prior to arrival of the depolarization wavefront at the ventricular pacing lead position) and oversensing of the paced atrial depolarization during the AV interval [97, 98]. Spurious mode switching can usually be eliminated by the use of bipolar atrial pacing leads, extending the postventricular atrial blanking period (PVAB) or reducing atrial sensitivity so as to reject far-field signals without compromising atrial sensing.

Loss of CRT Due to Prevention of Pacing on the T-wave

Theoretically, conduction delay could prevent a PVC initiated in the left ventricle from reaching the RV electrode (univentricular sensing) and inhibiting the scheduled biventricular pace triggered by a sensed (or paced) atrial event. In this situation, lack of LV sensing could result in competitive ventricular pacing outside the absolute myocardial refractory period. To prevent competitive pacing during the LV vulnerable period (including the T-wave), some Guidant CRTD systems incorporate a Left Ventricular Protection Period (LVPP). The LVPP is defined as the period after a left ventricular event, either paced or sensed when LV pacing is inhibited, and is programmable between 300 and 500 ms. The LVPP reduces the maximum LV pacing rate and theoretically could disrupt CRT by preventing LV stimulation when preceded by RV stimulation, depending on the programmed interventricular delay and the conduction time from the RV to LV electrode.

Loss of CRT Due to Competition with Native Ventricular Activation

Any situation that permits competition between the delivery of continuous ventricular pacing and native ventricular activation will degrade CRT efficacy. This is far more likely to occur among patients with intact AV conduction.

Atrial Tachyarrhythmias with Rapid Ventricular Conduction

Atrial tachyarrhythmias are the common cause of loss of CRT, accounting for 18% of all therapy interruptions in one study [91]. Paroxysmal AF in patients with dual-chamber CRT systems results in appropriate mode switching and loss of atrial synchronous ventricular pacing (see above). In the absence of mode switching, native ventricular activation due to rapidly conducted

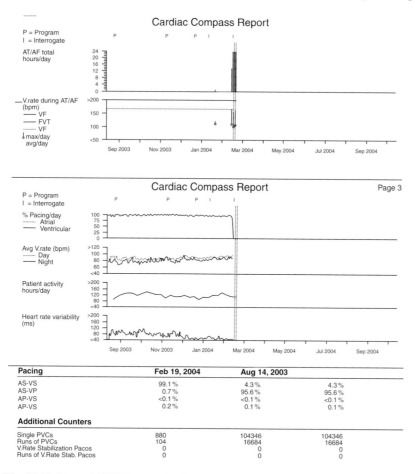

Fig. 21.39 Loss of CRT due to atrial fibrillation. Note high % ASVP counter prior to onset of atrial fibrillation. Onset of atrial fibrillation with rapid AV conduction results in sudden loss of CRT, indicated by high %ASVS counter.

paroxysmal AF may compete with continuous ventricular pacing (Figs. 21.39 and 21.40). Management should focus on pharmacologic suppression of AF and control of the conducted ventricular response.

The importance of rate control and regularization of the ventricular response during AF should not be underestimated. Historically, symptoms during AF have been attributed to a combination of loss of AV synchrony and rapid ventricular response (RVR), which may result in significant reductions in cardiac output. More recently, the independent effect of ventricular cycle length irregularity on adverse hemodynamic performance during AF has been recognized [99–101]. One study demonstrated acute improvement in hemodynamic performance and long-term improvement in symptoms and QoL among patients with chronic AF and a controlled ventricular response after AV junction ablation and VVIR pacemaker implantation [99].

These benefits were attributed to an independent effect of ventricular rate regularization, because loss of AV synchrony was constant and rapid ventricular rates were excluded by study design. These results contribute to the interpretation of prior studies that reported DDDR pacing with mode

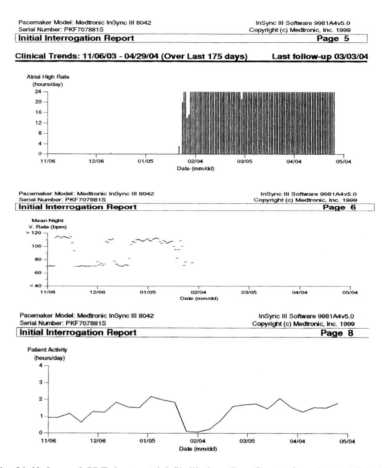

Fig. 21.40 Loss of CRT due to atrial fibrillation. *Top:* Onset of persistent AF in late January 2004. Note histogram showing 24 h/day of AF. *Middle:* Increase in mean ventricular rate at night corresponding with onset of AF. *Bottom:* Abrupt decline in patient activity hours/day corresponding with onset of persistent AF.

switching is preferred to VVIR pacing among patients who have undergone AV junction ablation for uncontrollable ventricular response during paroxysmal AF [102–105]. Such patients are rendered incapable of a rapid ventricular response during paroxysmal AF via mode switching; therefore, the symptomatic benefits are not surprising.

The importance of rate control and regularization of the ventricular response during AF to optimize CRT response should not be underestimated. For example, the relatively neutral effect of biventricular versus RVA pacing immediately after AV junction ablation among patients with systolic heart failure suggests that the benefits of rate control in AF are so large that it conceals the effect of asynchronous ventricular activation [6]. In patients with permanent AF and single-chamber CRT systems, continuous delivery of ventricular pacing and optimal CRT response may require ablation of the AV junction.

Specific features of pacing operation may increase the percentage of ventricular pacing during rapidly conducted AF and thereby prevent

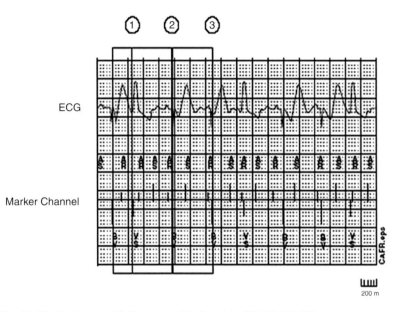

Fig. 21.41 Conducted AF Response (Medtronic). (**1**) BS-AR-VS sequence causes pacing rate to increase by 1 beat/min. (**2**) VS-BV sequence causes pacing rate to remain unchanged. (**3**) BV-BV sequence causes pacing rate to decrease by 1 beat/min.

disruptions to CRT. Conducted AF Response (Medtronic) increases the ventricular pacing rate in alignment with the native conducted ventricular response (Figs. 21.41–21.43). The intent is to regularize the ventricular rate by increasing the overall percentage of ventricular pacing while minimizing the increase in overall heart rate. This is achieved by adjusting the pacing escape interval after each ventricular event. The escape interval increases or decreases based on a contextual analysis of the preceding events. For example, a BV-AR-VS sequence will increment the pacing rate by 1 beat/min, whereas a BV-BV sequence will decrement the pacing rate by 1 beat/min. The result is a higher percentage of ventricular pacing at an average rate that closely matches the patient's own ventricular response. The maximum rate for Conducted AF Response pacing is programmable. The minimum rate derives from the otherwise-indicated (sensor rate, mode switch, or lower rate) pacing interval. When the otherwise-indicated pacing rate is faster than the programmed maximum rate, this feature is suspended and the device operates at the otherwise-indicated pacing rate. The use of Conducted AF Response necessitates interactions with other device operations. For example, in DDD and DDDR modes, Ventricular Rate Stabilization and Conducted AF Response cannot operate at the same time. When both are enabled, VRS operates only when the device is not mode switched. Conducted AF Response operates only in nontracking modes. Therefore, when DDD or DDDR mode is programmed, Conducted AF Response operates only during a mode switch. Conducted AF Response is suspended during automatic tachyarrhythmia therapies, arrhythmia inductions, manual therapies, and emergency fixed burst, cardioversion, and defibrillation.

Ventricular Rate Regulation (VRR; Guidant) is designed to reduce V-V cycle length variability during conducted atrial arrhythmias by moderating the

ON vs. OFF

12 hrs of CAFR ON

12 hrs of CAFR OFF

Each dot is a ventricular
beat:
Blue: intrinsic
Red: paced

Each line displays 2
hours of beats between
50–150 bpm

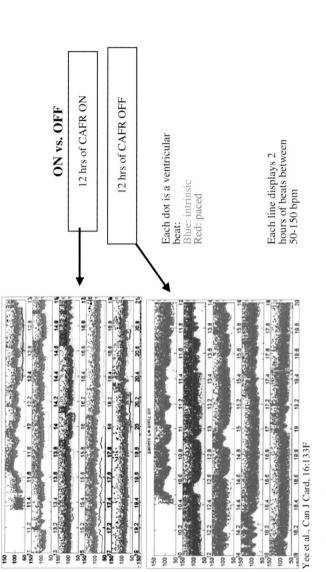

Yee et al., Can J Card, 16:133F

Fig. 21.42 Conducted AF Response (Medtronic). Plot of ventricular beats derived from Holter monitor of a patient with permanent AF. Top four lines show effect of CAFR therapy; bottom four lines show VVIR pacing (no CAFR therapy). Ventricular paced beats are shown in red; ventricular sensed beats in blue. Note the greater amount (and higher rate) of pacing (red dots) but also the apparent decrease in fast ventricular beats (blue dots) during CAFR operation. (From Yee et al. Can J Cardiol 16:133F.)

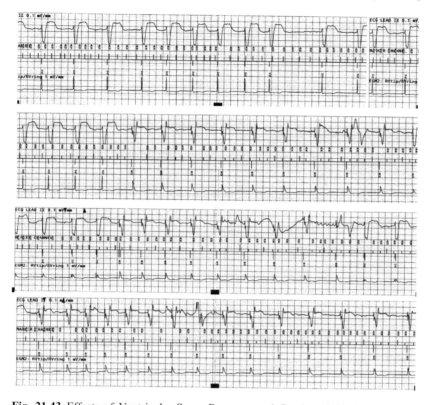

Fig. 21.43 Effects of Ventricular Sense Response and Conducted AF Response on ventricular pacing during AF with intact AV conduction. (**A**) Programmed mode is VVI 30 bpm. Note AF with intact AV conduction and absence of ventricular pacing. (**B**) Programmed mode is VVI 30 bpm with Ventricular Sense Response ON. Note delivery of biventricular pacing without any increase in ventricular rate. (**C**) Programmed mode is DDD 30 bpm with Conducted AF Response ON. Note increase in ventricular pacing rate immediately after mode switch (MS marker) occurs, which initiates Conducted AF Response operation. (**D**) Programmed mode is DDD 30 bpm with Ventricular Sense Response and Conducted AF Response ON. Note increase in ventricular pacing rate immediately after mode switch (MS marker) occurs, which initiates Conducted AF Response operation and also Ventricular Sense Response pacing during PVC (eighth complex from the left).

ventricular pacing rate based on a previous V-V average (Figs. 21.44–21.46). VRR provides ventricular regulation during conducted atrial arrhythmias, whereas Rate Smoothing (Guidant) is typically more useful for reducing pauses after PVCs. VRR operates in the DDD/R mode only during an AT/AF mode switch episode but is available all the time in the single-chamber VVI/R modes.

Unlike Rate Smoothing where changes are based on the most recent V-V interval, VRR uses a weighted ventricular average based on cycle lengths during the mode switch episode. This weighted average is made up of two parts: (1) the most recent V-V interval multiplied by 1.1 (if the most recent ventricular event was sensed) or 1.2 (if the event was paced). This calculation provides 6% of the next calculated VRR pacing rate value. (2) The calculated VRR interval value just prior to the most recent V event. This calculation provides 94% of the next calculated VRR pacing rate value. Therefore, the

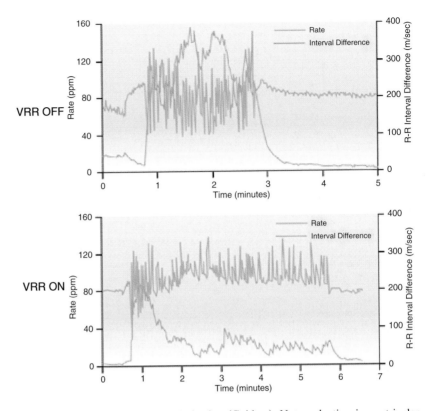

Fig. 21.44 Ventricular Rate Regularization (Guidant). Note reduction in ventricular interval variation but increase in pacing rate during VRR operation ON (*bottom*) versus VRR operation OFF (*top*).

next VRR pacing rate interval = 0.07 (recent V-V interval × 1.2 or 1.1) + 0.93 (previous VRR interval calculation). The calculated rates based on the weighted average yields a pacing rate that still adjusts on a cycle-by-cycle basis, but in much smaller increments than observed during Rate Smoothing. The frequency of VRR pacing is directly related to ventricular cycle length variability (i.e., pacing frequency increases with ventricular cycle length variability).

The use of VRR necessitates interactions with other device operations. The maximum VRR pacing rate is programmable between pacing rate and is limited between 60 and 150 beats/min. In dual-chamber modes, Rate Smoothing is temporarily disabled when VRR is active.

Frequent Ventricular Premature Beats

Frequent VPDs may disrupt CRT. Ventricular sense response (VSR; Medtronic) is intended to provide CRT when ventricular sensing occurs. Each right ventricular sensed event triggers a pace in one or both ventricles, as programmed.

When VSR is enabled in a nontracking or single-chamber pacing mode, a sensed ventricular event triggers an immediate ventricular pace. VSR pacing is delivered in one or both ventricles, according to the programmed ventricular pacing pathway. When VSR is enabled in an atrial tracking mode, a sensed ventricular event during the AV interval triggers an immediate pacing output

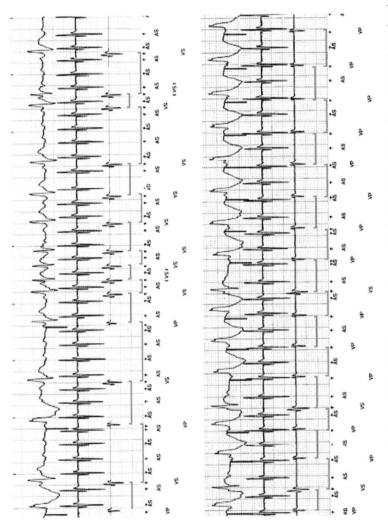

Fig. 21.45 Ventricular Rate Regularization (Guidant). *Top:* VRR OFF. Mean ventricular rate 167 ± 49 beats/min. Note wide ventricular interval variation (*horizontal bars*). *Bottom:* VRR ON. Mean ventricular rate 138 ± 37 beats/min. Note increase in ventricular pacing and reduction in ventricular interval variation (*horizontal bars*).

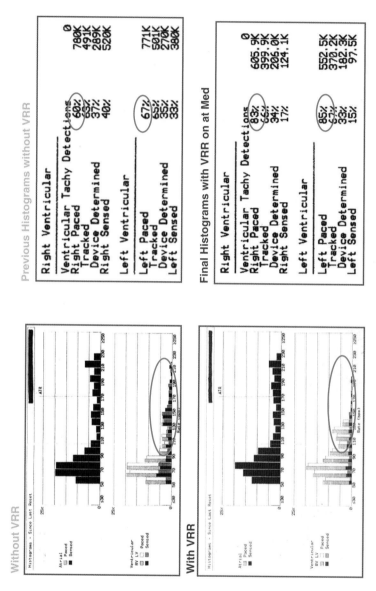

Fig. 21.46 Comparison of percent ventricular pacing histograms with VRR OFF (*top*) and VRR ON (*bottom*). VRR results in significantly higher frequency of ventricular pacing during AF with rapid ventricular conduction.

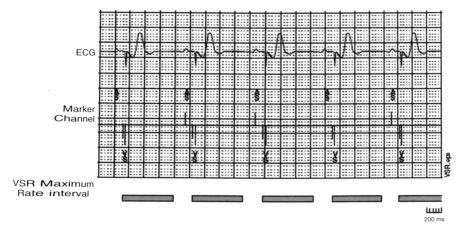

Fig. 21.47 Ventricular Sense Response (Medtronic).

to both ventricles (Fig. 21.47). The triggered output is rendered ineffectual in the chamber where sensing occurred due to ventricular refractoriness. Therefore, the triggered output "resynchronizes" ventricular activation by stimulating the chamber opposite the sensed event.

Some timing rules apply to prevent disruption of normal device operation. VSR pacing stimuli are delivered 1.25 ms after the ventricular sensed event only if the triggered pace does not violate the programmed VSR Maximum Rate. If the ventricular interval measured from the preceding ventricular event is shorter than the VSR Maximum Rate interval, no VSR pacing pulse is delivered. Ventricular sensing for VSR operation occurs via only the RV lead. Operating features of such algorithms designed to maximize cardiac resynchronization therapy such as VSR may result in pacing that occurs after QRS onset on surface ECG (Fig. 21.48).

VRS operation necessitates interactions with other device operations. When both VSR and Ventricular Safety Pacing (VSP) are enabled, VSP operation takes precedence during the VSP interval. If a ventricular event is sensed during the VSP interval, the device performs a safety pace at the end of the VSP interval. After the VSP interval expires, Ventricular Sense Response remains active for the remainder of the Paced AV interval. VSR pacing pulses are not considered in interval calculations for arrhythmia detection or pacing. VSR pacing pulses are not considered in the counts of consecutive sensed and paced events that define the beginning and end of ventricular sensing episodes storage. VSR operation is suspended during automatic tachyarrhythmia therapies, EP Study inductions, manual therapies, and emergency fixed burst, cardioversion, and defibrillation.

Loss of CRT Due to Differential LV Capture Threshold Rise

The principal limitation of the transvenous approach is that the selection of sites for pacing is entirely dictated by navigable coronary venous anatomy. A commonly encountered problem is that an apparently suitable target vein delivers the lead to a site where ventricular capture can be achieved at only very high output voltages or not at all. This presumably relates to the presence of scar on the epicardial surface of the heart underlying the target vein or

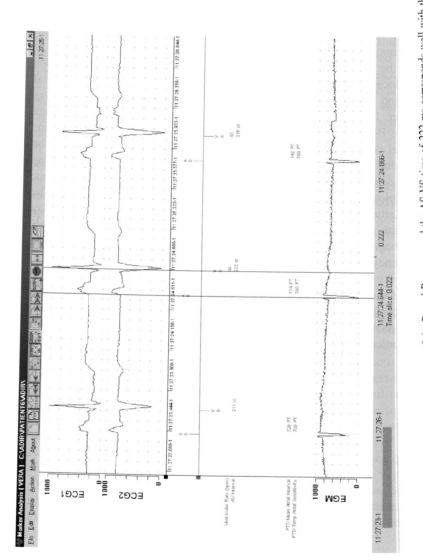

Fig. 21.66 AV intervals during atrial sensing. AS and VS occur at the start of the P- and R-waves, and the AS-VS time of 222 ms corresponds well with the surface ECG P-Q time measured by the cursors.

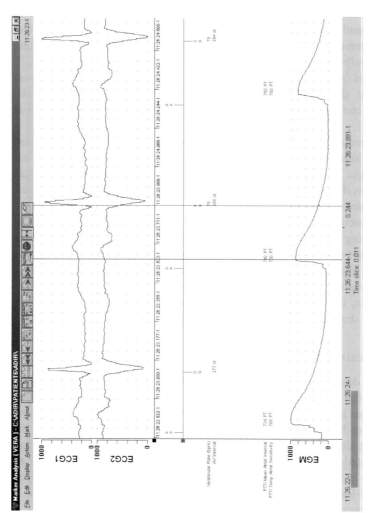

Fig. 21.67 Effect of atrial capture latency on AV interval during atrial pacing. AP occurs sooner than the P-wave is seen on the surface ECG. The AP–VS time is measured at 288 ms, but the time from the start of the P-wave–VS time is nearer to 244 ms. Thus, the AP–VS time is overreported by the device, versus the surface ECG.

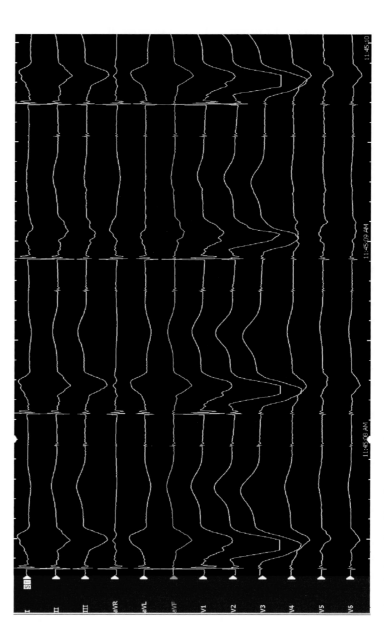

Fig. 21.74 Simultaneous biventricular pacing. Note the pattern of RV apical stimulation; there is no evidence of left ventricular capture based on the paced QRS morphology.

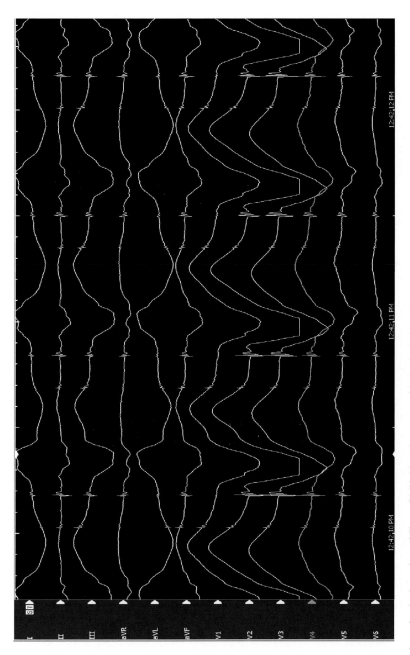

Fig. 21.75 RV only pacing in the patient of Figure 21.74. Note the pattern of RV apical stimulation.

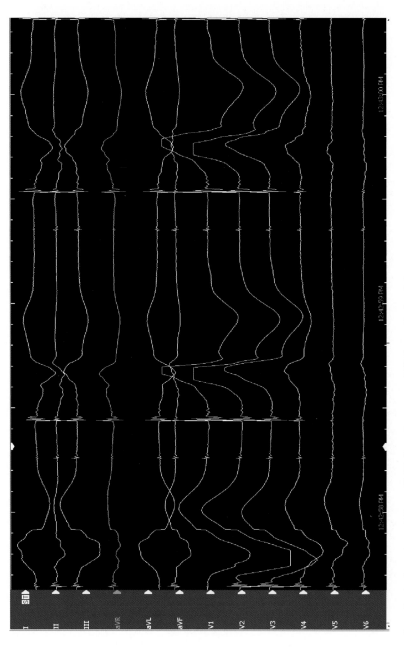

Fig. 21.76 LV only pacing in the patient of Figure 21.74. Note the pattern of LV free wall stimulation.

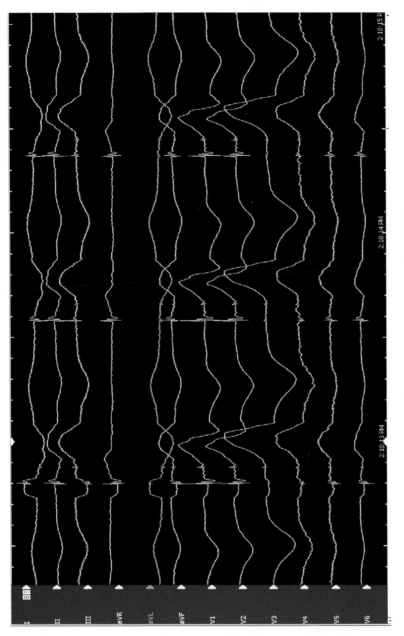

Fig. 21.77 Sequential ventricular stimulation with 80-ms offset (LV > RV). Note restoration of biventricular activation.

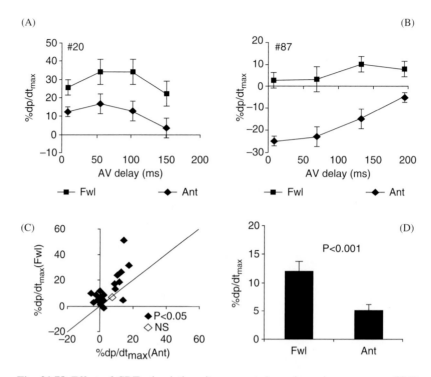

Fig. 21.78 Effect of CRT stimulation site on acute hemodynamic response to CRT. LV stimulation at free wall (FWL) sites yielded significantly larger LV +dP/dt and pulse pressure than anterior (ANT) sites. In one third of patients, stimulation at ANT sites worsened hemodynamic function, whereas FWL stimulation improved it. The opposite pattern was never observed. See text for details. (From Butter C, Auricchio A, Stellbrink C, et al., for the Pacing Therapy for Chronic Heart Failure II Study Group. Effect of resynchronization therapy stimulation site on the systolic function of heart failure patients. Circulation 2001;104(25):3026–3029.)

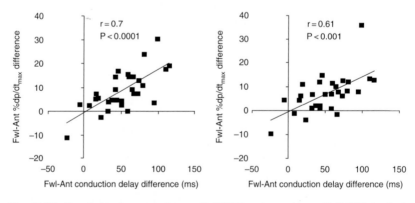

Fig. 21.79 Correlation between free wall (FWL) and anterior wall (ANT) intrinsic conduction delay differences and the LV +dP/dt$_{max}$ response differences during FWL and ANT stimulation for LV CRT (**A**) and BV CRT (**B**). Positive conduction delay differences correspond with more delayed FWL activation. Positive LV +dP/dt$_{max}$ differences correspond with a larger FWL stimulation response (percentage change from baseline). (From Butter C, Auricchio A, Stellbrink C, et al., for the Pacing Therapy for Chronic Heart Failure II Study Group. Effect of resynchronization therapy stimulation site on the systolic function of heart failure patients. Circulation 2001;104(25):3026–3029.)

systems, a suitable pacing site on the LV free wall cannot be achieved in 5–10% of patients. Even when the coronary venous anatomy is suitable and navigable, some free wall sites are rejected due to unacceptably high pacing thresholds related to epicardial scar or unavoidable phrenic nerve stimulation. Surgical placement of epicardial LV pacing leads or endocardial LV stimulation [174] are options when the coronary venous approach fails.

Approach to Avoiding or Correcting a Suboptimal LV Lead Position
Ideally, a suboptimal LV lead position should be identified and rejected at the time of implantation. The most common mistake of the uninformed or uncommitted implanter is to place the LV lead in the anterior vein and "see how the patient does." An example of the consequences of this thinking is shown in Figures 21.80 to 21.82. If a patient is not responding to CRT and the LV lead is in the anterior vein, an attempt to reposition the LV lead (or a different lead) in a lateral vein should be made. If this is not possible because of limitations in coronary venous anatomy or other insuperable technical obstacles (see below), the patient should be referred for surgical placement of the LV lead in an optimal location.

Experienced implanters using currently available tools and techniques can achieve optimal LV stimulation using a postero-basal or lateral coronary vein in >90% of cases. The techniques for transvenous delivery of CRT have been previously described [175]. However, some technical aspects merit special mention in order to increase the probability of achieving an optimal LV stimulation site.

Retrograde venography is essential to delineate optimal target veins for LV stimulation. Care must be taken to achieve a good seal within the main body of the coronary sinus in order to obtain maximal opacification of the distal vasculature. Underfilling the coronary venous system is a common mistake

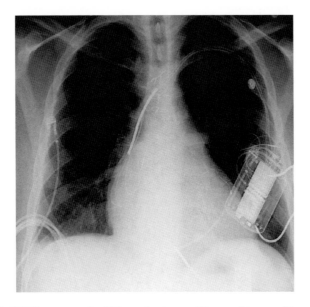

Fig. 21.80 CRT "nonresponder." The patient was a 35-year-old man with nonischemic dilated cardiomyopathy and LBBB in whom a CRTD was implanted February 5, 2002. Note position of LV lead in anterior interventricular vein.

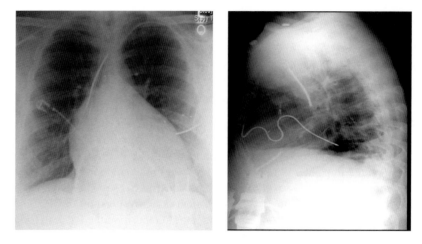

Fig. 21.81 Same patient as in Figure 21.80. The patient deteriorated subsequent to CRT and was rehospitalized on February 10, 2003, in cardiogenic shock, at which time a LVAD was implanted.

that may result in failure to identify potentially suitable targets for LV pacing lead placement. Occasionally, the inflated balloon will occlude the ostium of a suitable branch vessel for LV lead placement, therefore occlusive venography at multiple levels within the main CS are advisable.

Factors Limiting Optimal LV Lead Placement

Complex and unpredictable anatomic and technical considerations may preclude successful delivery of the LV lead to an optimal pacing site.

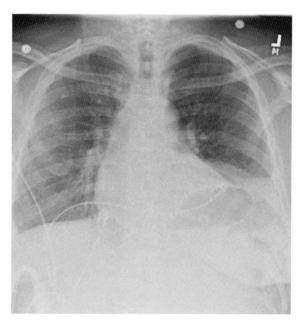

Fig. 21.82 Same patient as in Figures 21.80 and 21.81. Orthotopic heart transplant was performed on July 11, 2004.

Inability to Cannulate the Coronary Sinus

It is difficult to estimate the true percentage of cases in which the coronary sinus cannot be cannulated because this is clearly influenced by operator experience. It is probably in the range 1–5%. When the coronary sinus cannot be located by the superior approach, an adaptation of the inferior approach described for complex electrophysiology procedures is often successful in localizing the CS ostium.

Coronary Venous Anatomy: Absent or Inaccessible Target Veins

The coronary venous circulation demonstrates considerably more variability than the parallel arterial circulation. Careful studies of retrograde coronary venography have revealed that the anterior interventricular vein is present in 99% of patients and the middle cardiac vein is present in 100%. These veins are generally undesirable for LV preexcitation because they do not reach the late-activated portion of the LV free wall. Unfortunately, approximately 50% of patients have only a single vein serving the LV free wall. Anatomically, this is a lateral marginal vein in slightly more than 75% and a true posterior vein that ascends the free wall in approximately 50% of patients [176]. Thus, as many as 20% of patients may not have a vein that reaches the optimal LV free wall site for delivery of CRT. In some instances, target veins are present but too small for cannulation with existing lead systems or paradoxically too large to achieve mechanical fixation with reduced-diameter LV leads that rely primarily on "wedging" the lead tip into a distal site within the target vein for fixation such that the outer diameter of the lead closely approximates the inner luminal diameter of the vein.

Newer lead designs incorporate various self-retaining bends or cants that compress the distal segment of the lead against the outer wall of the vein and the epicardial surface of the heart. This permits fixation in larger-diameter veins and may be particularly useful for overcoming phrenic nerve stimulation or high pacing thresholds that would otherwise render optimal target veins unsuitable for use (see below).

Coronary Venous Tortuosity and Stenoses

Another commonly encountered difficulty in transvenous LV lead placement is tortuosity of the target vessel take-off or main segment. These anatomic constraints can be extremely difficult to overcome and often require the use of multiple LV lead designs and delivery systems. Larger-diameter stylet-driven leads are likely to fail in this situation unless they can be delivered with an inner guiding sheath that selectively cannulates and straightens the proximal segment of the tortuous target vein. Another approach utilizes coronary, renal, or other angiography catheters to selectively cannulate the small and tortuous target vein. A guide wire can then be placed deep into the target vein permitting delivery of an over-the-wire LV lead. In many instances, the guide wire itself will straighten the tortuous segment of the target vein permitting navigation of the LV lead. If significant resistance to lead advancement persists despite a guide wire, a second guide wire placed alongside the first ("buddy wire technique") may sufficiently straighten the vein to permit lead advancement.

Biventricular or LV Only Stimulation: Role in CRT Nonresponders?

It is important to note that uncertainty about the requirement of RV stimulation during CRT, uneasiness about long-term LV lead performance, and unavailability of pacing systems with separately programmable ventricular outputs influenced the use of biventricular pacing, as opposed to left univentricular pacing, in large RCTs. A particular concern is LV lead dislodgment that has a reported incidence of 5–10% in larger studies [48, 53, 108] and would impose risk for potentially lethal bradycardia. However, there is some scientific evidence that RV stimulation might not be necessary for optimal CRT response or even that LV pacing alone might be superior to biventricular pacing in some patients.

Left univentricular pacing alone has acute hemodynamic effects that are similar or superior to those achieved with biventricular pacing in some patients [27, 159, 177–179]. Blanc and co-workers recently extended these observations [180]. Functional capacity (6-min walk and maximal O_2 uptake), ventricular size and function, and blood norepinephrine levels prior to and after 12 months of left univentricular pacing were evaluated in 22 patients with dilated cardiomyopathy, LBBB NYHA class III or IV heart failure. The LV lead was placed in a lateral coronary vein when possible, and all patients had sinus rhythm to allow atrial synchronous left univentricular pacing with an AV delay initially programmed to 100 ms. Significant improvements in functional capacity, echocardiographic mitral regurgitation, and LV end diastolic diameter were observed with favorable trend toward improvement in EF. Thus, these results are encouraging and support persistent benefit (at least to 1 year) of left univentricular pacing in some patients.

Both LV and biventricular pacing synchronize LV contraction. This "retiming" effect was initially attributed to "preexcitation" of the delayed LV segments. However, insights from tissue Doppler studies have revealed that LV pacing from a late-activated site achieves synchronous contraction by simultaneously delaying all LV segments [56, 161]. This is a potentially critical observation because LV pacing reverses electrical activation and abolishes intraventricular dyssynchrony but with the result of a marked increase in LV activation time compared with biventricular pacing [6]. The consequences are a greater delay in RV contraction [159] and a shortened diastolic filling time that may have implications for ventricular pumping function, particularly at higher heart rates [161, 181].

Thus, it is theoretically possible that LV only pacing may achieve superior hemodynamic performance compared with biventricular pacing in some patients. For this reason, LV only pacing should probably be considered in the management of CRT nonresponders initially treated with biventricular pacing. This could be easily achieved noninvasively in the situation where a true bipolar LV lead is used with a pulse generator capable of separately programmable ventricular outputs. A similar effect could be achieved in the case of a unipolar LV lead (dual cathodal configuration) by programming RV output below the capture threshold. This could not be achieved in a dual cathodal configuration without separately programmable ventricular outputs unless the LV threshold was significantly lower than the RV threshold. In any event, it is not currently possible to identify patients who will respond better to LV alone compared with biventricular pacing.

Absence of Ventricular Mechanical Dyssynchrony

Finally, the lack of response to CRT may be due to the absence of intraventricular dyssynchrony despite patient selection according to existing guidelines (see above). The most critical realization is that the electrical and mechanical synchrony achieved with the "infinite electrode" of the specialized conduction system cannot be duplicated with any pacing technique (except His bundle pacing). Alternate site or biventricular pacing in hearts *without abnormal ventricular conduction* still results in abnormal activation patterns, albeit less than during RVA pacing [149]. In this situation, LV or biventricular pacing will cause a dyssynchronous ventricular contraction that may worsen pumping function. Therefore, if no other correctable causes of CRT nonresponse are identified, an echocardiographic evaluation for intraventricular dyssynchrony should be performed during inhibition of ventricular pacing. If the underlying native ventricular contraction is synchronous, ventricular pacing in any form should be eliminated. If bradycardia support is necessary, this should be provided in an atrial-based mode.

References

1. Auricchio A, Abraham WT. Cardiac resynchronization therapy: Current state of the art. Cost versus benefit. Circulation 2004;109:300–307.
2. Leclercq C, Kass DA. Retiming the failing heart: Principles and current clinical status of cardiac resynchronization. J Am Coll Cardiol 2002;39:194–201.
3. Wiggers C. The muscular reactions of the mammalian ventricles to artificial surface stimuli. Am J Physiol 1925;73:346–378.
4. Baldasseroni S, De Biase L, Fresco C, et al., Italian Network on Congestive Heart Failure. Cumulative effect of complete left bundle-branch block and chronic atrial fibrillation on 1-year mortality and hospitalization in patients with congestive heart failure. A report of the Italian network on congestive heart failure (In-CHF database). Eur Heart J 2002;23(2):1692–1698.
5. Grines CL, Boshore TW, Boudoulas H, Olson S, Shafer P, Wooley CF. Functional abnormalities in isolated left bundle branch block: The effect of interventricular asynchrony. Circulation. 1989;79:845–853.
6. Leclercq C, Faris O, Runin R, et al. Systolic improvement and mechanical resynchronization does not require electrical synchrony in the dilated failing heart with left bundle-branch block. Circulation 2002;106:1760–1763.
7. Verbeek XA, Vernooy K, Peschar M. Intra-ventricular resynchronization for optimal left ventricular function during pacing in experimental left bundle branch block. J Am Coll Cardiol 2003;42:558–567.
8. Baller D, Wolpers H-G, Zipfers J, Bretschneider H-J. Comparison of the effects of right atrial, right ventricular apex, and atrioventricular sequential pacing on myocardial oxygen consumption and cardiac efficiency: A laboratory investigation. Pacing Clin Electrophysiol 1988;11:394–403.
9. Prinzen FW, Peschar M. Relation between the pacing induced sequence of activation and left ventricular pump function in animals. Pacing Clin Electrophysiol 2002;25(4 Pt 1):484–498.
10. Park C, Little W. Effect of alteration of left ventricular activation sequence on the left ventricular end-systolic pressure-volume relationship in closed-chest dogs. Circ Res 1985;57:706–717.
11. Van Oosterhout MFM, Prinzen FW, Arts T, et al. Asynchronous electrical activation induces asymmetrical hypertrophy of the left ventricular wall. Circulation 1998;98:588–595.
12. Prinzen FW, Hunter WC, Wyman BT, et al. Mapping of regional myocardial strain and work during ventricular pacing: Experimental study using magnetic resonance imaging tagging. J Am Coll Cardiol 1999;33:1735–1742.

48. Bristow MR, Saxon LA, Boehmer J, et al., the Comparison of Medical Therapy P, and Defibrillation in Heart Failure (COMPANION) Investigators. Cardiac-resynchronization therapy with or without an implantable defibrillator in advanced chronic heart failure. N Engl J Med 2004;350(21):2140–2150.

49. Butter C, Stellbrink C, Belalcazar A, et al. Cardiac resynchronization therapy optimization by finger plethysmography. Heart Rhythm 2005;1:568–578.

50. Nishimura RA, Hayes DL, Holmes DR, Tajik AJ. Mechanism of hemodynamic improvement by dual-chamber pacing for severe left ventricular dysfunction: An acute Doppler and catheterization study. J Am Coll Cardiol 1995;25:281–288.

51. Auricchio A, Sommariva L, Salo RW, et al. Improvement of cardiac function in patients with severe congestive heart failure and coronary artery disease by dual chamber pacing with shortened AV delay. Pacing Clin Electrophysiol 1994;17:995–997.

52. Linde-Edelstam C, Nordlander R, Unden A-L, Orth-Gomer K, Ryden L. Quality-of-life in patients treated with atrioventricular synchronous pacing compared to rate modulated ventricular pacing: A long-term, double-blind, crossover study. Pacing Clin Electrophysiol 1992;15:1467–1476.

53. Abraham WT, Fisher WG, Smith AL, et al., for the MIRACLE Study Group. Cardiac resynchronization in chronic heart failure. N Eng J Med 2002;346(24):1845–1853.

54. Cazeau S, Leclercq C, Lavergne T, et al., The Multisite Stimulation in Cardiomyopathies (MUSTIC) Study Investigators. Effects of multisite biventricular pacing in patients with heart failure and intraventricular conduction delay. N Engl J Med 2001;344(12):873–880.

55. Sawhney NS, Waggoner AD, Garhwal S, Chawla MK, Osborn J, Faddis MN. Randomized prospective trial of atrioventricular delay programming for cardiac resynchronization therapy. Heart Rhythm 2004;1:562–567.

56. Yu CM, Chau E, Sanderson EJ, et al. Tissue Doppler echocardiographic evidence of reverse remodeling and improved synchronicity by simultaneous delaying regional contraction after biventricular pacing therapy in heart failure. Circulation 2002;105:438–445.

57. Bordachar P, Lafitte S, Reuter S, et al. Echocardiographic parameters of ventricular dyssynchrony validation in patients withheart failure using sequential biventricular pacing. J Am Coll Cardiol 2004;44:2157–2165.

58. Gregoratos G, Abrams J, Epstein AE, et al. ACC/AHA/NASPE 2002 Guideline Update for Implantation of Cardiac Pacemakers and Antiarrhythmia Devices: Summary Article: A Report of the American College of Cardiology/American Heart Association Task Force on Practice Guidelines (ACC/AHA/NASPE Committee to Update the 1998 Pacemaker Guideines). Circulation 2002;106:2145–2161.

59. Bardy GH, Lee KL, Mark DB, et al., for the Sudden Cardiac Death in Heart Failure Trial (SCD-HeFT) Investigators. Amiodarone or an implantable cardioverter-defibrillator for congestive heart failure. N Engl J Med 2005;352(3):225–237.

60. Fisher JD, Mehra R, Furman S. Termination of ventricular tachycardia with bursts of rapid ventricular pacing. Am J Cardiol 1978;41(1):94–102.

61. Sweeney MO. Antitachycardia pacing for ventricular tachycardia using ICDs: Substrates, methods and clinical experience. Pacing Clin Electrophysiol 2004;27(9):1292–1305.

62. Roberts WC, Siegel RJ. Idiopathic dilated cardiomyopathy: Analysis of 152 necropsy patients. Am J Cardiol 1987;60:1304–1315.

63. Lo YS, Billingham M, Rowan RA, Lee HC, Liem LB, Swerdlow CD. Histopathologic and electrophysiologic correlations in idiopathic dilated cardiomyopathy and sustained ventricular tachyarrhythmia. Am J Cardiol 1989;64:1063–1066.

64. de Bakker JM, van Capelle FJ, Janse MJ, et al. Fractionated electrograms in dilated cardiomyopathy: Origin and relation to abnormal conduction. J Am Coll Cardiol 1996;27:1071–1078.

65. Wu TJ, Ong JJC, Hwang C, et al. Characteristics of wavefronts during ventricular fibrillation in human hearts with dilated cardiomyopathy: Role of increased fibrosis in the generation of reentry. J Am Coll Cardiol 1998;32:187–196.

66. Cassidy DM, Vassallo JA, Miller JM, et al. Endocardial catheter mapping in humans in sinus rhythm: Relationship to underlying heart disease and ventricular arrhythmias. Circulation 1986;73:645–652.

67. Pogwizd SM, McKenzie JP, Cain ME. Mechanisms underlying spontaneous and induced ventricular arrhythmias in patients with idiopathic dilated cardiomyopathy. Circulation 1998;98:2404–2414.

68. Vermeulen JT, Tan HL, Rademaker H, et al. Electrophysiologic and extracellular ionic changes during acute ischemia in the failing and normal rabbit myocardium. J Mol Cell Cardiol 1996;28:123–131.

69. Sears SF, Todaro JF, Urizar G, Lewis TS, Sirois B, Wallace R. Assessing the psychosocial impact of the ICD: A national survey of implantable cardioverter defibrillator health care providers. Pacing Clin Electrophysiol 2000;23:939–945.

70. Sears SF, Conti JB. Understanding implantable cardioverter defibrillator shocks and storms: Medical and psychosocial considerations for research and clinical care. Clin Cardiol 2003;26:107–111.

71. Schron EB, Exner DV, Yao Q, Jenkins LS, Steinberg JS, Cook JR, for the AVID Investigators. Quality of Life in the Antiarrhythmics versus Implantable Defibrillators Trial. Impact of therapy and influence of adverse symptoms and defibrillator shocks. Circulation 2002;105:589–594.

72. Namerow PB, Firth BR, Heywood GM, Windle JR, Parides MK, for the CABG Patch Trial Investigators and Coordinators. Quality of Life six months after CABG surgery in patients randomized to ICD versus no ICD therapy: Findings from the CABG Patch Trial. Pacing Clin Electrophysiol 1999;22:1305–1313.

73. Irvine J, Dorian P, Baker B, et al., for the CIDS Investigators. Quality of life in the Canadian Implantable Defibrillator Study (CIDS). Am Heart J 2002;144:282–289.

74. Wathen MS, DeGroot PJ, Sweeney MO, et al., for the PainFREE Rx II Investigators. Prospective randomized multicenter trial of empirical antitachycardia pacing versus shocks for spontaneous rapid ventricular tachycardia in patients with implantable cardioverter defibrillators. PainFREE Rx II Trial Results. Circulation 2004;110:2592–2596.

75. Wilkoff B, Hess M, Young JD, Abraham WT. Differences in tachyarrhythmia detection and implantable cardioverter defibrillator therapy by primary or secondary prevention indication in cardiac resynchronization therapy patients. J Cardiovasc Electrophysiol 2004;15:1002–1009.

76. Russo AM, Nayak H, Verdino R, et al. Implantable cardioverter defibrillator events in patients with asymptomatic nonsustained ventricular tachycardia: Is device implantation justified? Pacing Clin Electrophysiol 2003;26(12):2289–2295.

77. Sweeney MO, Wathen MS, Volosin K, et al. Appropriate and inappropriate ventricular therapies, quality of life and mortality among primary and secondary prevention ICD patients: Results from PainFREE Rx II. Circulation 2005;111:2898–2905.

78. Bansch D, Castrucci M, Bocker D, Breithardt G, Block M. Ventricular tachycardias above the initially programmed tachycardia detection interval in patients with implantable cardioverter-defibrillators: Incidence, prediction and significance. J Am Coll Cardiol 2000;36(2):557–565.

113. Taieb J, Benchaa T, Foltzer E, et al. Atrioventricular cross-talk in biventricular pacing: A potential cause of ventricular standstill. Pacing Clin Electrophysiol 2002;25(6):929–935.

114. Oguz E, Akyol A, Okmen E. Inhibition of biventricular pacing by far-field left atrial activity sensing: Case report. Pacing Clin Electrophysiol 2002;25(10): 1517–1519.

115. Vollmann D, Luthje L, Gortler G, Unterberg C. Inhibition of bradycardia pacing and detection of ventricular fibrillation due to far-field atrial sensing in a triple chamber implantable cardioverter defibrillator. Pacing Clin Electrophysiol 2002;25(10):1513–1516.

116. Garrigue S, Barold SS, Clementy J. Double jeopardy in an implantable cardioverter defibrillator patient. J Cardiovasc Electrophysiol 2003;14:784.

117. Sweeney MO, Ellison KE, Shea JB. Provoked and spontaneous high frequency, low amplitude respirophasic noise transients in patients with implantable cardioverter-defibrillators. J Cardiovasc Electrophysiol 2001;12:402–410.

118. Zagrodzky JD, Ramaswamy K, Page RL, et al. Biventricular pacing decreases the inducibility of ventricular tachycardia in patients with ischemic cardiomyopathy. Am J Cardiol 2001;87:1208–1210.

119. Walker S, Levy T, Rex S, et al. Usefulness of suppression of ventricular arrhythmia by biventricular pacing in severe congestive cardiac failure. Am J Cardiol 2000;86:231–233.

120. Higgins SL, Yong P, Scheck D, et al. Biventricular pacing diminishes the need for implantable cardioverter defibrillator therapy. J Am Coll Cardiol 2000;36: 824–827.

121. Guerra J, Wu J, Miller JM, Groh WJ. Increase in ventricular tachycardia frequency after biventricular implantable cardioverter defibrillator upgrade. J Cardiovasc Electrophysiol 2003;14:1245–1124.

122. Medina-Ravell VA, Lankipalli RS, Yan GX, et al. Effect of epicardial or biventricular pacing to prolong QT interval and increase transmural dispersion of repolarization. Circulation 2003;107:740–746.

123. Fish JM, Di Diego JM, Nesterenko V, Antzelevitch C. Epicardial activation of left ventricular wall prolongs QT interval and transmural dispersion of repolarization: Implications for biventricular pacing. Circulation 2004;109:2136–2142.

124. Barold SS, Byrd CL. Cross-ventricular endless loop tachycardia during biventricular pacing. Pacing Clin Electrophysiol 2001;24(12):1821–1823.

125. Berruezo A, Mont L, Scalise A, Brugada J. Orthodromic pacemaker-mediated tachycardia in a biventricular system without an atrial electrode. J Cardiovasc Electrophysiol 2004;15:1100–1102.

126. Auricchio A, Stellbrink C, Sack S, et al. Long-term benefit as a result of pacing resynchronization in congestive heart failure: Results of the PATH-CHF Trial. Circulation 2000;102:II–693A.

127. Stellbrink C, Breithardt OA, Franke A, et al, PATH-CHF (PAcing THerapies in Congestive Heart Failure) Investigators, CPI Guidant Congestive Heart Failure Research Group. Impact of cardiac resynchronization therapy using hemodynamically optimized pacing on left ventricular remodeling in patients with congestive heart failure and ventricular conduction disturbances. J Am Coll Cardiol 2001;38(7):1957–1965.

128. Gorscan J, Kanzaki H, Bazaz R, Dohi K, Schwartzman D. Usefulness of echocardiographic tissue synchronization imaging to predict acute response to cardiac resynchronization therapy. Am J Cardiol 2004;93:1178–1181.

129. Abraham WT. Rationale and design of a randomized clinical trial to assess the safety and efficacy of cardiac resynchronization therapy in patients with advanced heart failure: The Multicenter InSync Randomized Clinical Evaluation (MIRACLE). J Card Fail 2000;6:369–380.

130. Packer M. Proposal for a new clinical end point to evaluate the efficacy of drugs and devices in the treatment of chronic heart failure. J Card Fail 2001;7:176–182.
131. Bax JJ, Mohoek SG, Marwick TJ, et al. Left ventricular dyssynchrony predicts benefit of cardiac resynchronization therapy in patients with end-stage heart failure before pacemaker implantation. Am J Cardiol 2003;92:1238–1240.
132. Reuter S, Garrigue S, Barold SS, et al. Comparison of characteristics in responders versus nonresponders with biventricular pacing for drug-resistant congestive heart failure. Am J Cardiol 2002;89(3):346–350.
133. Yu C-M, Fung W-H, Lin H, et al. Predictors of left ventricular reverse remodeling after cardiac resynchronization therapy for heart failure secondary to idiopathic dilated or ischemic cardiomyopathy. Am J Cardiol 2003;91(6):684–688.
134. Yu CM, Fung JWH, Chan CK, et al. Comparison of efficacy of reverse remodeling and clinical improvement for relatively narrow and wide QRS complexes after cardiac resynchronization therapy for heart failure. J Cardiovasc Electrophysiol 2004;15:1058–1065.
135. Yu CM, Lin H, Zhang Q, Sanderson JE. High prevalence of left ventricular systolic and diastolic asynchrony in patients with congestive heart failure and normal QRS duration. Heart 2003;89:54–60.
136. Pitzalis MD, Iacoviello M, Romito R, et al. Cardiac resynchronization therapy tailored by echocardiographic evaluation of ventricular asynchrony. J Am Coll Cardiol 2002;40:1615–1622.
137. Auricchio A, Kloss M, Trautmann SI, et al. Exercise performance following cardiac resynchronization therapy in patients with heart failure and ventricular conduction delay. Am J Cardiol 2002;89(2):198–203.
138. Linde C, Leclerc C, Rex S, et al. Long-term benefits of biventricular pacing in congestive heart failure: Results from the Multisite Stimulation in Cardiomyopathy (MUSTIC) Study. J Am Coll Cardiol 2002;40:111–118.
139. Linde C, Braunschweig F, Gadler F, Bailleul C, Daubert JC. Long-term improvement in quality of life by biventricular pacing in patients with chronic heart failure: Results from the MUSTIC Study. Am J Cardiol 2003;91:1090–1095.
140. Reynolds MR, Joventino LP, Josephson ME, Miracle ICD Investigators. Relationship of baseline electrocardiographic characteristics with the response to cardiac resynchronization therapy for heart failure. Pacing Clin Electrophysiol 2004;27(11):1513–1518.
141. Kadhiresan V, Vogt J, Auricchio A, et al. Sensitivity and specificity of QRS duration to predict acute benefit in heart failure patients with cardiac resynchronization. Pacing Clin Electrophysiol 2000;23(II):555 [abstract].
142. Moss AJ, Zareba W, Hall WJ, et al., for the Multicenter Automatic Defibrillator Implantation Trial II Investigators. Prophylactic implantation of a defibrillator in patients with myocardial infarction and reduced ejection fraction. N Engl J Med 2002;346(12):877–883.
143. Garrigue S, Reuter S, Labeque J-N, et al. Usefulness of biventricular pacing in patients with congestive heart failure and right bundle branch. Am J Cardiol 2001;88(12):1436–1441.
144. Aranda JM, Curtis AB, Conti JB, Stejskal-Peterson S. Do heart failure patients with right bundle branch block benefit from cardiac resynchronization therapy? Analysis of the MIRACLE Study. J Am Coll Cardiol 2002;39:96A [abstract].
145. Egoavil CA, Ho RT, Greenspon AJ, Pavri BB. Cardiac resynchronization therapy in patients with right bundle branch block: Analysis of pooled data from MIRACLE and ContakCD trials. Heart Rhythm 2005;2:611–615.
146. Bleeker GB, Schalij MJ, Molhoek SG, et al. Relationship between QRS duration and left ventricular dyssynchrony in patients with end-stage heart failure. J Cardiovasc Electrophysiol 2004;15(5):544–549.

Table 22.1 Causes of a dominant R-wave in lead V_1 during conventional right ventricular apical pacing.

- Ventricular fusion
- Pacing in the myocardial relative refractory period
- Left ventricular pacing from the coronary venous system
- Left ventricular endocardial or epicardial pacing
- Lead perforation of the right ventricle or ventricular septum with left ventricular stimulation
- Uncomplicated right ventricular pacing (lead V_1 recorded too high or in the correct place)

a pacemaker lead is most probably not in the right ventricle after excluding ventricular fusion from spontaneous AV conduction. However, LV pacing (endocardial or from the coronary venous system) that generates a positive complex in lead V_1 may not necessarily be accompanied by a positive QRS complex in leads V_2 and V_3.

RV outflow tract pacing does not cause a dominant R-wave in lead V_1 despite the following statement, which appeared in a recent book on resynchronization [3]: "Right ventricular leads placed in the right ventricular outflow tract, particularly in more leftward locations, produce a right bundle branch pattern because the right ventricular outflow tract is located on the left side of the body … ." Also: "… the relatively leftward location of a pacing site in the right ventricular outflow tract produces a positive deflection or right bundle branch block." RV outflow or septal pacing invariably generates a left bundle branch block (LBBB) pattern in the precordial leads. We have never seen a so-called RBBB pattern (defined as a dominant R-wave) in lead V_1 during RV outflow tract or septal pacing and it has never been reported so far. In this context, it is important to remember that right axis deviation of the ventricular paced beats in the frontal plane with a deep S-wave in leads I and aVL does not constitute a RBBB pattern without the presence of a dominant R-wave in lead V_1 [3].

Significance of a Small r-wave in Lead V_1 During Uncomplicated RV Pacing

A small early (r) wave (sometimes wide) may occasionally occur in lead V_1 during uncomplicated RV apical or outflow tract pacing. There is no evidence that this r-wave represents a conduction abnormality at the RV exit site. Furthermore, an initial r-wave during biventricular pacing does not predict initial LV activation [3].

Left Ventricular Endocardial Pacing

Passage of a pacing lead into the LV rather than the RV occurs usually via an atrial septal defect (patent foramen ovale) or less commonly via the subclavian artery [12–27]. The diagnosis of a malpositioned endocardial LV lead will be missed in a single-lead ECG. The problem may be compounded if the radiographic malposition of the lead is not obvious or insufficient projections are taken. A 12-lead paced ECG will show a RBBB pattern of

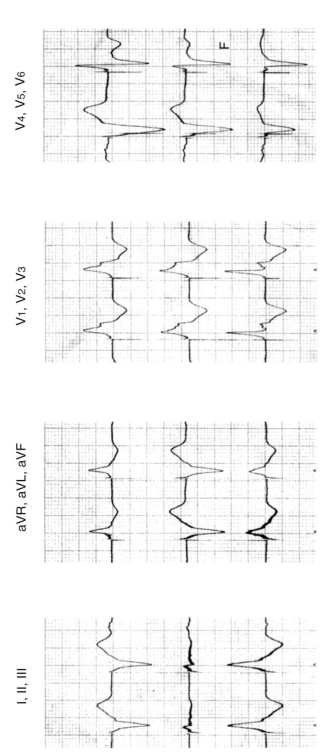

I, II, III   aVR, aVL, aVF   V1, V2, V3   V4, V5, V6

F

Fig. 22.1 Left ventricular endocardial pacing. ECG of a patient who received a dual-chamber pacemaker for sick sinus syndrome. Three years after pacemaker implantation, he presented with several transient ischemic attacks (TIAs). An ECG taken when the pacemaker was programmed to the VVI mode showed ventricular paced beats with a dominant R-wave in leads V_1–V_3 and right axis deviation in the frontal plane. There was a ventricular fusion beat in leads V_4–V_6. A transesophageal echocardiogram confirmed the position of the ventricular lead in the left ventricle passing from the right atrium to the left atrium and crossing the mitral valve. The lead was successfully extracted percutaneously without complications using a modified technique to prevent embolization. A new lead in the right ventricle produced ventricular paced beats with the typical left bundle branch pattern and left superior axis deviation in the frontal plane. (Reproduced with permission from Barold SS, Giudici MC, Herweg B, Curtis AB. Diagnostic value of the 12-lead electrocardiogram during conventional and biventricular pacing for cardiac resynchronization. Cardiol Clin 2006; 24:471–490).

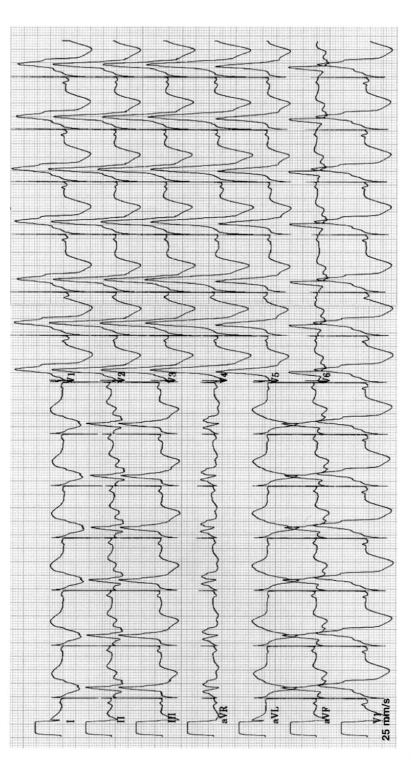

Fig. 22.2 Twelve-lead ECG showing monochamber LV pacing from the coronary venous system. There is typical right bundle branch pattern and right axis deviation. Note the dominant R-wave from V_1 to V_6 consistent with basal LV pacing. LV pacing shown in all the subsequent figures was performed from the coronary venous system. (Reproduced with permission from Barold SS, Herweg B, Giudici M. Electrocardiographic follow-up of biventricular pacemakers. Ann Noninvasive Electrocardiol 2005;10:231–255).

paced ventricular depolarization, commonly with preserved QRS positivity in the right precordial leads or at least V_1 (Fig. 22.1). The positive QRS complexes are unaltered when leads V_1 and V_2 are recorded one intercostal space lower. During LV pacing, the frontal plane axis of paced beats can indicate the site of LV pacing, but as a rule with a RBBB configuration, the frontal plane axis cannot differentiate precisely an endocardial LV site from one in the coronary venous system. The diagnosis of an endocardial LV lead is easy with transesophageal echocardiography. In the usual situation, it will show the lead crossing the atrial septum then passing through the mitral valve into the LV.

ECG Patterns Recorded During LV Pacing from the Coronary Venous System

Pacing from the lateral or posterolateral vein invariably produces a RBBB pattern in a correctly positioned lead V_1 [2–5, 7, 29] (Fig. 22.2). Leads V_2 and V_3 may or may not be positive. With apical sites, leads V_4–V_6 are typically negative. With basal locations, leads V_4–V_6 are usually positive as with the concordant positive R-waves during overt preexcitation in left-sided accessory pathway conduction in the Wolff–Parkinson–White syndrome [3]. During pacing from the correct site in the coronary venous system, the frontal plane axis often points to the right inferior quadrant (right axis deviation) and less commonly to the right superior quadrant. In an occasional patient with uncomplicated LV pacing with a typical RBBB pattern in lead V_1, the axis may point to the left inferior or left superior quadrant. The reasons for these unusual axis locations are unclear.

Pacing from the proximal part of the middle cardiac vein or the great (anterior) vein may produce a RBBB pattern, but stimulation from a more distal site yields a LBBB configuration. [28–36] (Fig. 22.3).

Negative QRS Complex in Lead V_1

When lead V_1 shows a negative QRS complex during LV pacing, one should consider incorrect ECG lead placement (lead V_1 too high as in Fig. 22.4), location in the middle or great (anterior interventricular) cardiac vein, or an undefined mechanism requiring elucidation [2].

Negative QRS Complex in Lead I

During RV apical pacing, the frontal plane axis points superiorly mostly to the left but occasionally to the right (superior quadrant). In the latter case, lead I shows a negative QRS deflection. This negativity (which is normal) has been erroneously interpreted as representing left-sided pacing [1].

ECG Patterns and Follow-up of Biventricular Pacemakers

So far, evaluation of the overall ECG patterns of biventricular pacing has focused mostly on simultaneous RV and LV stimulation [2, 5, 7, 37–40]. A baseline 12-lead ECG should be recorded at the time of implantation during

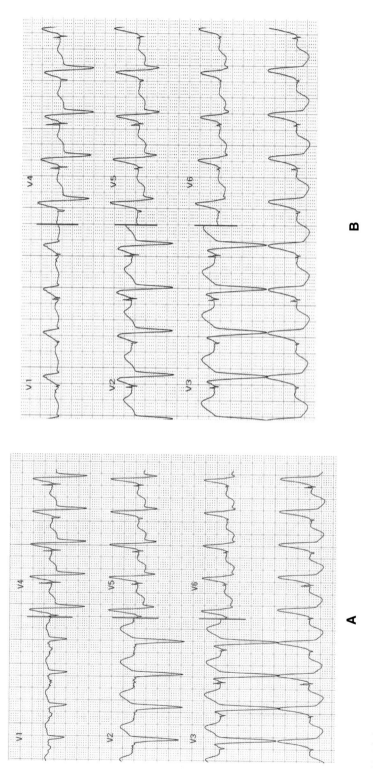

A

B

Fig. 22.4 (**A**) Twelve-lead ECG recorded during LV pacing with leads V_1 and V_2 placed at the level of the second intercostal space in a thin patient with an elongated chest. There is no dominant R-wave in lead V_1. Biventricular pacing also failed to show a dominant R-wave in V_1 at the same intercostal space. (**B**) The dominant R-wave in V_1 during LV pacing becomes evident only when lead V_1 is recorded in the 4th intercostal space. The R-wave in V_1 recorded in the 4th intercostal space during biventricular pacing also became dominant. (Reproduced with permission from Barold SS, Giudici MC, Herweg B, Curtis AB. Diagnostic value of the 12-lead electrocardiogram during conventional and biventricular pacing for cardiac resynchronization. Cardiol Clin 2006;24:471–490).

assessment of the independent capture thresholds of the right ventricle and left ventricle to identify the specific morphology of the paced QRS complexes in a multiplicity of leads [1]. This requires having the patient connected to a multichannel 12-lead ECG during the implantation procedure. A total of four 12-lead ECGs are required: [1] intrinsic rhythm and QRS complex prior to any pacing; [2] paced QRS associated with RV pacing; [3] paced QRS associated with LV pacing; [4] paced QRS associated with biventricular pacing. The four tracings should be examined to identify the lead configuration that best demonstrates a discernible and obvious difference between the four pacing states (inhibited, RV only, LV only, and biventricular). This ECG lead should then be used as the surface monitoring lead for subsequent evaluations. Loss of capture in one ventricle will cause a change in the morphology of ventricular paced beats in the 12-lead ECG similar to that of either single-chamber RV pacing or single-chamber LV pacing. A shift in the frontal plane axis may be useful to corroborate loss of capture in one of the ventricles [2,3,6,7]. If both the native QRS and the biventricular paced complex are relatively narrow, then a widening of the paced QRS complex will identify loss of capture in one chamber with effectual capture in the other.

Paced QRS Duration

The paced QRS during biventricular pacing is often narrower than that of monochamber RV or LV pacing. Thus, measurement of QRS duration during follow-up is helpful in the analysis of appropriate biventricular capture and fusion with the spontaneous QRS [3,4,7]. If the biventricular ECG is virtually similar to that recorded with RV or LV pacing alone and no cause is found, one should not automatically conclude that one of the leads does not contribute to biventricular depolarization without a detailed evaluation of the pacing system.

There is no correlation between QRS narrowing after ventricular resynchronization and the clinical response [41–43]. In some cases, the QRS complex after CRT may actually lengthen or remain unchanged despite substantial improvement in mechanical LV dyssynchrony. Increased QRS duration with CRT does not necessarily reflect the presence of ventricular areas with slow conduction resulting in more heterogeneous myocardial activation. With monochamber LV pacing, there is an obvious discrepancy between QRS duration (compared with baseline) and hemodynamic and clinical improvement [43]. Some patients with monochamber LV pacing exhibit an equal or superior degree of mechanical resynchronization compared with biventricular pacing despite a very wide paced QRS complex [44]. Thus, in CHF patients, the paced QRS duration cannot be assumed to reflect a more heterogeneous propagation pattern of LV activation and prolonged duration of mechanical activation.

Usefulness of the Frontal Plane Axis of the Paced QRS Complex

Table 22.2 and Figure 22.5 show the importance of the frontal plane axis of the paced QRS complex in determining the arrangement of pacing during testing of biventricular pacemakers [2,5,7]. The shift in the frontal plane QRS axis during programming the ventricular output is helpful in determining the

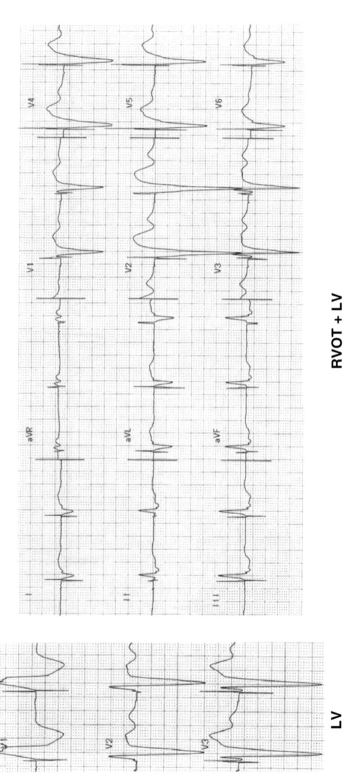

LV

RVOT + LV

Fig. 22.7 Biventricular pacing with the RV lead in the outflow tract. There was a very prominent R-wave in lead V_1 during monochamber left ventricular pacing. Note the typical absence of a dominant R-wave in lead V_1 and the presence of right axis deviation, an uncommon finding during biventricular pacing with the RV lead at the apex. The presence of ventricular fusion with the spontaneous conducted QRS complex was ruled out. (Reproduced with permission from Barold SS, Giudici MC, Herweg B, Curtis AB. Diagnostic value of the 12-lead electrocardiogram during conventional and biventricular pacing for cardiac resynchronization. Cardiol Clin 2006;24:471–490).

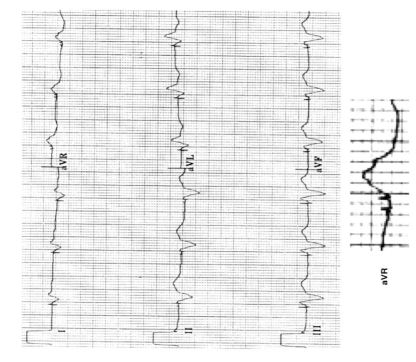

Fig. 22.8 *Top:* Uncomplicated biventricular pacing (right ventricular lead at the apex) in a patient with nonischemic cardiomyopathy. The interventricular (V-V) interval is 40 ms with left ventricular activation first. The 6-lead ECG shows a Qr complex in lead I and a QR complex in lead aVL. This pattern does not indicate an old myocardial infarction. The frontal plane axis lies in the right superior quadrant as expected with this pacing arrangement. *Bottom:* Magnified lead aVR showing separate right and left ventricular stimuli. (Reproduced with permission from Barold SS, Giudici MC, Herweg B, Curtis AB. Diagnostic value of the 12-lead electrocardiogram during conventional and biventricular pacing for cardiac resynchronization. Cardiol Clin 2006;24:471–490).

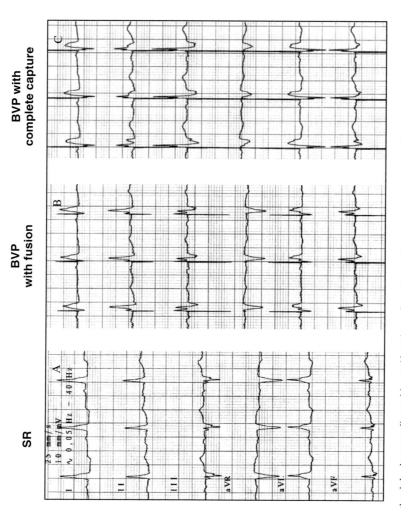

Fig. 22.10 Biventricular pacing with subtle electrocardiographic manifestations of ventricular fusion with the conducted QRS complex during biventricular pacing (BVP). (**A**) Spontaneous ventricular depolarization. Surface ECG from a patient with severe congestive heart failure showing sinus rhythm, complete left bundle branch block, and QRS duration of 125 ms. (**B**) Ventricular fusion. ECG from the same patient after receiving a biventricular device. The AV delay was fixed at 120 ms and the paced QRS shortened to 115 ms. The slight change in QRS morphology strongly suggests a fusion phenomenon with spontaneous ventricular depolarization. (**C**) Pure biventricular depolarization. The atrioventricular delay was programmed to 80 ms resulting in a longer QRS duration of 130 ms. The QRS morphology is different from that in (**B**) and similar to that obtained with biventricular VVI pacing, confirming complete biventricular capture. The shorter AV delay therefore eliminated ventricular fusion with spontaneous ventricular depolarization. (Reproduced with permission from Garrigue S, Barold SS, Clémenty J. Electrocardiography of multisite ventricular pacing. In: Barold SS, Mugica J, eds. The Fifth Decade of Cardiac Pacing. Elmsford, NY: Blackwell-Futura; 2004:84–100).

Fusion with Spontaneous Ventricular Activation: Beneficial or Harmful?

Van Gelder et al. [47] recently investigated the effect of intrinsic conduction over the right bundle branch (causing fusion) on the LV dP/dt_{max} index. LV pacing (biventricular activation with LV monochamber pacing) was compared with biventricular pacing in 34 patients with New York Heart Association (NYHA) functional class III or IV, sinus rhythm with normal AV conduction, left bundle branch block, QRS >130 ms, and optimal medical therapy. LV dP/dt_{max} was measured invasively during LV and simultaneous biventricular pacing. The AV interval was varied in four steps starting with an AV interval 40 ms shorter than the intrinsic PQ time and decreased with 25% for each step with ventricular fusion caused by intrinsic activation. LV dP/dt_{max} was higher with LV than biventricular pacing provided that LV pacing was associated with ventricular fusion caused by intrinsic activation via the right bundle branch.

The clinical implications of the study of Van Gelder et al. [47] are unclear. It is impossible to obtain sustained LV stimulation with fusion of right bundle branch depolarization because of variability of the PR interval related to autonomic factors. At present, it is best to program the AV delay to avoid all forms of ventricular fusion with spontaneous ventricular activity until more data are available, and a reliable way is found to synchronize right bundle branch activity (unpaced RV) with LV stimulation.

Influence of First-Degree AV Block

Pires et al. [48] studied the predictors of a CRT response in patients from the Multicenter InSync Randomized Clinical Evaluation (MIRACLE) and MIRACLE-ICD trials. Patients with an improvement of ≥ 1 NYHA class from baseline to the 6-month follow-up were considered responders, and those who had no change or worse NYHA class or died were classified as nonresponders. Based on improvement of ≥ 1 NYHA class, less than two thirds of patients enrolled in the MIRACLE or MIRACLE-ICD trials responded to CRT. One hundred forty-three (64%) of 224 and 190 (61%) of 313 patients in the MIRACLE and MIRACLE-ICD trials, respectively, responded to therapy. Using stepwise logistic regression methods, the study identified several differing factors that predicted CRT response in the two trials. One of these factors was the absence of first-degree AV block which was associated with a response to CRT (p = 0.005). Tedrow et al. [49], who evaluated 75 consecutive CRT patients, also found that patients with first-degree AV block have a poorer outcome than patients with a normal PR interval though the data were not quite statistically significant (hazard ratio = 1.01, p = 0.0650).

Enhanced hemodynamic response in patients with normal AV conduction by concealed resynchronization or fusion was suggested by Kurzidim et al. [50]. These workers studied 22 CHF patients, all in sinus rhythm with temporary multisite pacing prior to implantation of a CRT system. LV systolic function was evaluated invasively by the maximum rate of LV pressure increase (dP/dt_{max}). Sequential biventricular pacing was performed with preactivation of either ventricle at 20–80 ms. In 60% (6/10) of patients with a normal PR interval (≤ 200 ms), right atrial–triggered LV pacing produced a hemodynamic response superior to that of optimized sequential biventricular pacing and was equivalent to that of simultaneous biventricular pacing in time from right atrium to the QRS complex [52]. In the presence of inter-atrial conduction delay, one should consider placing the atrial lead in the interatrial septum where pacing produces a more homogeneous activation of both atria and abbreviates total atrial conduction time judged by a decrease of P-wave duration [53,54]. In the presence of established CRT with an atrial lead in the right atrial appendage, restoration of mechanical left-sided AV synchrony requires simultaneous biatrial pacing performed by the implantation of a second atrial lead either in the proximal coronary sinus or low atrium near the coronary sinus to preempt left atrial systole [55,56]. Difficult cases can be managed by AV nodal ablation to permit extension of the AV delay to promote mechanical left-sided AV synchrony, though biventricular ICDs may limit the maximum programmable AV delay.

Late Atrial Sensing (Intraatrial Conduction Delay)

In some patients with right intraatrial conduction delay, conduction from the sinus node to the right atrial appendage (site of atrial sensing) is delayed without significant conduction delay to the left atrium. In this situation, left atrial activation may take place or may even be completed by the time the device senses the right atrial electrogram (Fig. 22.11). In these circumstances, it may be difficult or impossible to program an optimal delay with CRT in the absence of ventricular fusion. A trial of ventricular-triggered biventricular pacing upon sensing the spontaneous QRS complex may be worthwhile.

Long-term ECG Changes

Many studies have shown that the paced QRS duration does not vary over time as long as the LV pacing lead does not move from its initial site [6,41,57]. Yet, surface ECGs should be performed periodically because the LV lead may become displaced into a collateral branch of the coronary sinus. Dislodgment of the LV lead may result in loss of LV capture with the ECG showing an RV pacing QRS pattern with an increased QRS duration and superior axis deviation. Ricci et al. [57] suggested that variation of the QRS duration over time may play a determinant role if correlated with remodeling of the ventricles by echocardiography. Finally, the underlying spontaneous ECG should be exposed periodically to confirm the presence of a LBBB type of intraventricular conduction abnormality. In this respect, turning off the pacemaker could potentially improve LV function and heart failure in patients who have lost their intraventricular conduction delay or block through ventricular remodeling. In other words, a spontaneous narrow QRS is better than biventricular pacing.

Anodal Stimulation in Biventricular Pacemakers

Although anodal capture may occur with high-output traditional bipolar RV pacing, this phenomenon is almost always not discernible electrocardiographically. Biventricular pacing systems may use a unipolar lead for LV pacing via a coronary vein. The tip electrode of the LV lead is the cathode and

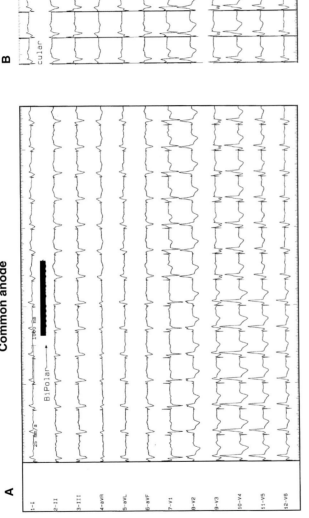

Common anode

B

Dual unipolar

Anodal capture ⟶ **No anodal capture**

Fig. 22.12 (**A**) On the left there is RV anodal capture during simultaneous biventricular pacing with a unipolar left ventricular lead in the coronary venous system and a bipolar RV lead. The proximal electrode of the RV lead provides a common anode. RV anodal capture disappears when the left ventricular output voltage is decreased. Note the change in QRS configuration when RV anodal capture is eliminated by reducing the left ventricular output on the right of the panel. (**B**) Same patient as in (**A**). Programming dual unipolar simultaneous biventricular pacing fails to produce RV anodal stimulation despite a high left ventricular output because the RV anode is now excluded from the circuit. Consequently, the ECG in (**B**) becomes identical to that in (**A**) on the right where there is no RV anodal capture.

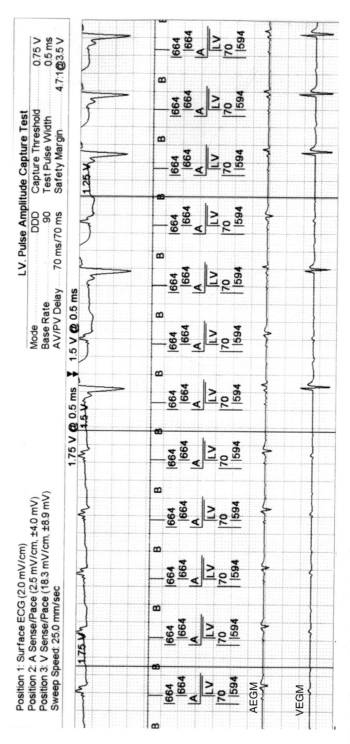

Fig. 22.13 Anodal pacing during monochamber left ventricular pacing. The left side shows the paced QRS morphology during monochamber LV pacular pacing. This was identical to the pattern previously recorded with pure biventricular pacing. This response was due to ventricular capture at the common anodal site (proximal or ring electrode of the right ventricular lead) in the right ventricle with consequent capture of both the left ventricle and the right ventricle simultaneously. Intermittent capture of the isolated left ventricle occurred only when the left ventricular output fell to 1.5 V at 0.5 ms. Monochamber left ventricular pacing became continual at 1.25 V and 0.5 ms. Thus, the threshold for anodal capture was 1.75 V at 0.5 ms. In other words, anodal capture disappeared at an output <1.75 V at 0.5 ms. A, atrial paced event; LV, LV paced event. P = atrial sensed event; BV = biventricular pacing.

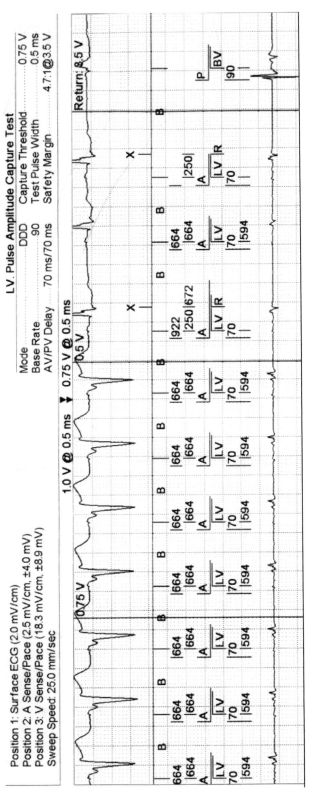

Fig. 22.14 Continuation of threshold testing from Figure 22.13. There was loss of LV capture at 0.5 V and 0.5 ms with emergence of the spontaneous rhythm. The first spontaneous QRS complex was sensed after an ineffectual LV stimulus and depicted as "R." This sensed event reset the timing cycle of the pacemaker. The second spontaneous QRS complex was unsensed because it fell into the postventricular blanking period initiated by the preceding ineffectual LV stimulus. The third spontaneous QRS complex behaved like the first one. *A*, atrial paced event; *LV*, LV paced event.

the proximal electrode of the bipolar RV lead often provides the anode for LV pacing. This arrangement creates a common anode for RV and LV pacing. A high current density (from two sources) at the common anode during biventricular pacing may cause anodal capture manifested as a paced QRS complex with a somewhat different configuration from that derived from pure biventricular pacing [58, 59] (Fig. 22.12). Anodal capture creates three distinct pacing morphologies exclusive of fusion with the spontaneous QRS complex: biventricular with anodal capture (at a high output), biventricular (at a lower output), and RV (with loss of LV capture) or rarely LV (with loss of RV capture).

A different form of anodal capture involving the ring electrode of the bipolar RV lead can also occur with contemporary biventricular pacemakers with *separately programmable ventricular outputs* (Figs. 22.13 and 22.14). During monochamber LV pacing at a relatively high output, RV anodal capture produces a paced QRS complex identical to that registered with biventricular pacing [60, 61]. Occasionally, this type of anodal capture prevents electrocardiographic documentation of pure LV pacing if the LV pacing threshold is higher than that of RV anodal stimulation. Such anodal stimulation may complicate threshold testing and should not be misinterpreted as pacemaker malfunction. Furthermore, if the LV threshold is not too high, appropriate programming of the pacemaker output should eliminate anodal stimulation in most cases. The use of true bipolar LV leads eliminates all forms of anodal stimulation.

Effect of Interventricular V-V Timing on the Electrocardiogram of Biventricular Pacemakers

The electrocardiographic consequences of temporally different RV and LV activation with programmable V-V timing in the latest biventricular devices have not yet been studied in detail (Fig. 22.15). Contemporary biventricular devices permit programming of the interventricular interval usually in steps from +80 ms (LV first) to –80 ms (RV first) to optimize LV hemodynamics. In the absence of anodal stimulation, increasing the V-V interval gradually to 80 ms (LV first) will progressively increase the duration of the paced QRS complex, alter its morphology with a larger R-wave in lead V_1 indicating more dominant LV depolarization [62] (Fig. 22.15). The varying QRS configuration in lead V_1 with different V-V intervals cannot be correlated with the hemodynamic response.

RV anodal stimulation during biventricular pacing interferes with a programmed interventricular (V-V) delay (often programmed with the LV preceding the RV) aimed at optimizing cardiac resynchronization because RV anodal capture causes simultaneous RV and LV activation (The V-V interval becomes zero) (Fig. 22.16). In the presence of anodal stimulation, the ECG morphology and its duration will not change if the device is programmed with V-V intervals of 80, 60, and 40 ms (LV before RV). The delayed RV cathodal output (80, 60, 40 ms) then falls in the myocardial refractory period initiated by the preceding anodal stimulation. At V-V intervals ≤20 ms, the paced QRS may change because the short LV–RV interval prevents propagation of activation from the site of RV anodal capture in time to render the

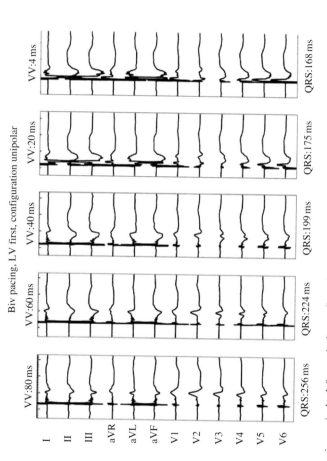

Fig. 22.15 Sequential biventricular pacing in a unipolar left ventricular configuration with varying V-V intervals. There is a gradual change in the morphology of the QRS complex, which is best reflected in the precordial leads. (Reproduced with permission from van Gelder BM, Bracke FA, Meijer A. The effect of anodal stimulation on V-V timing at varying V-V intervals. Pacing Clin Electrophysiol 2005;28:771–776).

cathodal site refractory (Fig. 22.17). Thus, the cathode also captures the RV and contributes to RV depolarization, which then takes place from two sites: RV anode and RV cathode [62,63].

Electrocardiography During Exercise

Exercise testing in CRT patients is technically difficult and inconvenient but helpful in the overall evaluation of CRT particularly in patients with a suboptimal CRT response where no obvious cause is found at rest [7]. An exercise test may reveal loss of capture, atrial undersensing, various arrhythmias, and the development of spontaneous AV conduction indicating that the upper rate should be reprogrammed to ensure consistent biventricular capture with effort. Exercise testing is important in patients with permanent atrial fibrillation who have not undergone ablation of the AV junction to determine the status of spontaneous AV conduction.

If the spontaneous PR interval on exercise becomes shorter than the programmed AV (atrial sensed–ventricular paced), CRT will be lost. There is preliminary evidence in acute studies suggesting that the short AV delay at rest should be prolonged during exercise to achieve optimal LV systolic performance [64]. This is in contrast with the proven benefit of programming rate-adaptive shortening of the AV delay in patients with conventional DDDR pacemakers. The dynamic changes of LV dyssynchrony on exercise may partially explain what appears to be paradoxical behavior of the AV delay on exercise in CRT patients [65]. If confirmed by other studies, it would be desirable to provide CRT devices with dynamic lengthening of the AV delay on exercise. In the meantime, it might be wise to program CRT devices without dynamic shortening of the AV delay in patients with normal sinus node function unless it is shown to be beneficial during an exercise study. At present, there are no chronic data available that provide insight regarding the optimal AV interval during activity states.

In CRT patients with severe chronotropic incompetence (defined by the failure to achieve 85% of the age-predicted heart rate (determined as 220 − the patient's age), rate-adaptive pacing DDDR with a rate-adaptive AV delay may provide incremental benefit on exercise capacity [66]. Therefore, an exercise test would be desirable to demonstrate the effect of a rate-adaptive AV delay if atrial pacing is likely to occur on exercise.

Latency

The delay from the pacing stimulus to the onset of ventricular depolarization is called *latency*. An isoelectric onset of QRS complex in one or only a few leads can mimic latency. Consequently, latency requires a 12-lead ECG taken at fast speed for diagnosis. In biventricular pacing, latency related to LV pacing may produce suboptimal hemodynamics associated with an ECG showing the pattern of RV pacing because LV depolarization is delayed and overshadowed by RV stimulation [67]. The electrical and hemodynamic problem can often be corrected by advancing LV stimulation by programming the interventricular (V-V) delay, a feature available only in contemporary devices as discussed in a special chapter on latency in this book.

Biventricular Pacing with a Conventional DDD Pacemaker

Some patients with permanent atrial fibrillation undergo CRT with conventional DDDR pacemakers. The "atrial" channel usually paces the left ventricle and the ventricular channel paces the right ventricle [68]. Two ventricular stimuli are often seen because such devices do not usually permit programming an AV interval of zero. The device is usually programmed to the DVI to prevent far-field atrial sensing by the ventricular lead.

References

1. Barold SS, Levine PA, Ovsyshcher IE. The paced 12-lead electrocardiogram should no longer be neglected in pacemaker follow-up. PACE 2001;24:1455–1458.
2. Barold SS, Herweg B, Giudici M. Electrocardiographic follow-up of biventricular pacemakers. Ann Noninvasive Electrocardiol 2005;10:231–255.
3. Asirvatham SJ. Electrocardiogram interpretation with biventricular pacing devices. In: Hayes DL, Wang PJ, Sackner-Bernstein J, Asirvatham SJ, eds. Resynchronization and Defibrillation for Heart Failure. A Practical Approach. Oxford: Blackwell-Futura; 2004:73–97.
4. Kay GN. Troubleshooting and programming of cardiac resynchronization therapy. In: Ellenbogen KA, Kay GN, Wilkoff BL, eds. Device Therapy for Congestive Heart Failure. Philadelphia: Saunders; 2004:232–293.
5. Steinberg JS, Maniar PB, Higgins SL, et al. Noninvasive assessment of the biventricular pacing system. Ann Noninvasive Electrocardiol 2004;9:58–70.
6. Garrigue S, Barold SS, Clémenty J. Electrocardiography of multisite ventricular pacing. In: Barold SS, Mugica J, eds. The Fifth Decade of Cardiac Pacing. Elmsford, NY: Blackwell-Futura; 2004:84–100.
7. Leclercq C, Mabo P, Daubert JC. Troubleshooting. In: Yu CM, Hayes DL, Auricchio A, eds. Cardiac Resynchronization Therapy. Malden, MA: Blackwell - Futura; 2006:259–290.
8. Barold SS, Falkoff MD, Ong LS, Heinle RA. Electrocardiographic analysis of normal and abnormal pacemaker function. In: Dreifus LS, ed. Pacemaker Therapy, Cardiovascular Clinics. Philadelphia: F.A.Davis; 1983:97–134.
9. Klein HO, Becker B, Sareli P, DiSegni E, Dean H, Kaplinsky E. Unusual QRS morphology associated with transvenous pacemakers. The pseudo RBBB pattern. Chest 1985;87:517–521.
10. Yang YN, Yin WH, Young MS. Safe right bundle branch block pattern during permanent right ventricular pacing. J Electrocardiol 2003;36:67–71.
11. Coman JA, Trohman RG. Incidence and electrocardiographic localization of safe right bundle branch block configurations during permanent ventricular pacing. Am J Cardiol 1995;76:781–784.
12. Ciolli A, Trambaiolo P, Lo Sardo G, Sasdelli M, Palamara A. Asymptomatic malposition of a pacing lead in the left ventricle: the case of a woman untreated with anticoagulant therapy for eight years. Ital Heart J 2003;4:562–564.
13. Paravolidakis KE, Hamodraka ES, Kolettis TM, Psychari SN, Apostolou TS. Management of inadvertent left ventricular permanent pacing. J Interv Card Electrophysiol 2004;10:237–240.
14. Ergun K, Tufekcioglu O, Karabal O, Ozdogan OU, Deveci B, Golbasi Z. An unusual cause of stroke in a patient with permanent transvenous pacemaker. Jpn Heart J 2004;45:873–875.

56. Doi A, Takagi M, Toda I, Yoshiyama M, Takeuchi K, Yoshikawa J. Acute haemodynamic benefits of biatrial atrioventricular sequential pacing: Comparison with single atrial atrioventricular sequential pacing. Heart 2004;90:411–418.

57. Ricci R, Pignalberi C, Ansalone G, et al. Early and late QRS morphology and width in biventricular pacing: Relationship to lead site and electrical remodeling. J Interv Card Electrophysiol 2002;6:279–285.

58. Van Gelder BM, Bracke FA, Pilmeyer A, Meijer A. Triple-site ventricular pacing in a biventricular pacing system. PACE 2001;24:1165–1167.

59. Bulava A, Ansalone G, Ricci R, et al. Triple-site pacing with biventricular device. Incidence of the phenomenon and cardiac resynchronization benefit. J Interv Card Electrophysiol 2004;10:37–45.

60. Herweg B, Barold SS. Anodal capture with second-generation biventricular cardioverter-defibrillator. Acta Cardiol 2003;58:435–436.

61. Thibault B, Roy D, Guerra PG, et al. Anodal right ventricular capture during left ventricular stimulation in CRT-implantable cardioverter defibrillators. Pacing Clin Electrophysiol 2005;28:613–619.

62. van Gelder BM, Bracke FA, Meijer A. The effect of anodal stimulation on V-V timing at varying V-V intervals. Pacing Clin Electrophysiol 2005;28:771–776.

63. Tamborero D, Mont L, Alanis R, Berruezo A, et al. Anodal capture in cardiac resynchronization therapy. Implications for device programming. Pacing Clin Electrophysiol 2006;29:940–945.

64. Scharf C, Li P, Muntwyler J, Chugh A, et al. Rate-dependent AV delay optimization in cardiac resynchronization therapy. Pacing Clin Electrophysiol 2005;28:279–284.

65. Bordachar P, Lafitte S, Reuter S, et al. Echocardiographic assessment during exercise of heart failure patients with cardiac resynchronization therapy. Am J Cardiol 2006;97:1622–1625.

66. Tse HF, Siu CW, Lee KL, et al. The incremental benefit of rate-adaptive pacing on exercise performance during cardiac resynchronization therapy. J Am Coll Cardiol 2005;46:2292–2297.

67. Herweg B, Ilercil A, Madramootoo C, et al. Latency during left ventricular pacing from the lateral cardiac veins: a cause of ineffectual biventricular pacing. Pacing Clin Electrophysiol 2006;29:574–581.

68. Barold SS, Gallardo I, Sayad D. The DVI mode of cardiac pacing: a second coming? Am J Cardiol 2002;90:521–523.

23

Cardiac Arrhythmias After Cardiac Resynchronization

S. Serge Barold and Bengt Herweg

Patients with devices for cardiac resynchronization therapy (CRT) can develop a variety of atrial and ventricular arrhythmias predominately related to poor left ventricular (LV) function. Less commonly, CRT patients may exhibit specific (long QT) ventricular proarrhythmias linked to altered ventricular repolarization resulting from reversed ventricular activation delivered by biventricular or left ventricular pacing.

Atrial Fibrillation

Atrial fibrillation/flutter occurs in up to 30% of patients with congestive heart failure and can be an important cause of decompensation after CRT. Atrial fibrillation (AF) interferes with the optimal delivery of CRT because the ventricular rhythm inhibits CRT or by the unfavorable hemodynamics associated with a fast ventricular rate. AV nodal ablation should always be considered in permanent AF but also in paroxysmal or persistent AF when it becomes troublesome and difficult to control [1].

In AF, some CRT devices provide some degree of ventricular resynchronization by attempting regularization of the paced beats up to the programmed maximum tracking rate. The overall ventricular rate remains undesirably high despite the automatic adjustment of the lower rate interval. Activation of this algorithm does not result in control of the ventricular rate and should not be a substitute for ablation of the AV junction in patients with substantial periods of drug-refractory rapid ventricular rates.

Impact of CRT on Incidence of Atrial Fibrillation

Despite reverse remodeling of the ventricle and left atrium provided by CRT together with its significant clinical benefit, the impact of CRT on the incidence of AF remains unclear because only a few studies have so far addressed this issue.

In one study, 84 CRT patients were assessed at baseline and at 3 months follow-up for AF burden (defined as time of AF per day, AF >30 s) [2]. AF was continuously measured by the device. In patients with AF episodes, the overall burden of AF was 9.88 ± 12.61 h/day in the first month of CRT and 4.20 ± 9.24 h/day in the third month of CRT (p = 0.001). The overall number of patients with AF also was significantly reduced from 26 of 84 (31%) patients in the first month to 18 of 84 (21%) patients in the second month and to 13 of 84 (15%) patients in the third month (p < 0.001, first vs. third month). One third of the patients were free of episodes although they had a history of AF before implantation. In contrast, half of the patients who presented with AF in the first 3 months of CRT had no prior history of AF, possibly due to asymptomatic episodes of AF before device implant. The study therefore showed a significant gradual reduction in AF burden and the number of patients experiencing AF episodes during CRT.

In the CArdiac REsynchronization in Heart Failure (CARE-HF) trial, 813 patients were randomly assigned to pharmacological therapy alone or with the addition of CRT [3]. The incidence of new-onset AF was assessed by adverse event reporting and by ECGs during follow-up at 1, 3, 6, 9, 12, and 18 months and every 6 months thereafter, or documented as a serious adverse event or during hospitalization. By the end of the study (mean duration of follow-up 29.4 months), AF had been documented in 66 patients in the CRT group compared with 58 who received medical therapy only [16.1% vs. 14.4%; hazard ratio (HR), 1.05; 95% confidence interval (CI), 0.73–1.50; p = 0.79]. There was no difference in the time until first onset of AF between groups.

Fung et al. [4] followed 36 consecutive patients (the CRT group) in sinus rhythm at baseline and no history of AF and a matched control group. Patients in the two groups were regularly seen every 6 to 8 weeks. Holter and event recorder examinations were performed if clinically indicated in the two groups. The detection of AF relied on electrocardiography, strips from event recorders, and 24-h Holter examination. After a follow-up of 3 years, three patients in the CRT group and 11 in the control group developed AF. The annual incidence of AF was 2.8% in the CRT group and 10.2% in the control group (p = 0.025). Two patients in the CRT group and seven in the control group had paroxysmal AF, and one patient in the CRT group and four in the control group had permanent AF. The mechanisms of the lower incidence of AF in the CRT group may be related to the significant improvement in LV systolic function and reduction in mitral regurgitation.

In a study from Leiden (The Netherlands), 74 consecutive CRT patients and AF (20 persistent and 54 permanent) were evaluated before and after 6 months of CRT for the restoration of sinus rhythm [5]. During implantation, 18 of 20 (90%) patients with persistent AF were cardioverted to sinus rhythm. At follow-up, 13 of 18 (72%) cardioverted patients had returned to AF; thus, only 5 of 74 patients (7%) were in sinus rhythm as none of the patients with permanent AF converted spontaneously to sinus rhythm.

Impact of CRT on Ventricular Tachyarrhythmias

CRT appears to produce favorable electrophysiologic benefits (electrical remodeling) that might diminish the susceptibility of potentially life-threatening ventricular arrhythmias. In this respect, Higgins et al. [6] first suggested that CRT may reduce antitachycardia therapy in patients with a CRT-D (D = defibrillator) device, though no reduction in mortality was found in this early study. Since then, a number of reports have provided growing evidence that CRT may indeed be antiarrhythmic and may prevent sudden death especially in association with an implantable cardioverter-defibrillator (ICD).

Does CRT Without an ICD Reduce All-Cause Mortality but Not Sudden Death?

In an extension of the of the already reported open-label randomized Cardiac Resynchronization–Heart Failure (CARE-HF) trial [7], the mean follow-up was 37.4 months (median, 37.6; interquartile range (IQR), 31.5–42.5; range, 26.1–52.6 months) [8]. There were 154 deaths (38.1%) in 404 patients assigned to medical therapy and 101 deaths (24.7%) in 409 patients assigned to CRT (HR, 0.60; 95% CI, 0.47–0.77; p < 0.0001) without evidence of heterogeneity in prespecified subgroups. A reduction in the risk of death due to heart failure (64 vs. 38 deaths; HR, 0.55; 95% CI, 0.37–0.82; p = 0.003) and sudden death was observed (55 vs. 32 sudden deaths or 4.3 vs.2.5% per annum hazard ratio 0.54, 95% CI 0.35–0.84; p = 0.005). The extended study highlighted that the prognostic benefits of CRT are maintained or increased with longer-term follow-up and are due to reductions in sudden death and death due to worsening heart failure in roughly equal proportion [8].

The influence of CRT alone on sudden death requires further investigation in view of a recent meta-analysis of a number of randomized controlled studies evaluating the effects of CRT (without an ICD) in patients with advanced heart failure and a depressed LV systolic performance [9]. Five studies met the criteria for inclusion, the Multisite Stimulation in Cardiomyopathies Study (MUSTIC), the Multicenter InSync Randomized Clinical Evaluation (MIRACLE), the MUSTIC AF, the Comparison of Medical Therapy, Pacing, and Defibrillation in Heart Failure (COMPANION) (CRT alone and control arms only), and the CARE-HF trials in its original form not involving the extended phase of this trial. Trials that did not independently report data on CRT alone or had a follow-up period of less than 3 months, were excluded. They included a total of 2,371 patients: 1,028 controls and 1,343 CRT-treated patients. Pooled analysis demonstrated that CRT alone, compared with optimal medical therapy, significantly reduced all-cause mortality by 29% [16.9% vs. 20.7%; odds ratio (OR), 0.71; 95% CI, 0.57–0.88] and mortality due to progressive heart failure by 38% (6.7% vs. 9.7%; OR, 0.62; 95% CI, 0.45–0.84). No effect on sudden cardiac death was observed with CRT (6.4% vs. 5.9%; OR, 1.04; 95% CI, 0.73–1.22).

Do CRT and ICD Reduce Mortality?

COMPANION trial

In the COMPANION trial, with regard to the all-cause mortality end point alone after 1 year of follow-up, CRT patients had a 24% risk reduction (p = 0.060), and CRT-ICD patients experienced a risk reduction of 36% (p < 0.003) when compared with optimal medical therapy [10]. Although COMPANION showed the impact of cardiac resynchronization plus ICD therapy in reducing early mortality in CRT patients, the mortality at 24 months of follow-up was the same in CRT alone patients vs. CRT- ICD patients.

VENTAK CHF and CONTAK CD trials

In the VENTAK CHF/CONTAK CD trial, 501 of the 581 patients enrolled received a CRT device [11]. Clinical characteristics included spontaneous or inducible (primary prevention, MADIT patient profile) sustained ventricular tachyarrhythmias and New York Heart Association (NYHA) class II (33%), III (58%), or IV (9%) congestive heart failure (CHF) symptoms. During 6 months of follow-up, 73 of 501 (14%) patients received an appropriate ICD therapy. Two independent predictors of appropriate therapy were identified: a history of a spontaneous, sustained ventricular arrhythmia (HR, 2.05; 95% CI, 1.31–3.20; p = 0.002) and NYHA class IV CHF (HR, 1.81; 95% CI, 1.10–2.96; p = 0.019). When patients with NYHA class II were excluded from analysis, a history of a sustained ventricular arrhythmia and the presence of NYHA class IV CHF symptoms remained as independent predictors of appropriate ICD therapy. Appropriate ICD therapy delivery was significantly greater in patients with NYHA class IV symptoms. Approximately one quarter of the patients with NYHA class IV CHF who received a CRT-D device received an appropriate ICD therapy within 3 months after implantation. The study found that patients with a prior history of spontaneous, sustained ventricular arrhythmias were twice as likely to receive an appropriate defibrillator therapy compared with patients who received a defibrillator for primary prevention [11].

MIRACLE Trial

In a retrospective review of 978 CRT-ICD patients of the MIRACLE-ICD (Multicenter InSync Implantable Cardioversion Defibrillation Randomized Clinical Evaluation) trial, it was reported that 28% of the secondary prevention patients experienced an appropriate shock at 12 months follow-up compared with only 14% of the primary prevention patients [12]. In other words, patients with a primary prevention indication for an ICD had a significantly lower incidence of appropriate ICD therapies (0.09 vs. 0.43 episodes/month) compared with patients with a secondary prevention indication. The appropriate use of the ICD in CRT patients with a primary ICD indication suggests that this arrangement may be potentially beneficial in such a patient population susceptible to life-threatening ventricular tachyarrhythmias.

Leiden Trial

A total of 191 consecutive patients with advanced heart failure, left ventricular ejection fraction (LVEF) <35%, and a QRS duration >120 ms received CRT-ICD device [13]. Seventy-one patients had a history of ventricular arrhythmias (secondary prevention); 120 patients did not have prior ventricular arrhythmias (primary prevention). During follow-up (18 ± 4 months), primary prevention patients experienced less appropriate ICD therapies than secondary prevention patients (21% vs. 35%, p < 0.05) [13]. Multivariate analysis revealed, however, no predictors of ICD therapy. Furthermore, a similar, significant, improvement in clinical parameters was observed at 6 months in both groups. Also, the mortality rate in the primary prevention group was lower than in the secondary prevention group (3% vs. 18%, p < 0.05).

The results obtained in the primary prevention group are in line with the results of the MADIT II (Multicenter Automatic Defibrillator Implantation) study (26% ICD therapy in ischemic cardiomyopathy patients, LVEF <30%) [14]. Also, the SCD-HeFT study (LVEF <35%, ischemic and nonischemic heart disease patients) reported an incidence of 21% ICD therapy, though the follow-up period was longer in the SCD-HeFT study [15].

Other Studies with CRT-D Devices

A number of smaller studies of patients with CRT-D devices have also confirmed that CRT reduces the need for ICD-delivered antitachycardia therapy (shocks) suggesting but not proving that ICD therapy prevent sudden arrhythmic deaths [16, 17].

Effect of Upgrading the Pacing Mode in ICD Patients with Ventricular Tachyarrhythmias

Eight consecutive ICD patients who underwent an upgrade to CRT-ICD were followed during two time periods: 47 ± 21 months (range, 24 to 70 months) before and 14 ± 2 months (range, 9 to 18 months) after CRT upgrade [18]. At time of upgrade, patient age was 69 ± 11 years and ejection fraction was $21 \pm 8\%$. During conventional ICD treatment, antitachycardia pacing was applied in 10 of 18 (56%) patients compared with 1 of 18 (3%) after CRT-ICD placement. Similarly, the number of patients receiving ICD shocks diminished after CRT. The frequency of shocks was 0.048 ± 0.085 episodes/month per patient with the conventional ICD versus 0.003 ± 0.016 episodes/month per patient after CRT-ICD ($p = 0.05$).

Inducibility of Ventricular Tachyarrhythmias

Three small studies involving 13 patients in two acute studies, and 15 patients with a CRT device in a long-term study suggest that biventricular pacing can prevent in about 60–80% of cases sustained monomorphic ventricular tachycardia (VT) that is inducible during right ventricular (RV) stimulation [19–21] (Table 23.1).

Table 23.1 Inducibility of sustained monomorphic ventricular tachycardia during biventricular pacing.

Reference	Year	Acute vs. chronic BiV pacing*	VT, no pts RV stim.	LVEF %	Testing stimulation	% noninducible VT
Zagrodzky et al. [19]	2001	Acute. CAD, old MI	7	<35	BiV drive, RV extrast	71% (5 pts), p < 0.05
Kowal et al. [20]	2004	Acute. CAD	6	30	BiV drive, RV extrast	80% (5 pts), p < 0.01
Kies et al. [21]	2005	7.1 ± 0.8 mths after CRT	15	I: 21 ± 4 NI: 24 ± 8	RV drive at apex	60% (9 pts), p < 0.01

CAD, coronary artery disease; MI, myocardial infarction; VT, sustained monomorphic ventricular tachycardia; RV, right ventricle; LVEF, left ventricular ejection fraction; BiV, biventricular; I, patients with inducible VT; NI, patients with noninducible VT; Stim, stimulation; extrast (premature), extrastimulation; CRT, cardiac resynchronization therapy; pts, patients; mths, months.
*Acute testing was performed in patients without an implanted device. Chronic testing involved patients with an implanted CRT device.

Proarrhythmic Effects of CRT

CRT Causes No Proarrhythmia in Two Major Trials

Of 1,041 subjects entering two trials, (CONTAK CD and InSync-ICD), 880 were randomized to CRT (N = 439) or control (N = 441). The data included 840 electrograms in 150 patients with ventricular tachyarrhythmias including 678 monomorphic VT episodes and 162 polymorphic VT episodes [22]. CRT was not found to be associated with a measurable increase in the incidence of polymorphic VT or in a reduction in monomorphic VT in the combined populations.

Despite the above negative studies, isolated cases of CRT-induced proarrhythmia have been reported because biventricular or LV pacing influences the myocardial electrophysiology in a way that may occasionally result in malignant ventricular arrhythmias.

Disturbed Myocardial Electrophysiology by CRT

The ventricular myocardium is not uniform and exhibits electrical heterogeneity in that it comprises three electrophysiologically distinct cell types, epicardial, endocardial, and M (mid-myocardial) cells differing mainly with respect to repolarization characteristics [23–27]. The hallmark of M cells is the tendency for their action potentials to prolong disproportionately compared with epicardium or endocardium during bradycardia or in the presence of QT prolonging drugs or in response to agents that normally prolong the action potential. Hence, M cells (which have a different ionic basis) are thought to play an important role in delayed ventricular repolarization as in the long QT syndrome.

Normally, ventricular activation starts with the endocardium via a subendocardial Purkinje network and spreads across the ventricular wall. Although the epicardium is activated last, it repolarizes first because of its shorter action potential duration, producing a repolarization sequence opposite to activation. On the ECG, such an activation and repolarization sequence produces an upright T-wave with the same polarity as the QRS. In other words, the QT interval is normally determined by the myocardial layers with the longest action potential duration located in subendocardium or endocardium. Full repolarization of the epicardial action potential coincides with the peak of the T-wave and repolarization of the M cells is coincident with the end of the T-wave. It follows that the duration of the M-cell action potential determines the QT interval, whereas the duration of the epicardial action potential determines the QT_{peak} interval [23–27]. Because QRS duration determines QT interval duration, the QT interval should be interpreted cautiously during RV endocardial pacing and LV epicardial pacing when it is longer than during biventricular pacing.

The $T_{peak}-T_{end}$ interval on the surface ECG may not be absolutely equivalent to transmural dispersion of repolarization (TDR), but this interval provides an index of TDR (electrical heterogeneity) if the measurements are limited to precordial leads [23–27]. A great deal of evidence has accumulated in support of the concept that amplification of TDR rather than QT prolongation underlies the substrate responsible for the creation of reentry and the development of polymorphic VT or torsades de pointes (TdP). Thus, TDR may be prognostic of arrhythmic risk under a variety of conditions. Enhanced TDR increases the risk for the development of TdP, probably via two mechanisms. It facilitates early afterdepolarization (EAD) propagation leading to R-on-T ventricular extrasystoles capable of initiating TdP, and it could serve as a reentrant substrate for the maintenance of TdP.

Amplification of the TDR does not cause monomorphic VT because of different underlying mechanisms [23–27]. Most monomorphic VT can be initiated by any type of ventricular beat and can be maintained via a fixed reentrant circuit, for example, ventricular scar. Polymorphic VT or TdP from increased TDR is often initiated by an R-on-T extrasystole in the setting of a functional reentrant circuit. However, not all agents that prolong the QT interval increase TDR. Amiodarone is rarely associated with TdP. Chronic administration of amiodarone produces a greater prolongation of action potential duration (APD) in epicardium and endocardium, but less of an increase, or even a decrease at slow rates, in the M region, thereby reducing TDR.

Experimental Considerations

Using arterially perfused rabbit LV wedge preparation, transmembrane action potentials were recorded simultaneously from several sites using separate intracellular floating microelectrodes [28,29]. A transmural ECG was recorded concurrently. Action potential duration was measured at 90% repolarization. TDR was defined as the difference between the longest and shortest repolarization times across LV wall, which closely approximated $T_{peak}–T_{end}$ interval. Shifting the stimulation site from endocardium to epicardium resulted in a change in activation sequence between epicardium and endocardium with delayed activation and repolarization of the M cells coupled with earlier activation of repolarization of epicardial cells. This was associated with an increase in QT interval and TDR and $T_{peak}–T_{end}$ interval without a parallel increase in endocardial and epicardial transmembrane action potential duration (Fig. 23.1). Although reversal of the direction of activation causes a substantial increase in TDR in both the canine and rabbit LV wedge models under control conditions, this increase is not enough to permit the development of TdP (Fig. 23.2). However, an increase in TDR facilitates the occurrence of polymorphic VT under conditions that prolong ventricular repolarization. Thus, under long QT conditions (class III agent), the shift from endocardial to epicardial pacing at the same cycle length was sufficient to increase the TDR ($T_{peak}–T_{end}$ interval) to the threshold for reentry (which in the canine ventricular wedge is approximately 90 ms) and the resultant development of polymorphic VT with the application of an epicardial extra stimulus with a short coupling interval.

Clinical Evidence

Medina-Ravell et al. [28] measured the TDR in 29 CRT patients during RV endocardial (Endo) pacing and LV epicardial (Epi) pacing but not during biventricular (BiV) pacing (P) because of flattened T-waves in most of the patients. TDRc (c = corrected) was significantly greater during LV epicardial pacing than during RV endocardial pacing (197 ± 26 vs. 163 ± 25 ms, n = 29, p < 0.01). In 4 of 29 patients, BiVP/LVEpiP, which caused a marked increase in TDR (149 ± 19 ms in RVEndoP vs. 220 ± 33 ms in LVEpiP) resulted in frequent R-on-T ventricular extrasystoles (presumably phase 2

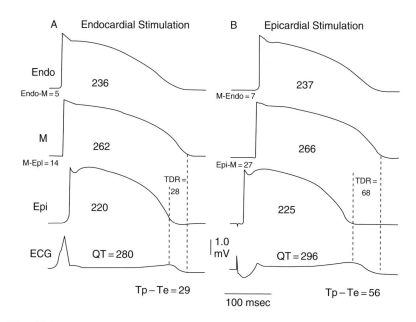

Fig. 23.1 Effect of reversal of transmural sequence of activation in canine left ventricular wedge preparation. Epicardial (*Epi*), endocardial (*Endo*), and M cell action potentials and a transmural ECG were simultaneously recorded during endocardial (**A**) and epicardial (**B**) pacing at a basic cycle length of 2,000 ms. All numbers are in milliseconds. (Reproduced with permission from Fish JM, Brugada J, Antzelevitch C. Potential proarrhythmic effects of biventricular pacing. J Am Coll Cardiol 2005;46:2340–7).

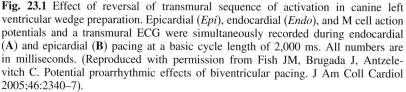

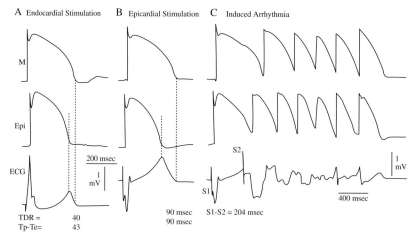

Fig. 23.2 Cisapride [(0.2 μmol/L), a drug with a propensity to cause torsades de pointes because it blocks Ikr] the rapid-delayed rectifying potassium current] induces torsades de pointes during epicardial (*Epi*) but not endocardial stimulation in a LV wedge preparation. Epicardial and M-cell action potentials and a transmural ECG were simultaneously recorded during endocardial (**A**) and epicardial (**B**) pacing of the canine LV wedge preparation at a basic cycle length of 2,000 ms. A polymorphic ventricular tachycardia was induced by an extrastimulus delivered to epicardium at an S_1–S_2 interval of 204 ms (**C**). (Reproduced with permission from Fish JM, Brugada J, Antzelevitch C. Potential proarrhythmic effects of biventricular pacing. J Am Coll Cardiol 2005;46:2340–7).

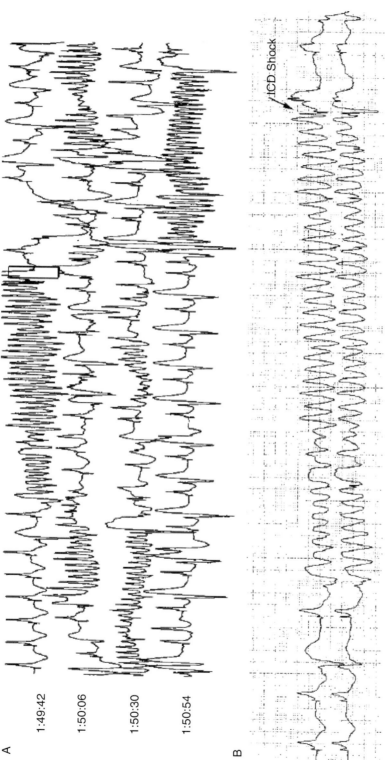

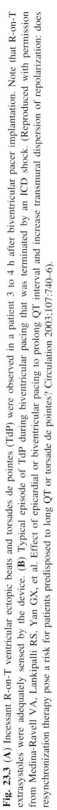

A

1:49:42

1:50:06

1:50:30

1:50:54

B

tICD Shock

Fig. 23.3 (A) Incessant R-on-T ventricular ectopic beats and torsades de pointes (TdP) were observed in a patient 3 to 4 h after biventricular pacer implantation. Note that R-on-T extrasystoles were adequately sensed by the device. **(B)** Typical episode of TdP during biventricular pacing that was terminated by an ICD shock. (Reproduced with permission from Medina-Ravell VA, Lankipalli RS, Yan GX, et al. Effect of epicardial or biventricular pacing to prolong QT interval and increase transmural dispersion of repolarization: does resynchronization therapy pose a risk for patients predisposed to long QT or torsade de pointes? Circulation 2003;107:740–6).

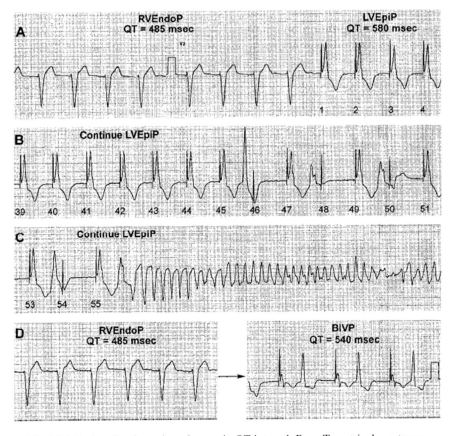

Fig. 23.4 Pacing site–dependent changes in QT interval, R-on-T ventricular extrasystoles, and the onset of torsades de pointes (TdP). Right ventricular (RV) endocardial pacing (RR interval of 840 ms) yielded a QT interval of 485 ms. Immediately after switching to left ventricular (LV) epicardial pacing (mode VOO), the QT interval increased to 580 ms (**A**). Ventricular extrasystoles started at the 46th beat of LV epicardial pacing (**B**) and initiated one episode of TdP at the 55th beat (**C**) that was terminated by an ICD shock. Switching from RV endocardial pacing to biventricular pacing resulted in an increase in QT interval by 55 ms accompanied by R-on-T ventricular extrasystoles (**D**). (Reproduced with permission from Medina-Ravell VA, Lankipalli RS, Yan GX, et al. Effect of epicardial or biventricular pacing to prolong QT interval and increase transmural dispersion of repolarization: does resynchronization therapy pose a risk for patients predisposed to long QT or torsade de pointes? Circulation 2003;107:740–6).

early after depolarizations) that were completely inhibited by RVEndoP. One developed recurrent nonsustained polymorphic VT, another suffered incessant TdP requiring multiple electrical shocks (Figs. 23.3 and 23.4). No new episodes of TdP occurred overnight during RVEndoP. BiVP was resumed the next morning after an event-free night. Numerous episodes of sustained TdP and nonsustained TdP reoccurred 4 h later. Again, switching to RVEndoP completely and immediately suppressed TdP and extrasystoles. The patient was then discharged from the hospital with RVEndoP and returned for follow-up 10 days later without any TdP events. When the device was reprogrammed from RVEndoP to BiVP and to LVEpiP, marked QT prolongation occurred and frequent R-on-T extrasystoles, leading to the development of TdP.

Reference	No pts	Previous smVT	Type VT after CRT	VT control
DiCori et al. [30]	1	No	smVT	D/C LV pacing
Guerra et al. [31]	1	VT ablation No VT in 3 mths	smVT	BiV pacing + amiodarone
Mykytsey et al. [32]	1	VT suppressed by drugs	smVT	D/C LV pacing
Bortone et al. [33]	1	No	smVT	D/C LV pacing
Medina-Ravell et al. [29]	1	Yes	TdP	D/C LV pacing
Turitto et al. [34]	1	No	TdP	D/C LV pacing
Rivero-Ayerza et al. [35]	1	No	TdP	BiV pacing induced no TdP
Shukla et al. [36]	5	Yes in all 5 pts	smVT in 4, polymVT in 1	Temporary control: D/C BiV or LV pacing Long-term control: ablation, amiodarone and resumption of BiV pacing

VT, ventricular tachycardia; smVT = sustained monomorphic VT; TdP, torsades de pointes; LV, left ventricular; BiV, biventricular; pts, patients; mths, months; D/C, discontinuation; polym, polymorphic.

Table 23.2 outlines the documented cases of CRT ventricular proarrhythmia that presented either as sustained monomorphic VT or polymorphic VT (torsades de pointes) precipitated by mainly by epicardial LV and to a lesser degree biventricular pacing [28, 30–36] (Figs. 23.5 and 23.6). VT induced by LV pacing alone could be eliminated by turning off LV pacing, but some cases of LV-induced VT failed to occur during biventricular pacing. The opposite situation was reported by Tanabe et al. [37], who controlled an electrical storm in an ICD patient (with right bundle branch block) by upgrading the system to biventricular pacing.

In some patients, the induction of monomorphic VT by LV or biventricular pacing represents an exacerbation of a previously controlled arrhythmia but in others it appears de novo. The mechanism may involve the early arrival of LV wavefront at a site of slow conduction with resultant unidirectional block, and initiation of reentry. The prevention of VT by biventricular pacing in some cases may be due to the collision of two wavefronts preventing penetration of the reentrant circuit. In contrast, TdP is caused by a different mechanism related to amplified transmural dispersion of repolarization.

Transmural Dispersion of Repolarization Harada et al. [38] showed in man that epicardial LV pacing produces a pronounced prolongation of JTc (interval from the end of depolarization to the end of repolarization in the ventricle) and with a parallel prolongation of $Tc_{peak-end}$ interval. The increases in JTc and $Tc_{peak-end}$ intervals were similar to the enhancement of transmural dispersion of repolarization demonstrated in the experimental studies using LV wedge

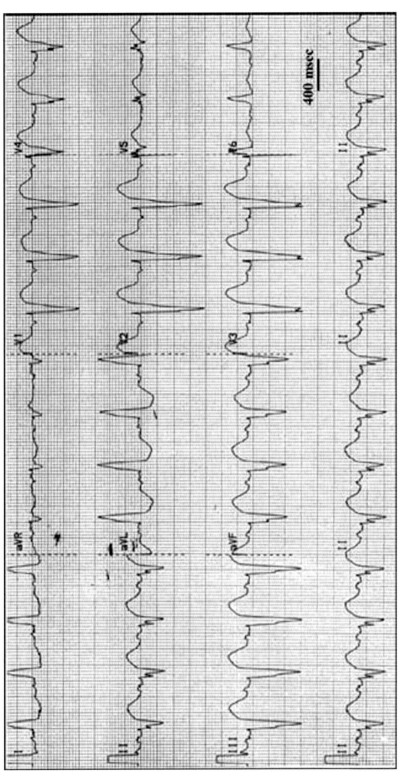

Fig. 23.5 ECG before implantation of a biventricular pacing system (see Fig. 23.6). Heart rate, 92/min; QRS duration, 150 ms; QT interval, 414 ms; corrected QT interval, 468 ms. (Reproduced with permission from Turitto G, Haq S, Benson D, El-Sherif N. Torsade de pointes: an electrophysiological effect of cardiac resynchronization? Pacing Clin Electrophysiol 2006;29:520–2).

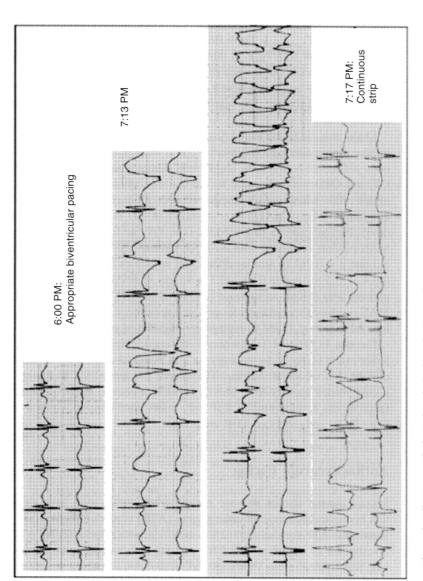

Fig. 23.6 Marked QT prolongation and malignant ventricular tachyarrhythmias a few hours after implantation of a biventricular pacing system in the patient whose preoperative ECG is shown in Figure 23.5. (Reproduced with permission from Turitto G, Haq S, Benson D, El-Sherif N. Torsade de pointes: an electrophysiological effect of cardiac resynchronization? Pacing Clin Electrophysiol 2006;29:520–2).

15. Bardy GH, Lee KL, Mark DB, et al.; Sudden Cardiac Death in Heart Failure Trial (SCD-HeFT) Investigators. Amiodarone or an implantable cardioverter-defibrillator for congestive heart failure. N Engl J Med 2005;352:225–37.

16. Voigt A, Barrington W, Ngwu O, Jain S, Saba S. Biventricular pacing reduces ventricular arrhythmic burden and defibrillator therapies in patients with heart failure. Clin Cardiol 2006;29:74–7.

17. Arya A, Haghjoo M, Dehghani MR, et al. Effect of cardiac resynchronization therapy on the incidence of ventricular arrhythmias in patients with an implantable cardioverter-defibrillator. Heart Rhythm 2005;2:1094–8.

18. Ermis C, Seutter R, Zhu AX, et al. Impact of upgrade to cardiac resynchronization therapy on ventriculararrhythmia frequency in patients with implantable cardioverter-defibrillators. J Am Coll Cardiol 2005;46:2258–63.

19. Zagrodzky JD, Ramaswamy K, Page RL, et al. Biventricular pacing decreases the inducibility of ventricular tachycardia in patients with ischemic cardiomyopathy. Am J Cardiol 2001;87:1208–10.

20. Kowal RC, Wasmund SL, Smith ML, et al. Biventricular pacing reduces the induction of monomorphic ventricular tachycardia: a potential mechanism for arrhythmia suppression. Heart Rhythm 2004;1:295–300.

21. Kies P, Bax JJ, Molhoek SG, et al. Effect of cardiac resynchronization therapy on inducibility of ventricular tachyarrhythmias in cardiac arrest survivors with either ischemic or idiopathic dilated cardiomyopathy. Am J Cardiol 2005;95:1111–4.

22. McSwain RL, Schwartz RA, DeLurgio DB, Mera FV, Langberg JJ, Leon AR. The impact of cardiac resynchronization therapy on ventricular tachycardia/fibrillation: an analysis from the combined Contak-CD and InSync-ICD studies. J Cardiovasc Electrophysiol 2005;16:1168–71.

23. Fish JM, Brugada J, Antzelevitch C. Potential proarrhythmic effects of biventricular pacing. J Am Coll Cardiol 2005;46:2340–7.

24. Antzelevitch C, Oliva A. Amplification of spatial dispersion of repolarization underlies sudden cardiac death associated with catecholaminergic polymorphic VT, long QT, short QT and Brugada syndromes. J Intern Med 2006;259:48–58.

25. Antzelevitch C. Cardiac repolarization. The long and short of it. Europace 2005; 7:Suppl 2:3–9.

26. Antzelevitch C. Modulation of transmural repolarization. Ann N Y Acad Sci 2005; 1047:314–23.

27. Antzelevitch C. Cellular basis and mechanism underlying normal and abnormal myocardial repolarization and arrhythmogenesis. Ann Med 2004;36(Suppl 1): 5–14.

28. Fish JM, Di Diego JM, Nesterenko V, Antzelevitch C. Epicardial activation of left ventricular wall prolongs QT interval and transmural dispersion of repolarization: implications for biventricular pacing. Circulation 2004;109:2136–42.

29. Medina-Ravell VA, Lankipalli RS, Yan GX, et al. Effect of epicardial or biventricular pacing to prolong QT interval and increase transmural dispersion of repolarization: does resynchronization therapy pose a risk for patients predisposed to long QT or torsade de pointes? Circulation 2003;107:740–6.

30. Di Cori A, Bongiorni MG, Arena G, et al. New-onset ventricular tachycardia after cardiac resynchronization therapy. J Interv Card Electrophysiol 2005;12:231–5.

31. Guerra JM, Wu J, Miller JM, Groh WJ. Increase in ventricular tachycardia frequency after biventricular implantable cardioverter defibrillator upgrade. J Cardiovasc Electrophysiol 2003;14:1245–7.

32. Mykytsey A, Maheshwari P, Dhar G, et al. Ventricular tachycardia induced by biventricular pacing in patient with severe ischemic cardiomyopathy. J Cardiovasc Electrophysiol 2005;16:655–8.

33. Bortone A, Macia JC, Leclercq F, Pasquie JL. Monomorphic ventricular tachycardia induced by cardiac resynchronization therapy in patient with severe nonischemic dilated cardiomyopathy. Pacing Clin Electrophysiol 2006;29:327–30.

34. Turitto G, Haq S, Benson D, El-Sherif N. Torsade de pointes: an electro-physiological effect of cardiac resynchronization? Pacing Clin Electrophysiol 2006;29:520–2.

35. Rivero-Ayerza M, Vanderheyden M, Verstreken S, de Zutter M, Geelen P, Brugada P. Images in cardiovascular medicine. Polymorphic ventricular tachy-cardia induced by left ventricular pacing.Circulation 2004;109:2924–5.

36. Shukla G, Chaudhry GM, Orlov M, Hoffmeister P, Haffajee C. Potential proar-rhythmic effect of biventricular pacing: fact or myth? Heart Rhythm 2005;2:951–6.

37. Tanabe Y, Chinushi M, Washizuka T, et al. Suppression of electrical storm by biventricular pacing in a patient with idiopathic dilated cardiomyopathy and ventricular tachycardia. Pacing Clin Electrophysiol 2003;26:101–2.

38. Harada M, Osaka T, Yokoyama E, Takemoto Y, Ito A, Kodama I. Biven-tricular pacing has an advantage over left ventricular epicardial pacing alone to minimize proarrhythmic perturbation of repolarization. J Cardiovasc Electro-physiol 2006;17:151–6.

39. Berger T, Hanser F, Hintringer F, et al. Effects of cardiac resynchronization therapy on ventricular repolarization in patients with congestive heart failure. J Cardiovasc Electrophysiol 2005;16:611–7.

40. Bai R, Yang XY, Song Y, et al. Impact of left ventricular epicardial and biventricular pacing on ventricular repolarization in normal-heart individuals and patients with congestive heartfailure. Europace 2006;8:1002–10.

41. van Huysduynen BH, Swenne CA, Bax JJ, et al. Dispersion of repolarization in cardiac resynchronization therapy. Heart Rhythm 2005;2:1286–93.

42. Chalil S, Yousef ZR, Muyhaldeen SA, et al. Pacing-induced increase in QT dispersion predicts sudden cardiac death following cardiac resynchronization therapy. J Am Coll Cardiol 2006;47:2486–92.

43. Garrigue S, Barold SS, Hocini M, Jais P, Haissaguerre M, Clementy J. Treatment of drug refractory ventricular tachycardia by biventricular pacing.Pacing Clin Electrophysiol 2000;23:1700–2.

44. Byrd IA, Rogers JM, Smith WM, Pollard AE. Comparison of conventional and biventricular antitachycardia pacing in a geometrically realistic model of the rabbit ventricle. J Cardiovasc Electrophysiol 2004;15:1066–77.

45. Kuhlkamp V; InSync 7272 ICD World Wide Investigators. Initial experience with an implantable cardioverter-defibrillator incorporating cardiac resynchronization therapy. J Am Coll Cardiol 2002;39:790–7.

46. Fernandez Lozano I, Higgins S, Escudier Villa JM, et al. Antitachycardia pacing efficacy significantly improves with cardiac resynchronization therapy. Rev Esp Cardiol 2005;58:1148–54.

Parasympathetic nervous system mediates its chronotropic effect by acetyl-choline release from the postganglionic neurons arising from the vagus nerve. Its effect is mainly on increasing the beat-to-beat cycle length in response to cardiopulmonary afferents via the respiratory center. The strong vagal input accounts for the high-frequency cyclic fluctuations in heart rate during ventilations [7]. In addition to positive chronotropic effect, sympathetic stimulation would increase cardiac inotropy by stimulating beta-adrenergic receptors. However, sympathetic stimulation would preferentially induce a low-frequency effect on heart rate and eventually reduce HRV [8]. The observed heart rate changes are the balance between these two autonomic systems. Apart from the autonomic modulation, HRV, especially the circadian changes during day and night, is also mediated through a complex and poorly understood neurohormonal mechanism (e.g., angiotensin II) [9].

The balance between the sympathetic and parasympathetic systems can be measured by the heart rate changes over certain period of time (i.e., HRV). It reflects the response of the neural control on the cardiovascular system when facing physiologic stress (e.g., myocardial infarction or heart failure exacerbation). There is a shift of HRV to an increase in sympathetic input and/or parasympathetic withdrawal in the presence of stressors. As a matter of fact, HRV has been evaluated in large-scale clinical trials and was a predictor of mortality after myocardial infarction and heart failure [10–12].

In simple terms, HRV can be arbitrarily classified as high or low. A low HRV usually refers to the condition of sympathetic predominance and represents the presence of stress, and indicates a high risk of lethal events. Patients are in relatively higher heart rate with little change over time. A high HRV is characterized by strong vagal tone and usually associates with lower risk of death or significant arrhythmia. However, acute changes in HRV can be a response to physiologic condition (e.g., exercise and posture). Therefore a continuous recording of heart rate changes over time is necessary to avoid these acute influences. The most common method to collect heart rate changes is a 24-h recording by Holter, and the ways to quantify HRV would include time domain, frequency domain, geometric, and nonlinear methods. There are obvious limitations to collect HRV information from 24-h Holter. It requires the clear acquisition of R-R interval by surface ECG in order to calculate time domain HRV. ECG with poor quality would definitely limit its utility. Moreover, HRV is a dynamic process and does not just vary over a 24-h period of time but rather over days or weeks indeed. A snapshot of HRV in 1 day may not be precise enough to predict an acute event, for example, heart failure decompensation, which is considered an important objective in heart failure management nowadays. A continuous monitoring is the most desirable method. However, it is not practical to ask the patients to have repeated daily measurement. HRV measurements based on intracardiac electrograms recorded in an implantable device seem to be the solution to the limitation by Holter recording. The R-R or P-P intervals (i.e., time domain analysis of HRV) can then be retrieved from the device for further analysis. In a CRT device, P-P interval obviously is the parameter of choice to determine continuous HRV in these patients with advanced heart failure.

Time Domain Analysis of HRV

In time domain analysis, the intervals of adjacent normal R-waves (NN interval) are measured over a period of time. In CRT, the intrinsic or sensed

P-waves would be used instead as continuous biventricular pacing is necessary for obvious reasons. A variety of statistical variables can be calculated from these NN intervals and other parameters can then be derived from the differences between these intervals.

SDNN, the standard deviation of measured NN interval over period of time, is the most commonly used time domain measure of HRV in general. Accurate measurements of SDNN require vigorous editing to exclude artifacts, ectopic or missed beats. Otherwise, SDNN may be substantially increased by these events. It is probably not the most appropriate and convenient parameter to reflect device-based HRV assessment. The SDANN, the standard deviation of average intrinsic interval over 5-min [13], and SDAAM, the standard deviation of the 5-min median A-A interval [14], are the two more practical and useful parameters to assess device-based HRV. They smooth out the acute changes and minimize the adverse effect of artifacts or ectopic beats on estimated HRV.

Effect of CRT on HRV

The recipients of CRT are, in general, in the advanced stage of heart failure with worse functional class and low LV ejection fraction. Diminished HRV and high mean heart rates in these patients were associated with poor prognosis [15, 16]. Previous beta-blocker trials in patients with severe heart failure have shown that the time domain parameters of HRV and the mean heart rates were improved together with the prognosis [17]. It is of great clinical interest to know whether a comparable change in HRV or autonomic control can be observed in these patients after CRT.

The standard deviation of the atrial cycle length using 10 beats/min device-based histogram resolution over a 2-month period was used in early study to assess HRV in patients with CRT [18]. In the pilot phase of the Multicenter InSync Randomized Clinical Evaluation trial [1], patients were randomized to pacing therapy ON and OFF mode and the time domain parameters of HRV were compared between the two groups. The HRV in those randomized to pacing ON group was significantly higher than that of the pacing OFF group. Furthermore, the mean atrial cycle length had no difference between the two groups suggesting that CRT favorably shifted the cardiac autonomic balance toward less sympathetic dominance. This is the first study measuring HRV from the data collected via CRT in patients with severe heart failure. This study also formed the basis for HRV assessment in CRT device to delineate autonomic control over cardiovascular system in high-risk patients. However, the parameter chosen in this study may not be sensitive enough in recording small but meaningful changes of mean heart rates and time domain parameters of HRV. Moreover, it only reflected the early changes in HRV by CRT but did not provide any information about long-term effect and prognostic value of device-based HRV.

With advances in technology and increased storage capability, continuous sampling of heart rate changes and automatic calculation of time domain parameters of HRV become feasible in the recent generation of CRT devices. The SDANN of the 288 5-min segments of a day and heart rate profiles in 113 patients with CRT devices were evaluated in a long-term study [13]. The results confirmed that CRT induced a reduction of minimum and mean heart rates and an increase in SDANN at 3 months time. Interestingly, the improvement in SDANN reached a plateau at an earlier stage than those of mean and minimum heart rates. The most salient finding of this particular study was that lack of HRV improvement as early as 4 weeks after the implantation could identify patients at higher risk for major cardiovascular events. The 2-year event-free survival rate for those with improved or no change in SDANN was 94% compared with 62% in those with worsened SDANN. When classifying responders to CRT as those with favorable SDANN changes, those with an increase in HRV were associated with significant improvement in peak oxygen consumption, LV ejection fraction, and LV end-diastolic diameter. In other words, HRV changes showed a strong and significant correlation with the structural and physiologic improvements in these patients with advanced heart failure after CRT (Fig. 24.1).

Prognostic Value of HRV in CRT

It is well-known that patients with severe heart failure are associated with significant morbidity and mortality. Apart from the high mortality due to pump failure or ventricular arrhythmic events, these patients also had frequent cardiovascular or heart failure–related hospitalizations. Prevention of hospitalization due to decompensation is one of the many goals in heart failure management nowadays. In fact, among the huge health-care burden for the management of heart failure, more than two-thirds of the expenses were spent on the treatment of acute heart failure exacerbation [19]. Hospital admission does not only increase the health care cost but, most importantly, also adversely affects the quality of life and possibly results in a worse long-term outcome. Therefore, when determining the prognostic value of certain parameters, they can grossly be divided into short-term and long-term, which represent the predictability of acute decompensation (e.g., hospitalization) and significant cardiovascular events (e.g., death), respectively.

As mentioned in previous section, Fantoni et al. reported the long-term prognostic value of device-based HRV in identifying patients at higher risk for major cardiovascular events [13]. Patients with lack of favorable changes in SDANN at 4 weeks after implantation were at significant risk of all-cause mortality, cardiovascular hospitalization, and heart transplantation than those with improved or no change in SDANN. Adamson et al. also reported the usefulness of SDAAM from the device to predict long-term prognosis [14]. The parameter was collected as an average over 4 weeks time 1 month after the implantation. Of the 397 patients in the clinical trial, those with SDAAM <50 ms had significantly higher all-cause and cardiovascular mortality with a hazard ratio of 3.2 and 4.43, respectively. When averaging the SDAAM from week 5 to 52 after device implantation, patients who died or were hospitalized had lower SDAAM than those with minor or no clinical events. It is now quite clear that the continuous or long-term autonomic assessment by HRV derived from CRT device can provide valuable information about the neural control on the cardiovascular system and should be considered as a clinical tool helping to risk-stratify patients with end-stage heart failure. In patients with persistently low HRV after CRT, repositioning of suboptimal LV lead [13] or other methods to optimize the resynchronization therapy, aggressive intervention, or early planning for heart transplantation are deemed appropriate.

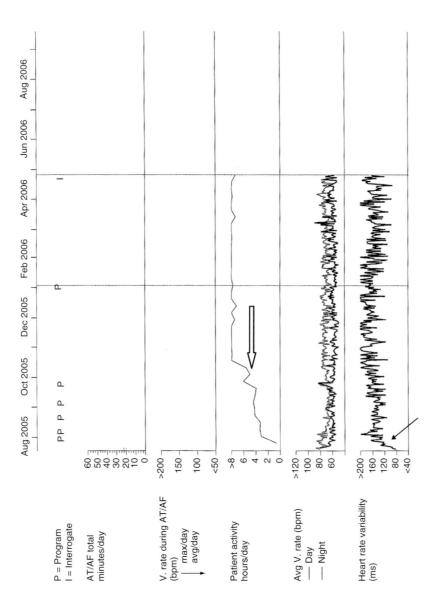

Fig. 24.1 The short- and long-term changes of heart rate variability (HRV) and activity log in a patient with CRT-D are shown. The patient was 56-year-old male with the device implanted in July 2005. There was a gradual increase in HRV as early as 4 weeks after the procedure (*arrow*) from 80 ms to 160 ms in August 2005. Parallel improvement in activity log (*open arrow*) was also observed with a plateau reached 3 months after CRT-D. The patient had no hospitalization or major cardiovascular events throughout the 7-month period. Echocardiographic examination showed significant improvement in ejection fraction, and the patient was a responder to CRT.

Determining short-term prognosis for heart failure hospitalization or precise prediction of upcoming heart failure decompensation is a clinical challenge. However, the clinical benefit of such prediction is obvious and valuable as early and appropriate intervention, for example, titrating up the dose of diuretic, may be able to abort symptomatic heart failure decompensation or even hospitalization. It does not only improve the morbidity but also potentially helps to reduce health care cost. HRV may have an important role in predicting such events. There was a significant decline in SDAAM in 34 patients who were hospitalized during the study period from 76 ± 27 ms to 64 ± 26 ms at the time of hospitalization [14]. The change in SDAAM was apparent around 3 weeks before hospital admission. With a threshold of 200 ms day, a 70% sensitivity rate was associated with a 2.4 false-positive events per patient-year follow-up. In addition, the true positive detection was not affected by the use or not of beta-blockers. Night heart rate changes (75 ± 11 bpm to 78 ± 11 bpm) were also observed in this study, but the magnitude of changes and estimated sensitivity were not comparable with that of SDAAM. It seems that continuous HRV assessment from the device is able to provide early warning signs to clinicians for more frequent follow-up and volume management in these high-risk patients. However, its role in preventing hospitalization or improving morbidity is still not clear, and whether its predictability for heart failure decompensation is comparable with other established parameters (e.g., intrathoracic impedance or central hemodynamic sensors) remain undetermined. A prospective clinical trial is needed to determine the role of HRV in preventing hospitalization in the future.

Limitations of Device-Based HRV

Device-based HRV assessment requires detection of intrinsic or sensed P-wave for calculation. A minimum of 20% of sinus rhythm over a 24-h period of time is required for estimation of SDAAM. Therefore, the most obvious limitation of its application is in those with atrial fibrillation and atrial pacing dependence. A lower atrial pacing rate (e.g., 40 bpm) is necessary in the MIRACLE trial in order to collect meaningful HRV data. Around 15–30% of patients with severe dilated cardiomyopathy were in atrial fibrillation [20], and the use of beta-blockers in heart failure may further aggravate the issue of atrial pacing dependency. Other parameters apart from HRV are needed to risk-stratify these patients.

Summary of Clinical Utility of Device-Based HRV

Device-based HRV is an important marker of autonomic condition in patients with severe heart failure. The short- and long-term prognostic value of device-based HRV in these patients is well established. It can help identify patients at significantly higher risk for major clinical events or even mortality. Furthermore, HRV can provide early warning signs and help to determine how intensively the patients should come back for clinical assessment and receive appropriate interventions. Continuous HRV now becomes feasible due to technological advances. Transmission of HRV data via the Internet may provide additional clinically relevant information to facilitate decision-making even when patients are staying at home. Appropriate interventions based on this information may help to reduce the probability of frequent hospitalization so that the morbidity of patients can be improved substantially and the health care cost may be reduced.

Activity Status

Exercise intolerance is a common feature in patients with heart failure. Various tests to assess the exercise tolerance in a laboratory-controlled setting have confirmed their prognostic value in patients with systolic heart failure. Six-minute corridor walking distance and exercise capacity measured as metabolic equivalent by modified Bruce protocol during treadmill tests are valuable tools to assess submaximal exercise tolerance in these patients with advanced heart failure. Interestingly, the severity of heart failure as measured by LV ejection fraction had little correlation with maximal exercise capacity [21], and changes in maximal exercise tolerance also did not have any relationship with the changes in quality of life in patients receiving specific heart failure treatment [22]. Perhaps tests in which patients decide their own workload can reflect the degree of symptomatic impairment. Normal daily activity levels measured by pedometers were dramatically reduced in patients with chronic heart failure and were predictive of mortality [23]. In this early study, patients were requested to wear the pedometers around the hips. These pedometers were designed to display output as proportional to the movements of a vertically placed pendulum. The output measured by the pedometers represented the cumulated number of footsteps by the patients. Reduced levels of daily activity measured by the pedometers were even more predictive of death in chronic heart failure than the conventional exercise tolerance parameters. Although the role of daily activity to predict survival in these patients is established, the implication of this parameter for heart failure exacerbation is still unclear. Theoretically, patients with upcoming heart failure decompensation should have reductions in daily activity, and it may be a useful early warning sign for necessary intervention. However, such hypothesis has not been evaluated in a prospective trial.

Nowadays, patients' activity level can be measured by an activity sensor or accelerometer sensors in an implanted device. Rather than measuring number of footsteps, a mean daily physical activity (MDPA) index was established to measure the time in minutes per day with physical activity greater than 70 steps per minute walk rate. A sustained increase in MDPA was observed in a clinical trial assessing the effect of CRT on this index in 56 patients with NYHA class II to IV [24]. There was significant improvement in daily activity levels irrespective of baseline NYHA class after CRT. The most dramatic improvement, however, was observed in those with baseline NYHA class II patients as early as 2 weeks after CRT. The results were not entirely unexpected as the other parameters evaluating the exercise tolerance of these patients have already confirmed the beneficial of role of CRT in this aspect. More importantly, the MDPA index retrieved from the device correlated with the improvement in heart failure and may have the potential to monitor patients' response to the therapy received (Fig. 24.1). This measurement may also be applicable in other devices (e.g., conventional pacemaker or defibrillators) as well.

As mentioned, it is even more beneficial for any parameters that are predictive of upcoming heart failure decompensation or hospitalization. The role of MDPA index to predict such events has been evaluated and compared with SDAAM, the time domain measure of HRV, and the nigh heart rate changes in one study [14]. MDPA decreased significantly from 188 ± 109 to 164 ± 118 min/day at the time of hospitalization. However, the sensitivity of MDPA was lower than that of SDAAM to predict hospitalization over the entire range of false-positive rates. Its role in predicting heart failure exacerbation is probably complementary to other parameters (e.g., HRV or intrathoracic impedance).

Intrathoracic Impedance

Heart failure exacerbation and hospitalization accounts for a significant proportion of health care budget and adversely affects quality of life in patients with systolic heart failure. Factors leading to heart failure decompensation are diverse (e.g., progression of the disease, suboptimal medical therapy, drug noncompliance, failure or inability to detect worsened heart failure). Symptoms of heart failure exacerbation include shortness of breath, ankle edema, paroxysmal nocturnal dyspnea and orthopnea, and so forth, and pulmonary congestion is one of the important clinical features. Prevention of heart failure hospitalization is one of the many goals in current heart failure management. In theory, early and accurate prediction of upcoming deterioration and delivery of appropriate intervention may be able to reverse the decompensation and abort the hospitalization. Monitoring of symptoms, volume status, body weight, or change in ventricular performance by means of frequent visit and physical examination for heart failure patients is recommended as part of the management program. However, none of these measures showed promising impact on heart failure morbidity [25,26]. In addition, both symptoms and physical signs are not reliable or early enough for prediction of heart failure exacerbation [27,28]. Search for other parameters is necessary for precise prediction and prevention of hospitalization.

In general, fluid accumulates when heart failure decompensation is developing. Elevated left atrial pressure would lead to pulmonary interstitial congestion and eventually pulmonary edema. As the conductance of fluid is much higher than air in the alveoli, the transthoracic impedance would decrease as heart failure worsens. As a result, measurement of transthoracic impedance may be able to detect early stage of heart failure exacerbation. This concept was first evaluated by the noninvasive transthoracic setting in animal studies [29,30]. Preliminary data showed that such measurement was proportional to the degree of pulmonary congestion and confirmed its feasibility. In human studies, the transthoracic impedance correlated well with the changes in clinical and radiologic evidence of pulmonary edema [31]. It has also been suggested that transthoracic impedance measurement can be a valuable tool in the emergency department for diagnosis of fluid overload [32]. However, transthoracic impedance measured transcutaneously has several limitations including lack of reproducibility, poor sensitivity and specificity, unpredictable effect of different skin impedance with different electrode placements, and so forth [33,34].

Feasibility of Intrathoracic Impedance Measurement

Intrathoracic measurement may circumvent the limitations by transcutaneous route. Intrathoracic impedance measured by implanting a modified pacemaker in a heart failure canine model correlated well with the level of pulmonary congestion and hemodynamic parameter [35]. An implantable cardioverter-defibrillator (ICD) lead was positioned into the right ventricle and connected to a modified pacemaker capable of measuring impedance. Impedance was measured from the ICD lead using the pathway of right ventricular (RV) ring electrode to device case for current stimulation and RV coil to device case for voltage measurement. The LV end-diastolic pressure in the canine was measured by the pressure sensor lead in the left ventricle, which was connected to an implantable hemodynamic device. Both the intrathoracic impedance and LV end-diastolic pressure data were collected before, during, and after heart failure as induced by rapid RV pacing. There was a significant correlation between the measured intrathoracic impedance and the hemodynamic parameters in all phases, confirming the feasibility of such measurement in an animal setting and the potential role in detecting pulmonary congestion in early stage of exacerbation.

Prediction of Heart Failure Exacerbation

The relationship between measured intrathoracic impedance and degree of pulmonary congestion in humans was assessed in a clinical trial with 34 patients who were in NYHA functional class III or IV with a history of recurrent heart failure hospitalization [36]. Similar to the animal study, a conventional ICD lead was inserted transvenously to the RV apex and was connected into a modified pacemaker. A constant current was sent via the RV coil electrode to the device case, and the voltage was then measured to calculate the intrathoracic impedance. Instead of direct measurement of LV end-diastolic pressure, pulmonary capillary wedge pressure was determined by transvenous Swan–Ganz catheter once patients were hospitalized for decompensated heart failure. There were a total of 24 hospitalizations in 9 patients in this study. Intrathoracic impedance started to decrease and provided early warning with a mean lead time of 18 days prior to admission while the symptom onset occurred only 3 days before hospitalization (Fig. 24.2). A significant reduction of impedance from the reference baseline was noted on the day before hospitalization. During the hospitalization period, the intrathoracic impedance correlated significantly with the pulmonary capillary wedge pressure and net fluid loss with diuretic therapy. The device-measured intrathoracic impedance may also serve as a surrogate measure of pulmonary fluid status in heart failure patients. Using 60 Ω-day as the nominal threshold, the device has a sensitivity of 76.9% at the cost of 1.5 false-positives per patient-year of monitoring and gives an early warning of 13.4 ± 6.2 days before heart failure hospitalization.

This is the first landmark study confirming the strong relationship between intrathoracic impedance measurement and degree of pulmonary congestion and its predictive potential for heart failure decompensation. A 13.4-day early warning by intrathoracic impedance monitoring ahead of the symptom onset for heart failure hospitalization may allow clinical intervention such as fluid restriction or medication adjustment to prevent hospital admission. Furthermore, the measurement may act as a guide to therapy

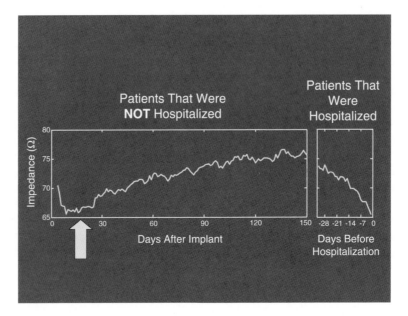

Fig. 24.2 The mean changes in intrathoracic impedance between the patients hospitalized or not are shown [36]. For those without hospitalization (*left*), there was a drop in the impedance measured right after the implantation due to pocket edema (*arrow*). It rose above 70 Ω 30 days after the procedure. The mean changes in impedance 28 days before the hospitalization are shown on the *right* side. At around 14 days before hospitalization, the mean impedance dropped below 70Ω

after hospitalization to ensure optimal volume status and avoid overdiuresis (Fig. 24.3). From the technical point of view, the intrathoracic impedance can be measured via the conventional ICD or CRT system without the need of additional lead implantation. The latter issue seems to be superior to the central hemodynamic monitor [37].

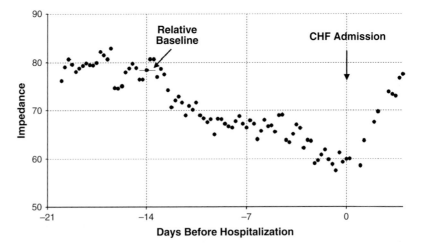

Fig. 24.3 An example of the changes in intrathoracic impedance around 14 days before heart failure hospitalization is shown. With diuretic therapy and resolution of pulmonary edema, the impedance was gradually increased back to the baseline reference.

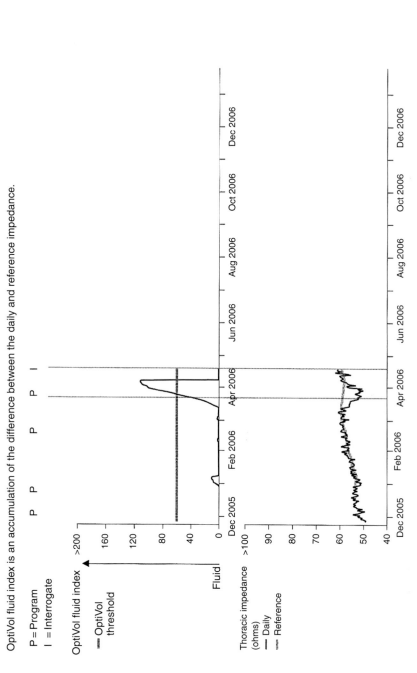

Fig. 24.4 The changes in fluid index and thoracic impedance in a 70-year-old male with CRT-D are shown. The patient received the device in November 2005. There was an episode of heart failure hospitalization in April 2006. A dramatic increase in fluid index above the threshold (60 Ω·days) was noted. The fluid index and the measured intrathoracic impedance returned to baseline or reference ranges after diuretic therapy.

The intrathoracic impedance measurement is now one of the key diagnostic parameters in the recent generation of CRT with defibrillator function (CRT-D). A *reference impedance* value was established as the average of daily impedance measurements. The reference impedance was used to quantify the magnitude and duration of any transient impedance reductions leading up to hospitalization. An automated algorithm for detection of transient decreases in impedance prior to heart failure admission was developed. On days when the measured impedance was less than the reference impedance, the difference between the measured impedance and the reference impedance was accumulated to produce the output of the algorithm, the *fluid index* (Fig. 24.4). Although this index has now been incorporated in daily use when interrogating the device, its value in aborting heart failure hospitalization by appropriate intervention has not yet been tested in prospective clinical trials. There are at least two multicenter clinical trials planned to recruit more than 1,000 patients to assess the efficacy of intrathoracic impedance monitoring with the alert algorithm on the prediction of heart failure events in patients with ICD indication.

Limitations of Intrathoracic Impedance

There are several conditions other than pulmonary congestion that would lead to a decrease in intrathoracic impedance measured by the device (i.e., false-positive events). As the measured impedance reflects the conductivity of the tissue between right ventricle and the device case, conditions that change the conduction property would potentially affect this diagnostic parameter. Thus, chronic lung disorder, chest infection, pocket infection, or even pulmonary embolism in patients may cause erroneous measurement. Cautious interpretation and careful consideration of a patient's coexisting medical condition is necessary in order to make a correct diagnosis. However, not all of the false detections occurred in the absence of the need for intervention. Anecdotally, "false-positive" detections by diuretic changes, pneumonia, and dietary noncompliance may in fact be worthy of medical attention.

Summary of Device Diagnostics

The relative merits and limitations of the three diagnostic parameters in CRT devices are displayed in Table 24.1. The mean and night heart rates are also the diagnostic features of CRT devices that may be able to monitor heart failure progression though their specificity and sensitivity are still not satisfactory. It is apparent that intrathoracic impedance and HRV can provide relatively reliable and early warning parameters to alert clinicians for upcoming heart failure exacerbation or hospitalization. The window provided by both parameters is sufficiently early to allow appropriate intervention to abort the deterioration, though data from prospective clinical trials are still pending. On the other hand, the sensitivity of activity log seems to be suboptimal. With regard to guiding therapy after heart failure hospitalization, supporting data by impedance method is available while HRV may have a potential role. It is very unlikely that activity log plays a key role in this particular aspect during the inpatient period. However, HRV has the most convincing data to support

Table 24.1 Summary of merits and limitations of the three diagnostic parameters in CRT.

	Heart rate variability	Activity log	Intrathoracic impedance
Parameters measured	SDAAM/SDANN	MDPA measured as time (min) per day with walk rate >70 steps/min	Intrathoracic impedance between RV apex and left pectoral device case across the left lung
Measuring tools	Sensed P-wave by atrial lead	Accelerometer sensor	Conventional ICD RV lead
HF exacerbation detection performance (per patient-year follow up)	70% sensitivity/2.4 false-positive events	50% sensitivity/approx. 2.2 false-positive events	77% sensitivity/1.5 false-positive events
Early alert capability	Median of 16 days [14]	NA	15.3 ± 10.6 days [36]
Conditions other than HF that may potentially affect the measurement	Any physiologic stress, e.g., major cardiovascular events, sepsis	Any conditions resulting in impairment in physical activity, e.g., major cardio/ cerebrovascular or respiratory disorders	Chronic lung disorder, chest infection, pocket infection, pulmonary embolism
Guide for therapy after HF hospitalization	NA, possible	NA, but unlikely	Yes
Monitor response to CRT	Yes	Yes	NA, but unlikely
Long-term prognostic value after CRT	Yes	NA	NA

SDANN, the standard deviation of average intrinsic interval over 5-minute; SDAAM, the standard deviation of the 5-min median A-A interval; MDPA, mean daily physical activity; RV, right ventricle; HF, heart failure; ICD, implantable cardioverter-defibrillator; NA, not available.

its role as a long-term prognosticator after CRT. It may even be a significant marker of response to CRT [13].

Device Diagnostics in Clinical Practice

Care of heart failure patients is never an easy task. The disease itself is a complex and dynamic condition characterized by marked morbidity and mortality. Even though proven pharmacological therapy has been available for a long time, underuse of these medications in the community is still rather common [38]. It has been shown that patients with suboptimal medical therapy were associated with less improvement by CRT [39]. Poor drug and fluid compliance, natural progression of the disease, development of atrial or ventricular arrhythmia, and exacerbation of other comorbid conditions are some of the common causes leading to decompensation or hospitalization. Failure to reduce hospitalization rates was still observed despite adopting a structured community-based heart failure program [40]. Methods to closely monitor, predict, and prevent heart failure exacerbation are imminently necessary to reduce the hospitalization, morbidity, or even mortality in these high-risk patients. As a matter of fact, the concepts of predicting the deterioration and long-term prognosis by heart rate changes, physical activity, or lung impedance are not really contemporary issues. The major limitation is how to provide a convenient, safe, and reliable platform for continuous monitoring. CRT does not just open a new treatment area for a subset of heart failure patients with significant electromechanical dyssynchrony but also, as an implantable device, provides such a platform to capture, analyze, and transfer this vital information for better patient care.

Apart from conventional device interrogation to ensure its integrity, follow-up visits for every CRT patient become more complex than ever due to advances in technology and device diagnostics. Cumulative data on HRV or activity log can help to monitor the response to CRT in addition to NYHA class assessment, symptom score, and echocardiographic examination. Lack of improvement in HRV and other parameters should alert the clinician to the possibility of suboptimal LV placement/performance or RV-LV timing in the device. Proper interventions (e.g., LV lead reposition or epicardial placement) should be considered accordingly. For those at ultrahigh risk as suggested by lack of sustained HRV improvement, early revision of aggressive therapy or even heart transplantation should also be considered. Detection of both symptomatic and asymptomatic arrhythmic events is also part of device interrogation nowadays. Development of atrial fibrillation (AF) is a common cause of hemodynamic deterioration in these patients (Fig. 24.5). Even though the incidence of AF appears lower in patients with CRT [41], proper treatment especially anticoagulation is absolutely necessary to prevent thromboembolism. In addition, monitoring the response to therapy for AF (e.g., antiarrhythmic drugs or ablation) can now also be retrieved from the device, the so-called AF burden.

Although detectable changes in device-derived HRV and intrathoracic impedance monitoring have been shown to occur around 2 weeks before hospitalization, the ways to alert physicians is a particular challenge. In other words, transmission of these continuously collecting data to clinicians' attention is necessary in order to decide the nature of the events and delivery of appropriate intervention to prevent the exacerbation. Telemonitoring via Internet is now the working direction. The idea of home telemonitoring allows frequent assessment of patients' clinical status and provides diagnostic information. Early signs of heart failure exacerbation may be detected by telemonitoring. The mean duration of hospital stay has been shown to be reduced by this approach in a recent study [42]. Application of this remote patient management by modern technology may further enhance the efficacy of hemodynamic and impedance monitoring systems in these implantable devices to improve the quality of life, reduce hospitalization and even mortality rates in patients with heart failure. Such application has been tested in the implantable hemodynamic monitoring system. The stored hemodynamic data in the device was read-out by radiofrequency transmission to a secure centralized server where data are maintained and reviewed by

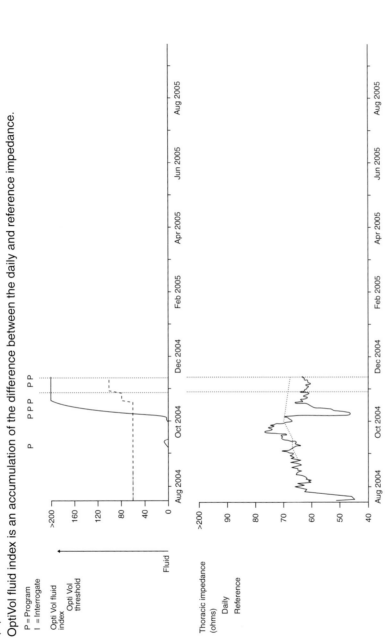

Fig. 24.5 An episode of heart failure exacerbation due to development of atrial fibrillation. There was surge in fluid index over 200 Ω-days in October 2004 (**A**). The cause of decompensation and pulmonary edema was due to the episode of atrial fibrillation and fast ventricular response, as shown in (**B**). Note there was a corresponding decrease in activity level during the exacerbation.

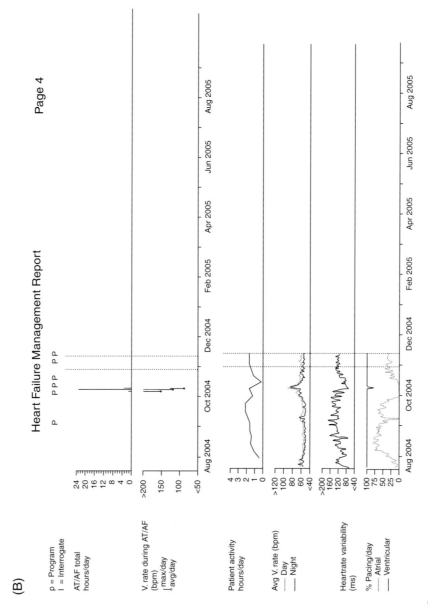

Fig. 24.5 (*Continued*)

clinicians through the Internet [43]. Further exploration and evaluation of applying the telemonitoring concept in impedance monitoring for heart failure management program is warranted.

With telemonitoring via the Internet, HRV may have a role to determine the frequency of follow-up [44]. For those with high HRV, clinic visit once in 3–4 months is acceptable with remote monitoring. In those with HRV less than 50 ms, close monitoring in 2–4 weeks time is needed. In case there is a persistent decline in HRV for a week, patients should be called back, and adjustment of the medical therapies may be necessary. Similarly, when the intrathoracic impedance drops below the reference baseline or the fluid index is persistently above 60 Ωdays, patients should come back for detailed assessment. Furthermore, the impedance derived from the device can also act as a guide to titrate the dose of diuretic therapy to relieve pulmonary congestion and minimize the risk of overdiuresis or even to help decide the proper date of discharge in addition to clinical assessment.

Conclusion

Device diagnostic parameters from the cutting-edge CRT have revolutionized the management program for patients with advanced heart failure. Continuous HRV, activity log, and intrathoracic impedance monitoring provide the opportunity to monitor patients' heart failure status, determine the response to CRT, detect significant arrhythmic events, predict upcoming heart failure hospitalization, guide medical therapy to relieve decompensation, and estimate the long-term prognosis in these high-risk patients. Telemonitoring via the Internet makes the idea of home monitoring feasible. With advances in technology, comprehensive assessment of autonomic status, accurate measurement of pulmonary congestion, and devotion of all health care providers, an even better care for these unfortunate patients is expected in the very near future.

References

1. Abraham WT, Fisher WG, Smith AL, et al. MIRACLE Study Group. Multicenter InSync Randomized Clinical Evaluation. Cardiac resynchronization in chronic heart failure. N Engl J Med 2002;346:1845–1853.
2. Bristow MR, Saxon LA, Boehmer J, et al. Comparison of Medical Therapy, Pacing, and Defibrillation in Heart Failure (COMPANION) Investigators. Cardiac-resynchronization therapy with or without an implantable defibrillator in advanced chronic heart failure. N Engl J Med 2004;350:2140–2150.
3. Young JB, Abraham WT, Smith AL, et al. Multicenter InSync ICD Randomized Clinical Evaluation (MIRACLE ICD) Trial Investigators. Combined cardiac resynchronization and implantable cardioversion defibrillation in advanced chronic heart failure. JAMA 2003;289:2685–2694.
4. Cleland JG, Daubert JC, Erdmann E, et al. Cardiac Resynchronization-Heart Failure (CARE-HF) Study Investigators. The effect of cardiac resynchronization on morbidity and mortality in heart failure. N Engl J Med 2005;352:1539–1549.
5. Hunt SA, Abraham WT, Chin MH, et al. ACC/AHA 2005 Guideline Update for the Diagnosis and Management of Chronic Heart Failure in the Adult: A report of the American College of Cardiology/American Heart Association Task Force

on Practice Guidelines (Writing Committee to Update the 2001 Guidelines for the Evaluation and Management of Heart Failure): Developed in collaboration with the American College of Chest Physicians and the International Society for Heart and Lung Transplantation: endorsed by the Heart Rhythm Society. Circulation 2005;112:e154–235.

6. Lombardi F. Clinical implications of present physiological understanding of HRV components. Card Electrophyiol Rev 2002;6:245–249.

7. Billman GE, Dujardin JP. Dynamic changes in cardiac vagal tone as measured by time-series analysis. Am J Physiol 1990;258:H896.

8. Pagani M, Mallini A. Interpreting oscillations of muscle sympathetic nerve activity and heart rate variability. J Hypertens 2000;18:1709–1719.

9. Molgaard H, Sorensen KE, Bjerregaard P. Circadian variation and influence of risk factors on heart rate variability in healthy subjects. Am J Cardiol 1991;68:777.

10. Malik M, Camm AJ, Janse MJ, et al. Depressed heart rate variability identifies postinfarction patients who might benefit from prophylactic treatment with amiodarone: a substudy of EMIAT (The European Myocardial Infarct Amiodarone Trial). J Am Coll Cardiol 2000;35:1263–1275.

11. Adamson PB, Vanoli E. Early autonomic and repolarization abnormalities contribute to lethal arrhythmias in chronic ischemic heart failure: Characteristics of a novel heart failure model in dogs with post myocardial infarction left ventricular dysfunction. J Am Coll Cardiol 2001;37:1741–1748.

12. La Rovere MT, Pinna GD, Hohnloser SH, et al. Baroreflex sensitivity and heart rate variability in the identification of patients at risk for life-threatening arrhythmias: Implications for clinical trials. Circulation 2001;103:2072–2077.

13. Fantoni C, Raffa S, Regoli F, et al. Cardiac resynchronization therapy improves heart rate profile and heart rate variability of patients with moderate to severe heart failure. J Am Coll Cardiol 2005;46:1875–1882.

14. Adamson PB, Smith AL, Abraham WT, et al. Continuous autonomic assessment in patients with symptomatic heart failure: prognostic value of heart rate variability measured by an implanted cardiac resynchronization device. Circulation 2004;110:2389–2394.

15. Nolan J, Batin PD, Andrews R, et al. Prospective study of heart rate variability and mortality in chronic heart failure: results of the United Kingdom heart failure evaluation and assessment of risk trial (UK heart). Circulation 1998;98:1510–1516.

16. La Rovere MT, Pinna GD, Maestri R, et al. Short-term heart rate variability strongly predicts sudden cardiac death in chronic heart failure patients. Circulation 2003;107:565–570.

17. Mortara A, La Rovere MT, Pinna GD, et al. Nonselective beta-adrenergic blocking agent, carvedilol, improves arterial baroreflex gain and heart rate variability in patients with stable chronic heart failure. J Am Coll Cardiol 2000;36:1612–1618.

18. Adamson PB, Kleckner KJ, VanHout WL, et al. Cardiac resynchronization therapy improves heart rate variability in patients with symptomatic heart failure. Circulation 2003;108:266–269.

19. Stewart S, Jenkins A, Buchan S, et al. The current cost of heart failure to the National Health Service in the UK. Eur J Heart Fail 2002;4:361–371.

20. Carson PE, Johnson GR, Dunkman WB, et al. The influence of atrial fibrillation on prognosis in mild to moderate heart failure. Circulation 1993;87(Suppl VI);VI-102–VI-110.

21. Cohn JN, Johnson GR, Shabetai R, et al. Ejection fraction, peak exercise oxygen consumption, cardiothoracic ratio, ventricular arrhythmias, and plasma norepinephrine as determinants of prognosis in heart failure. Circulation 1993;87(Suppl VI):VI-5–VI-16.

22. Francis GS, Rector TS. Maximal exercise tolerance as a therapeutic end point in heart failure—are we relying on the right measure? Am J Cardiol 1994;73:304–306.

23. Walsh JT, Charlesworth A, Andrews R, Hawkins M, Cowley AJ. Relation of daily activity levels in patients with chronic heart failure to long-term prognosis. Am J Cardiol 1997;79:1364–1369.

24. Braunschweig F, Mortensen PT, Gras D, et al. Monitoring of physical activity and heart rate variability in patients with chronic heart failure using cardiac resynchronization devices. Am J Cardiol 2005;95:1104–1107.

25. Goldberg LR, Piette JD, Walsh MN, et al. Randomized trial of a daily electronic home monitoring system in patients with advanced heart failure: The weight monitoring in heart failure (WHARF) trial. Am Heart J 2003;46:705–712.

26. Louis AA, Turner T, Gretton M, et al. A systematic review of telemonitoring for the management of heart failure. Eur J Heart Fail 2003;5:583–590.

27. Friedman MM. Older adults' symptoms and their duration before hospitalization for heart failure. Heart Lung 1997;26:169–176.

28. Stevenson LW, Perloff JK. The limited reliability of physical signs for estimating hemodynamics in chronic heart failure. JAMA 1989;261:884–888.

29. Luepker RV, Michael JR, Warbasse JR. Transthoracic electrical impedance; quantitative evaluation of a non-invasive measure of thoracic fluid volume. Am Heart J 1973;85:83–93.

30. Baker LE, Denniston JC. Noninvasive measurement of intrathoracic fluids. Chest 1974;65(Suppl):37S.

31. Fein A, Grossman RF, Jones JG, et al. Evaluation of transthoracic electrical impedance in the diagnosis of pulmonary edema. Circulation 1979;60:1156–1160.

32. Saunders CE. The use of transthoracic electrical bioimpedance in assessing thoracic fluid status in emergency department patients. Am J Emerg Med 1988;6:337–340.

33. Ramos MU, LaBree JW, Remole W, Kubicek WG. Transthoracic electric impedance. A clinical guide of pulmonary fluid accumulation in congestive heart failure. Minn Med 1975;58:671–676.

34. Yamamoto T, Yamamoto Y, Ozawa T. Characteristics of skin admittance for dry electrodes and the measurement of skin moisturisation. Med Biol Eng Comput 1986;24:71–77.

35. Wang L, Lahtinen S, Lentz L, et al. Feasibility of using an implantable system to measure thoracic congestion in an ambulatory chronic heart failure canine model. Pacing Clin Electrophysiol 2005;28:404–411.

36. Yu CM, Wang L, Chau E, et al. Intrathoracic impedance monitoring in patients with heart failure: Correlation with fluid status and feasibility of early warning preceding hospitalization. Circulation 2005;112:841–848.

37. Adamson PB, Magalski A, Braunschweig F, et al. Ongoing right ventricular hemodynamics in heart failure: Clinical value of measurements derived from an implantable monitoring system. J Am Coll Cardiol 2003;41:565–571.

38. Komajda M, Follath F, Swedberg K, et al; Study Group on Diagnosis of the Working Group on Heart Failure of the European Society of Cardiology. The EuroHeart Failure Survey programme – a survey on the quality of care among patients with heart failure in Europe. Part 2: treatment. Eur Heart J 2003;24: 464–474.

39. Fung JW, Chan JY, Leo CC, et al. Suboptimal medical therapy in patients with systolic heart failure is associated with less improvement by cardiac resynchronization therapy. Int J Cardiol 2007;115:214–9.

40. Galbreath AD, Krasuski RA, Smith B, et al. Long-term healthcare and cost outcomes of disease management in a large, randomized, community-based population with heart failure. Circulation 2004;110:3518–3526.

41. Fung JW, Yu CM, Chan JY, et al. Effects of cardiac resynchronization therapy on incidence of atrial fibrillation in patients with poor left ventricular systolic function. Am J Cardiol 2005;96:728–731.

triggering interventions before actual deterioration of the clinical situation occurs. It can be expected that future devices will evolve into multimodality treatment and monitoring platforms and that more monitoring-only systems will become available for patients without an indication for CRT.

Thus, since the introduction of CRT, now more than 10 years ago, significant technical progress has been achieved in implantation tools and device technology [1]. However, with the increasing complexity of the devices and the growing number of heart failure patients receiving these devices, follow-up and monitoring of the technical and clinical status has become a challenging task. In this overview, some of the most important device-related issues encountered during CRT follow-up are addressed.

Device Programming

Lower and Upper Rate Programming

Although atrial pacing has potential beneficial effects on stabilizing atrial rhythm, the hemodynamic effects of atrial pacing may be unfavorable [6, 7]. Because of the intraatrial conduction delay, left atrial activation may be delayed, with consequent adverse hemodynamic effects on diastolic left ventricular filling. Therefore, programming a low lower rate to avoid atrial pacing seems reasonable, unless the patient is chronotropic incompetent.

The upper rate should be programmed higher than the maximum sinus rate to ensure tracking with biventricular pacing at high intrinsic sinus rates. In CRT-D devices, the upper rate will be limited by the cutoff value programmed for detection of ventricular arrhythmias in the lowest ventricular tachycardia zone, as current devices do not incorporate the possibility of bradycardia pacing in the ventricular tachycardia zone(s).

In order to achieve optimal resynchronization therapy, the percentage of ventricular pacing should be maximized. However, the percentage pacing provided by the device counters and the resulting histograms may not reflect the real percentage of ventricular pacing, due to intrinsic conduction, which may cause fusion and pseudo-fusion ventricular stimulation. The location of the RV lead influences the timing of ventricular sensing. To ensure early sensing by the RV lead, the lead should be placed in a more proximal position than the RV apex. Such a proximal position may decrease the amount of fusion/pseudo-fusion pacing and may contribute to a better outcome [8].

Atrioventricular Delay

It is well recognized that the programmed atrioventricular delay (AV delay) of crucial importance in optimizing the benefit of CRT [9]. Several studies have demonstrated that relatively short AV delays should be programmed to improve LV systolic function. Because CRT patients usually have intact intrinsic AV conduction, short AV delays may help to increase the percentage of biventricular pacing and to decrease the number of fusion beats. However, a short AV delay may also have a negative effect on cardiac performance. Although a short AV delay permits enough time for diastolic filling, the active filling phase may be terminated prematurely thus leading to a suboptimal preload of the LV (Fig. 25.1). Right to left intraatrial conduction

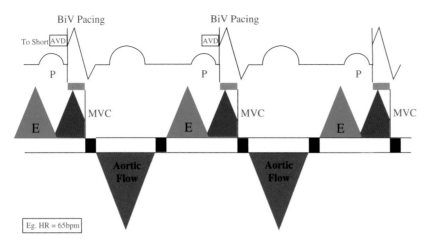

Fig. 25.1 Programming a short AV delay advances the mitral valve closure (*MVC*) and terminates the active filling phase prematurely, resulting in a suboptimal preload of the left ventricle.

time varies between patients but the impact of sensed versus paced atrial rhythms on intraatrial conduction time may be even more pronounced. AV offset programming, which increases AV delay during atrial stimulation, compensates for this phenomenon, but augments the possibility of fusion beats. Automatic shortening of the AV delay is programmed in regular DDD pacemakers because of the positive effect on upper rate programmability. In CRT patients, this feature overcomes the inherent shortening in rate-dependent intrinsic AV conduction time and thus has a positive effect on the percentage of biventricular pacing. However, in a recent publication, Scharf et al. demonstrated that lengthening of the AV delay during exercise led to a more favorable LV systolic performance at higher atrial rates [10]. In summary, optimizing the AV delay in CRT patients is a complex issue in which pacemaker parameters, intrinsic conduction and conduction times, and hemodynamic effects are intricately linked.

Ventricle-to-ventricle Timing

Because transvenous positioning of the LV lead is limited by the anatomy of the coronary sinus and the venous system of the heart, the final LV pacing site may be suboptimal with respect to the hemodynamic effects. Optimization ventricle-to-ventricle (V-V timing) is therefore usually desirable to compensate for these anatomical limitations and may enhance the clinical outcome of CRT. Optimization of V-V timing has been shown to have beneficial acute effects on dyssynchrony, systolic function, ejection fraction, and mitral regurgitation, although no chronic effects have been demonstrated [9, 11, 12]. The optimal sequence of right and left ventricular stimulation and the optimal V-V delay vary widely between individual patients, and lead positions and may change over time due to LV reverse remodeling induced by CRT [13]. Several noninvasive methods have been proposed of which the aortic velocity-time interval (VTI) may be the method of choice [14].

The relationship between V-V and AV delay is complex, because programming the V-V delay has a direct effect on the right versus the left

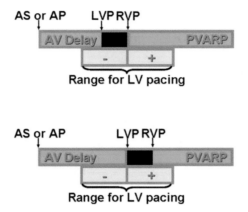

Fig. 25.2 The effect of programming the V-V delay on the AV delay varies between device manufacturers. *Upper panel*: Programming the left before right shortens the effective left-sided AV delay (Guidant). *Lower panel*: Programming of left before right increases the right-sided AV delay (Medtronic).

AV delay and is further complicated by the fact that different manufacturers offer different tools to handle this issue. For example, programming the left before right may shorten the effective left-sided AV delay (Boston Scientific) or increase the right-sided AV delay (Medtronic) (Fig. 25.2).

When programming left before right, unintentionally occurring anodal stimulation of the RV may abolish the programmed V-V delay. Anodal stimulation most commonly occurs at higher output settings when the RV lead serves as the anode, especially in case of a small anodal surface area and thus a higher currency density. Therefore, when the RV ventricular lead anode is used in the pacing circuit, one should be aware of the possible presence of anodal stimulation and this should be evaluated before optimizing the V-V delay.

Arrhythmias

Atrial Arrhythmias

Atrial fibrillation (AF) is the most common atrial arrhythmia in heart failure patients, occurring in 20–40% of patients with a significant correlation with the severity of the heart failure [15]. The loss of AV synchrony, the irregular ventricular rate causing varying left ventricular filling times, and a decrease in biventricular stimulation during atrial fibrillation may lead to a deteriorating functional status. In a subanalysis of the MUSTIC-AF study, the importance of a high percentage of biventricular pacing was demonstrated [16]. Patients with >95% biventricular pacing showed significantly more improvement of clinical parameters and a reduction of the number of all-cause and heart failure–related hospitalizations than those with a low percentage (<50%) of biventricular pacing. A subanalysis of the CARE-HF study reported that although CRT improved the outcome of the patient regardless of whether AF developed, CRT per se did not reduce the incidence of AF [17].

Algorithms used to increase the percentage of biventricular pacing during AF like ventricular rate regulation may be helpful (Fig. 25.3). The effect of RV sensed-triggered pacing warrants further investigation.

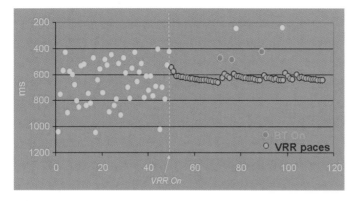

Fig. 25.3 Variation in V-V intervals during atrial fibrillation before (*left*) and after (*right*) switching on the "Ventricular Rate Regularization" (*VRR*) algorithms. VRR stabilizes the ventricular rate during atrial fibrillation.

Although modern mode switch algorithms are well capable of recognizing atrial fibrillation and react appropriately by switching to a nontracking mode, regular atrial tachycardias can lead to intermittent underdetection caused by unfortunate timing relations (Fig. 25.4).

In patients with therapy resistant or permanent atrial arrhythmias in whom rate control by drugs is not sufficient to achieve a high percentage of biventricular pacing, AV node ablation should be considered without reluctance [18]. In patients with paroxysmal AF, all efforts should be directed to maintain sinus rhythm.

Ventricular Arrhythmias

The increased risk of ventricular arrhythmias and sudden death is well recognized in patients with LV dysfunction and low ejection fraction (LVEF) [2–5, 19, 20]. Several large, randomized trials demonstrated that implantation of an ICD in patients with a low LVEF has a positive effect on all-cause mortality [3, 19, 20]. Recently, the SCD-HeFT trial demonstrated that ICD therapy in patients with symptomatic heart failure and a low LVEF, regardless of the underlying cause, has a positive effect on all-cause mortality [3].

It is therefore challenging to speculate that combining CRT with ICD therapy may have a significant additional mortality effect and should be considered in all patients with a depressed LV function [5]. However, until now no large, randomized trials comparing the efficacy of CRT only with CRT-D have been conducted. Although the COMPANION trial reported only a significant mortality effect in the CRT-D group compared with optimal medical therapy, the difference between CRT-D and CRT-P patients was not significant [4].

Ventricular arrhythmias with a cycle length of <500 ms are also relatively common in patients with low ejection fraction, especially when antiarrhythmic drugs such as amiodarone are used (Fig. 25.5). In the current ICD generation, no overlap between bradycardia and tachycardia zones is allowed. Consequently, this results in limited possibilities to program the upper tracking rate and the lowest tachycardia rate.

The choice of antitachycardia therapy, antitachycardia pacing only, or antitachycardia pacing followed by shocks is ambiguous. Antitachycardia

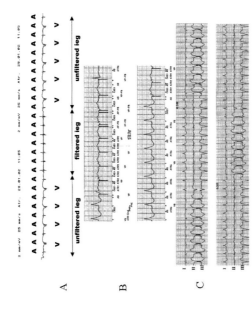

Fig. 25.4 (**A**) Intracardiac atrial electrocardiogram, unfiltered and filtered, as recorded by an external recording system. The atrial electrogram (**A**) reveals an atrial tachycardia. Far-field R-waves (*V*) can be discerned in the unfiltered parts of the registration. Note the simultaneous occurrence of every second atrial deflection with the far-field ventricular signal. (**B**) Pacemaker tracing (continuous): surface ECG lead I and marker annotations. Note the cyclic character of the tracing. After two intrinsic beats, nine ventricular beats are paced in DDD mode with tracking of the atrium in a 2:1 fashion. Sensing of the atrial tachyarrhythmia is reflected in the marker annotations as (*as*) and as, referring to an atrial sensed event or not in the postventricular atrial refractory period (PVARP). The markers show *ATR↑*, reflecting the process of counting up until the programmed number of atrial deflections fulfill the onset criteria for atrial tachycardia (programmed to 8). When the duration is also reached (*ATR-Dur*), pacing in the fallback mode is started (*ATR-FB*). The pacemaker now switches to DDI pacing in the fallback mode, slowly decelerating to its programmed rate (similar to rate smoothing), with dynamic AV delay on. The first two beats in the fallback mode show atrial pacing (*AP-FB*) as well as ventricular pacing (*VP-FB*), because the sensed atrial events fall in the PVARP [(*as*)]. The fourth *VP-FB* is a fusion beat of ventricular pacing and intrinsic conduction and therefore has a different configuration. From that beat on, the intrinsic rate is higher than the pacemaker rate, inhibiting DDI pacing. The atrial rhythm is misinterpreted as sinus rhythm, because due to their nearly simultaneous occurrence, every second flutter wave falls in the blanking period of the ventricular deflection. The other atrial deflections are sensed and followed by the ventricle (*Vs*). The marker channel shows *ATR↓* representing the counting down of atrial deflections, after which sinus rhythm is supposedly present (*ATR-End*). Inappropriate back switching to the DDD mode occurs during which the atrial tachyarrhythmia is sensed again (*ATR↑*). (**C**) Surface ECG leads I, II, and III. This continuous tracing illustrates the unusual cyclic character of repeatedly mode switching. After appropriate mode switching, the atrial tachyarrhythmia was conducted to the ventricle in a 2:1 fashion. Due to simultaneous occurrence of each second atrial flutter wave and the intrinsic ventricular deflection, the atrial channel was blanked at the second flutter wave. The atrial rate was interpreted by the pacemaker as being below the cutoff rate for mode switching. This led to inappropriate mode switching to DDD mode after at least eight conducted beats. (Adapted from van Erven L, Molhoek SG, van der Wall EE, Schalij MJ. Cyclic appropriate mode switching and inappropriate back switching of a biventricular pacemaker during atrial tachycardia. Pacing Clin Electrophysiol 2004;27:249-51).

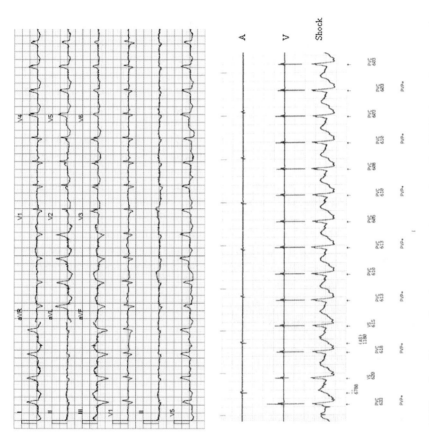

Fig. 25.5 Twelve-lead ECG (*upper panel*) and ICD tracing of intracardiac electrograms and annotations of a CRT-D device (*lower panel*), showing a very slow VT of less than 100 bpm. *A*, atrial electrogram; *V*, ventricular electrogram; *Shock*, shock electrogram.

pacing may be ineffective or may accelerate the slow VT, whereas shock therapy may be troublesome for the patient. In some cases, catheter ablation of the slow VT may be necessary to allow optimization of the device settings.

Device- and Lead-Related Issues

Pacemaker-Mediated Tachycardia

CRT patients are prone to the occurrence of pacemaker-mediated tachycardia (PMT) due to their often intact retrograde conduction through the AV node. A PMT can be initiated by retrograde activation of the atrium that occurs beyond the PVARP (Post Ventricular Atrial Refractory Period). The presence of slow intrinsic retrograde conduction, amplified by drugs used for heart failure, may result in a slow PMT that may be difficult to discriminate from sinus rhythm with the use of intracardiac signals and device annotations. PMT exhibits relatively stable heart rates (within the boundaries of lower and upper rate limits). The surface ECG may be helpful, as during PMT the P-wave axis is changed compared with regular sinus rhythm (Fig. 25.6).

In CRT patients, the effects of PMT are often more dramatic than in the normal bradycardia pacing population. During a PMT, the patient suffers from a nonphysiologic high heart rate, loss of normal AV synchrony, and reversed atrial activation. In combination with the already compromised left ventricular systolic function, this may lead to worsening symptoms of heart failure. PMT break algorithms are indispensable but are limited by their PMT recognition possibilities, which vary from manufacturer to manufacturer. Because in most devices, PMT break algorithms operate at a rate near the programmed upper tracking rate, underdetection of PMT by the device may occur especially in case of a relatively slow PMT.

Phrenic Nerve Stimulation

Phrenic nerve stimulation (PNS) is one of the most common complications of CRT, with an important impact on the patient's well-being. The inadvertent manifestation of PNS in relation to the target vessel during implant cannot be predicted, although some efforts have been made [21], and may necessitate relocation of the electrode. On the other hand, the absence of PNS during implant does not ensure the nonappearance during daily life because a significant postural-dependency may exist. Phrenic nerve stimulation has been reported to occur in up to 12% of the patients during follow-up in earlier studies. PNS can often be resolved noninvasively. Some newer devices have the possibility of programming a different vector, using either the LV tip or the LV ring electrode as a cathode either or not in combination with different anode poles [22]. This "electronic repositioning" of the vector and/or the pacing site may be successful in the majority of the patients. Programming the output closer to the LV threshold may also be of help but compromises the threshold margin with its possible negative effects on the percentage of effective biventricular pacing. Widening the pulse width is another method to lower the amplitude threshold, thereby compensating for the decreased threshold margin.

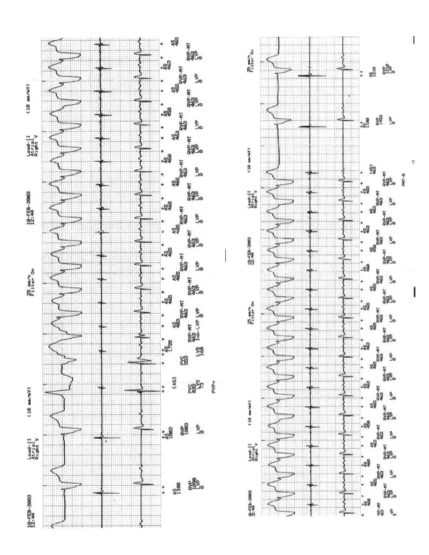

Fig. 25.6 Pacemaker mediated tachycardia in a CRT device. *Upper panel*: After two sinus beats, two PVC occurred. Retrograde atrial activation followed after the second PVC, starting the PMT. *Lower panel*: The PMT was ended with a PMT-break (PMT-B) algorithm, which prolonged the PVARP; the atrial activity falls in the refractory period [annotated as (AS)] and was therefore not followed by a ventricular paced event.

LV Lead Failures

Mechanical lead problems like lead fractures or insulation defects occur both in LV and RV pacing leads [21]. However, long-term LV lead performance data are not available yet due to the relatively short period of time these leads are used. Lead dislocation is a more common problem, with a reported incidence of 4–10%. In our own series of >500 patients, lead dislodgment occurred in 3% of patients, whereas a significant rise in pacing threshold up to submaximal levels, suggesting microdislocation, occurred in another 1.5%. In our series, we observed significant increases in pacing threshold up to 4 years after implantation, whereas macrodislocations of the LV lead were observed up to 10 months after implantation. Endovascular repositioning of the LV lead was successful in 87% of these cases. This suggests that epicardial lead placement in case of endovascular LV lead dysfunction should not be the first-choice solution for these problems in most patients.

Conclusion

Since the introduction of cardiac resynchronization therapy, technical progress has been impressive. With all options offered by the current devices, patient-tailored therapy has become possible. It can be expected that CRT devices will evolve into multimodality diagnostic and therapeutic platforms offering the possibility to detect and treat a variety of different cardiac conditions. However, the complexity of the current CRT devices requires profound knowledge and comprehension of all technical aspects. Furthermore, it is of importance to understand the possible effects of different settings on cardiac performance.

References

1. Bakker PF, Meijburg HW, de Vries JW, et al. Biventricular pacing in end-stage heart failure patients improves functional capacity and left ventricular function. J Interv Card Electrophysiol 2000;4:395–404.
2. Kadish A, Dyer A, Daubert JP, et al. Defibrillators in Non-Ischemic Cardiomyopathy Treatment Evaluation (DEFINITE) Investigators. A randomized study of the prevention of sudden death in patients with coronary artery disease. Multicenter Unsustained Tachycardia Trial Investigators. N Engl J Med 1999;341:1882–90.
3. Bardy GH, Lee KL, Mark DB, et al. Sudden Cardiac Death in Heart Failure Trial (SCD-HeFT) Investigators.. Amiodarone or an implantable cardioverter-defibrillator for congestive heart failure. N Engl J Med 2005;352:225–37.
4. Bristow MR, Saxon LA, Boehmer J, et al. Comparison of Medical Therapy, Pacing, and Defibrillation in Heart Failure (COMPANION) Investigators. Cardiac-resynchronization therapy with or without an implantable defibrillator in advanced chronic heart failure. N Engl J Med 2004;350:2140–50.
5. Ypenburg C, van Erven L, Bleeker GB, et al. Benefit of combined resynchronization and defibrillator therapy in heart failure patients with and without ventricular arrhythmias. J Am Coll Cardiol 2006;48:464–70.
6. Hemels ME, Wiesfeld AC, Inberg B, et al. Right atrial overdrive pacing for prevention of symptomatic refractory atrial fibrillation. Europace 2006;8:107–12.
7. Bernheim A, Ammann P, Sticherling C, et al. Right atrial pacing impairs cardiac function during resynchronization therapy: acute effects of DDD pacing compared to VDD pacing. J Am Coll Cardiol 2005;45:1482–7.

8. Riedlbauchová L, Čihák R, Bytešník J, et al. Optimization of right ventricular lead position in cardiac resynchronisation therapy. Eur J Heart Fail 2006;8:609–14.

9. Auricchio A, Stellbrink C, Block M, et al. Effect of pacing chamber and atrioventricular delay on acute systolic function of paced patients with congestive heart failure. The Pacing Therapies for Congestive Heart Failure Study Group. The Guidant Congestive Heart Failure Research Group. Circulation 1999;99: 2993–3001.

10. Scharf C, Li P, Muntwyler J, et al. Rate-dependent AV delay optimization in cardiac resynchronization therapy. PACE 2005;28:279–84.

11. Sogaard P, Egeblad H, Pedersen AK, et al. Atrial versus simultaneous biventricular resynchronization for severe heart failure: Evaluation by tissue Doppler imaging. Circulation 2002;106:2078–84.

12. Bordachar P, Lafitte S, Reuter S, et al. Echocardiographic parameters of ventricular dyssynchrony validation in patients with heart failure using sequential biventricular pacing. J Am Coll Cardiol 2004;44:2157–65.

13. Porciani MC, Dondina C, Macioce R, et al. Echocardiographic examination of atrioventricular and interventricular delay optimization in cardiac resynchronization therapy. Am J Cardiol 2005;95:1108–10.

14. Bax JJ, Abraham T, Barold SS, et al. Cardiac resynchronization therapy: Part 2–issues during and after device implantation and unresolved questions. J Am Coll Cardiol 2005;46:2168–82.

15. Maisel W, Stevenson L. Atrial fibrillation in heart failure: epidemiology, pathophysiology and rationale for therapy. Am J Cardiol 2003;91:2D–8D.

16. Leclercq C, Walker S, Linde C, et al. Comparative effects of permanent biventricular and right-univentricular pacing in heart failure patients with chronic atrial fibrillation. Eur Heart J 2002;23:1780–7.

17. Hoppe UC, Casares JM, Eiskjaer H, et al. Effect of cardiac resynchronization on the incidence of atrial fibrillation in patients with severe heart failure. Circulation 2006;114:18–25.

18. Gasparini M, Auricchio A, Regoli F, et al. Four-year efficacy of cardiac resynchronization therapy on exercise tolerance and disease progression the importance of performing atrioventricular junction ablation in patients with atrial fibrillation. J Am Coll Cardiol 2006;48:734–43.

19. Moss AJ, Hall WJ, Cannom DS, et al. Improved survival with an implanted defibrillator in patients with coronary disease at high risk for ventricular arrhythmia. Multicenter Automatic Defibrillator Implantation Trial Investigators. N Engl J Med 1996;335:1933–40.

20. Buxton AE, Lee KL, Fisher JD, et al. A randomized study of the prevention of sudden death in patients with coronary artery disease. Multicenter Unsustained Tachycardia Trial Investigators. N Engl J Med 1999;341:1882–90.

21. Albertsen AE, Nielsen JC, Pedersen AK, et al. Left ventricular lead performance in cardiac resynchronization therapy: Impact of lead localization and complications. PACE 2005;28:483–8.

22. Gurevitz O, Nof E, Carasso S, et al. Programmable multiple pacing configurations help to overcome high left ventricular pacing thresholds and avoid phrenic nerve stimulation. Pacing Clin Electrophysiol 2005;28:1255–9.

Recurrent Heart Failure and Appropriate Evaluation After Cardiac Resynchronization Therapy

Juan M. Aranda, Jr.

Introduction

Heart failure (HF) continues to be a significant cause of morbidity and mortality in the United States with an estimated 5 million patients now affected [1]. Despite the advancement of neurohormonal blockade with angiotensin-converting enzyme (ACE) inhibitors, beta blockade, and aldosterone antagonists [2–4], more than 271,000 patients with HF in the United States have received cardiac resynchronization therapy (CRT) since 2001 when the U.S. Food and Drug Administration approved this therapy for moderate to severe HF [5].

Indications for the use of CRT have included New York Heart Association (NYHA) functional class III or IV HF refractory to pharmacologic therapy, QRS duration greater than 120 ms, left ventricular (LV) ejection fraction less than or equal to 35%, and LV end-diastolic dimension greater than or equal to 55 mm (level of evidence IIA). These indications are reviewed and emphasized in the guidelines of the American College of Cardiology, American Heart Association, and Heart Rhythm Society published in 2001 [6].

There are now seven major randomized trials of CRT involving more than 3,000 patients with HF of both ischemic and nonischemic origins [6–13]. These trials have consistently shown improvement in functional class, exercise capacity, ejection fraction, and LV systolic and diastolic volumes in the presence of CRT. They have also shown a reduction in hospitalization and mortality with CRT. The benefits of CRT have been shown to occur as early as 1 month after initiation of CRT and to continue for as long as 18 months [7, 12].

The nonresponder rate for this therapy has been reported to be as high as 30% [15]. This is a subjective number that is derived from several clinical trials that showed that about 30% of patients failed to reduce their functional class by at least one class. There is no standardized definition of who should be considered a true CRT nonresponder, only various interpretations accounting for lack of improvement in functional class or exercise capacity. Nevertheless, the 30% nonresponder rate brings up the issue that we can have continued

HF in patients who received CRT and recurrent HF in patients who had a previous response to CRT.

The purpose of this chapter is to review and describe clinical and device issues that can contribute to early nonresponse to CRT or later reoccurrence of HF in those patients who had initially benefited from this therapy.

Clinical Expectations After CRT

After a patient with HF receives CRT, a series of hemodynamic and clinical events can be expected over the next several months (Table 26.1). These clinical and hemodynamic events must be recognized because they can be used to further optimize medical therapy that may help prevent the reoccurrence of HF during long-term follow-up after CRT. Immediately after implant—assuming adequate lead position and device function—systolic blood pressure, cardiac output, and dp/dt usually increase while end-systolic volume, pulmonary capillary wedge pressure, and mitral regurgitation usually decrease [16, 17]. This improvement in cardiac function is the result of correction of ventricular dyssynchrony. The change in hemodynamic parameters is important to recognize because it may require reduction in diuretics. Failure to reduce diuretics in a HF patient receiving CRT with optimal filling pressure may result in prerenal azotemia, masking or delaying the symptom improvement related to CRT. After CRT, diuretic adjustment is required both early on and during long-term follow-up as this device is maintaining ventricular synchrony and improving cardiac function. Volume status is a continuous variable, which depends on diet and compliance to medical regimen among other factors. Volume status can be independent of adequate device function and requires chronic assessment to avoid dehydration or reoccurrence of HF symptoms caused by increased filling pressures.

As the clinical benefits unfold during the first year after CRT, other interventions can be performed to decrease the chances of HF reoccurring. These interventions involve the optimization of neurohormonal blockade. After CRT, systolic blood pressure increases and continues to increase during many months of follow-up [11, 12]. This increase offers a unique opportunity to optimize neurohormonal blockers to evidence-based clinical trial

Table 26.1 Clinical and hemodynamic changes after CRT therapy.

Early response

1. Improvement in systolic blood pressure, cardiac output, and dp/dt
2. Reduction in mitral regurgitation
3. Improvement in exercise capacity and NYHA function class
4. Improvement in quality of life

Late response

1. Reduction in hospitalization and mortality
2. Improvement in ejection fraction
3. Reduction in left ventricular systolic and diastolic volume
4. Reverse cardiac remodeling

doses. Pharmacologic therapy with beta-blockers and ACE inhibitors has dramatically reduced HF mortality, sudden death, and HF hospitalizations [2, 3, 18, 19]. Despite these benefits, the use of beta blockade in recent randomized clinical trials is only around 60% to 70%. Doses of beta-blockers are often subtherapeutic. Many physicians hesitate regarding initiation of beta-blocker therapy or aggressive up-titration of beta-blocker therapy because of hypotension, bradycardia, and worsening HF [20]. CRT improves HF symptoms and systolic blood pressure while correcting ventricular dyssynchrony by pacing both ventricles. Therefore, the clinical problems that are related to beta-blocker administration are decreased by CRT. Several small retrospective analyses demonstrate that beta-blocker dose can be increased after CRT [21, 22]. We have demonstrated that beta-blocker therapy can be reinitiated after CRT in 50% of patients with a history of intolerance to these drugs [22]. The issue of device therapy and beta blockade cannot be overemphasized. Both CRT and defibrillator HF trials have shown that device use with concomitant beta-blocker therapy leads to better outcomes compared with device use without beta-blocker therapy [11, 23]. Beta-blockers can reduce the incidence of atrial fibrillation and ventricular arrhythmias. These arrhythmias can alter or reduce device function and increase antitachycardiac right ventricular (RV) pacing and defibrillator shocks, which can worsen HF. The combination of CRT and enhanced medical management may provide synergistic effects regarding reverse LV remodeling and improved systolic and diastolic function. This may prevent or reduce the reoccurrence of HF far beyond the follow-up periods currently reported in CRT trials.

Reoccurrence of Heart Failure

The reoccurrence of HF after CRT can be divided into patients who had an initial response to CRT and now have reoccurring HF and those patients who have simply not improved after CRT (nonresponders). It is important to note that when it comes to reoccurrence of HF in a patient who previously responded to CRT, we simply do not know how long this benefit lasts. Published reports have shown the benefit of CRT up to 18 months after implantation [12]. We have all had clinical experiences of patients receiving benefit long after the first 18 months of CRT, and we have all had individual patients who required advanced HF management after CRT. Systolic HF secondary to ischemic heart disease is a progressive disease that may improve with CRT. However, recurrent cardiac ischemia or myocardial infarction may cause HF symptoms to reoccur in the presence of CRT. Although initial nonresponders and patients who have reoccurrence of HF after an initial response may be considered two separate patient populations, several clinical events must be investigated in both types of patients. Table 26.2 describes clinical and mechanical issues that could affect device function and cause recurrent or continued HF early or late after CRT therapy.

We have previously described a potential troubleshooting algorithm that takes into account common problems that occur in HF and can effect CRT device function [24]. This algorithm describes the process of advanced HF management after CRT. The first step in evaluating worsening HF in a patient with CRT involves interrogating the device for adequate function. Is the device providing biventricular pacing 100% of the time? Is there loss of RV

Table 26.2 Clinical and device issues that can contribute to reoccurrence of heart failure after CRT.

A. Cardiac resynchronization therapy device function

    1. Loss of right ventricular capture
    2. Loss of left ventricular capture

B. Clinical issues affecting device function

    1. Development of atrial fibrillation
    2. Pre-renal azotemia (volume status)
    3. Cardiac ischemia (patients with ischemic cardiomyopathy)
    4. Mitral regurgitation

C. Evaluation of atrioventricular–interventricular delay
D. Presence of dyssynchrony after cardiac resynchronization therapy

or LV capture that could account for worsening or reoccurring HF? The rate of lead dislodgment in CRT trials is about 5%, but this involves 6 months to 1 year of follow-up. Although the chance of lead dislodgment decreases over time, its presence should be ruled out early in the troubleshooting process.

If there is adequate device function, then clinical issues that frequently occur in HF and can affect device function should be ruled out. Is the patient having intermittent atrial fibrillation affecting the ability of the device to maintain 100% biventricular pacing? It is known that patients with permanent atrial fibrillation benefit from CRT [25]. However, if the device is not programmed correctly with optimal mode switching and adequate rate control not exceeding the upper pacing rate of the CRT device, atrial fibrillation can affect device function leading to less CRT and worsening or reoccurring HF. Many of these devices provide downloadable summary cardiac reports that give an analysis of the number of episodes of atrial fibrillation, ventricular rates, duration of atrial fibrillation, and percent of biventricular pacing during episodes of atrial fibrillation. As we enter the era of chronic hemodynamic monitoring and diagnostic utilities provided by these devices, we are starting to find out that atrial fibrillation is extremely common in our HF population and can affect the function of an incorrectly programmed device.

If atrial fibrillation is ruled out, volume status should be addressed. As mentioned previously in this chapter, volume status reflecting filling pressures is a continuous variable that can be affected by many other issues regardless of adequate device function. Both prerenal azotemia (low filling pressures) and volume overload can cause the same constellation of HF symptoms. Simple management of diuretic agents may solve the immediate problem, but a search for the underlying reason (diet, compliance, cardiac ischemia, atrial fibrillation) should be performed. The important message is that advanced HF management is required and should be continued after CRT, especially as our patients live longer and pass the follow-up periods that have been reported in CRT trials.

Patients with ischemic cardiomyopathy present interesting problems. Up to 50% of patients enrolled in CRT trials have ischemic heart disease as the etiology of their HF. Ischemic heart disease is a progressive disease. We are introducing the CRT device in a heart that has scar tissue with complete or incomplete revascularization. Some of the CRT trials have shown that patients with ischemic cardiomyopathy did not show as much improvement in HF symptoms and exercise capacity as patients with nonischemic cardiomyopathy [8]. This may be one of the issues regarding initial nonresponder rates. In a patient with ischemic cardiomyopathy who develops recurrent HF after initial response to CRT, cardiac ischemia or myocardial infarction can develop, potentially altering the ventricular dyssynchrony pattern that was being corrected by the CRT device. Reoccurrence of HF after CRT in a patient with ischemic cardiomyopathy should lead to consideration and reevaluation of the patient's ischemic heart disease.

The presence of mitral regurgitation (MR) continues to be problematic in our HF population. Causes of functional MR can be multifactorial. There is evidence to suggest that CRT can reduce MR [26, 27]. Correction of ventricular dyssynchrony results in earlier activation of the posterior medial papillary muscle, thus reducing MR. However, if the mechanism of MR is not caused by ventricular dyssynchrony (i.e., cardiac ischemia or enlarged mitral annulus restricting leaflet motion), then the continued presence or progression of MR can mask the effects of CRT and cause reoccurrence of HF.

There is much work on atrioventricular (AV) and interventricular (V-V) optimization in the early management of the CRT patient to improve hemodynamics and maintain adequate device function. Optimal AV intervals may vary among HF patients and may improve hemodynamic effects of the device [28]. Optimization of RV and LV activation is a new feature of CRT devices. Most of the CRT clinical trials have provided simultaneous RV–LV pacing. RV–LV optimization can further improve dp/dt and has recently been shown to provide greater exercise capacity compared with simultaneous CRT pacing [29, 30].

There are several important observations that should be considered regarding RV–LV optimization that have clinical relevance to the reoccurrence of HF after CRT. Optimal sequence of CRT may be difficult to predict in some individuals and may vary according to the etiology of HF. Patients with ischemic cardiomyopathy may require longer RV–LV intervals necessitating more preexcitation of the left ventricle due to the presence of scar tissue resulting in slower conduction velocities [31]. RV and LV delays are currently being optimized to improve device function and responder rates despite a lack of long-term follow-up data on the association between these intervals and the reoccurrence of HF. Although there is no clinical evidence to support it, AV and RV–LV delays should be considered in the evaluation of a patient with late reoccurrence of HF after CRT. Progression of ischemic heart disease can easily affect RV–LV delays, which may necessitate the reprogramming of the CRT device in order to provide optimal ventricular activation.

The presence of ventricular dyssynchrony prior to implant of a CRT device is currently one of the best predictors of response to CRT [32,33]. Ventricular dyssynchrony should decrease after CRT. In the MIRACLE study, interventricular dyssynchrony was reduced by 19 ms. In CARE-HF, interventricular dyssynchrony was reduced from 50 to 29 ms after 18 months of follow-up. The presence of significant ventricular dyssynchrony in an early CRT nonresponder indicates inadequate lead placement [32]. We can only speculate about the reoccurrence of significant ventricular dyssynchrony in an initial responder who now has reoccurring heart failure. In the presence of adequate device function, reoccurrence of ventricular dyssynchrony may represent disease progression regardless of the etiology of HF. There is still much about chronic CRT that we simply do not know. As we continue to follow CRT patients for longer periods, clinical experience will help clarify these issues.

Conclusion

The use of CRT has developed and helped solve electrical mechanical issues that can affect cardiac function and cause progression of HF. Most of the clinical trials of CRT have evaluated the sole effect of restoring ventricular synchrony on clinical outcomes without significant change or intervention on other clinical issues that can affect CRT function. As our HF patients feel better and live longer with CRT, we are quickly passing the follow-up periods that are provided in the current evidence-based clinical trials.

The CRT device has been introduced in a clinical HF syndrome that includes many factors that can affect device function. Reoccurrence of HF symptoms after CRT is the last clinical manifestation of subclinical HF events (atrial fibrillation, cardiac ischemia, volume overload, noncompliance, or inadequate device function) leading to elevated filling pressures. Whether in an initial nonresponder or a responder who has reoccurring HF, an integrated approach between the HF specialist and the electrophysiologist will be needed to develop new strategies and algorithms to reduce the chance of reoccurrence of HF after CRT [34].

Acknowledgment

The author thanks Lisa A. Hamilton, M.A., for editorial assistance and manuscript preparation.

References

1. Hunt SA, Abraham WT, Chin MH, et al. ACC/AHA 2005 Guideline Update for the Diagnosis and Management of Chronic Heart Failure in the Adult: a report of the American College of Cardiology/American Heart Association Task Force on Practice Guidelines. Circulation 2005;112:e154–235.
2. MERIT-HF Study Group. Effect of metoprolol CR/XL in chronic heart failure: Metoprolol CR/XL Randomized Intervention Trial in Congestive Heart Failure. Lancet 1999;353:2001–7.
3. Cohn JN, Johnson G, Ziesche S, et al. A comparison of enalapril with hydralazine-isosorbide dinitrate in the treatment of chronic congestive heart failure. N Engl J Med 1991;325:303–10.
4. Pitt B, Zannad F, Remme WJ, et al for the Randomized Aldactone Evaluation Study Investigators. The effect of spironolactone on morbidity and mortality in patients with severe heart failure. N Engl J Med 1999;341:709–717.
5. Reicin G, Miksic M, Yik A, Roman D. Hospital Supplies and Medical Technology 4Q05 Statistical Handbook: Growth Moderating But Outlook Remains Strong. New York: Morgan Stanley Equity Research North America; 2005:44.

6. Gregoratos G, Abrams J, Epstein AE, et al. ACC/AHA/NASPE 2002 guidelines update for implantation of cardiac pacemakers and antiarrhythmia devices: Summary article. Circulation 2002;106:2145–61.

7. Abraham WT, Fisher WG, Smith AL, Delurigic DB, et al. Cardiac resynchronization in chronic heart failure. N Engl J Med 2002;346:1845–53.

8. Young JB, Abraham WT, Smith AL, et al. Combined cardiac resynchronization and implantable cardioversion defibrillation in advanced chronic heart failure. JAMA 2003;289:2685–94.

9. Cazeau S, Leclercq C, Lavergne T, et al. Effects of multisite biventricular pacing in patients with heart failure and intraventricular conduction delay. N Engl J Med 2001;344:873–80.

10. Auricchio A, Stellbrink C, Sack S, et al. Long-term clinical effect of hemodynamically optimized cardiac resynchronization therapy in patients with heart failure and ventricular conduction delay. J Am Coll Cardiol 2002;39:2026–33.

11. Bristow MR, Saxon LA, Boehmer J, et al. Cardiac-resynchronization therapy with or without an implantable defibrillator in advanced heart failure. N Engl J Med 2004;350:2140–50.

12. Cleland JGF, Daubert JC, Erdmann E, et al., for the Cardiac Resynchronization-Heart Failure (CARE-HF) Study Investigators. The effect of cardiac resynchronization on morbidity and mortality in heart failure. N Engl J Med 2005;352:1539–49.

13. Saxon LA, DeMarco T, Schafer J, Chatterjee K, Kumar UN, Foster E. Effects of long-term biventricular stimulation for resynchronization of echocardiographic measures of remodeling. Circulation 2002;105:1304–10.

14. Leclercq C, Kass DA. Retiming the failing heart: principle and clinical status of cardiac resyncrhonization. J Am Coll Cardiol 2002;39:194–201.

15. Mehra MR, Greenberg BH. Cardiac resynchronization therapy: caveat medicus! J Am Coll Cardiol 2004;43:1145–8.

16. Kass DA, Chan CH, Curry C, et al. Improved left ventricular mechanics from acute VDD pacing in patients with dilated cardiomyopathy and ventricular conduction delay. Circulation 1999;99;1567–73.

17. Leclercq C, Cazeau S, Le Breton H, et al. Acute hemodynamic effects of biventricular DDD pacing in patients with end-stage heart failure. J Am Coll Cardiol 1998;32:1825–31.

18. Packer M, Coats AJ, Fowler MB, et al. Carvedilol Prospective Randomized Cumulative Survival Study Group. Effect of carvedilol on survival in severe chronic heart failure. N Engl J Med 2001;344:1651–8.

19. CIBIS-II Investigators and committees. The Cardiac Insufficiency Bisoprolol Study II (CIBIS-II). Lancet 1999;353:9–13.

20. Wikstrand J, Hjalmarson A, Waagstein F, et al. MERIT-HF Study Group. Dose of metoprolol CR/XL and clinical outcomes in patients with heart failure: analysis of the experience in the Metoprolol CR/XL Randomized Intervention Trial in Chronic Heart Failure. J Am Coll Cardiol 2002;40:491–8.

21. Gasparini M, Mantica M, Galimberti P, et al. Is the outcome of cardiac resynchronization therapy related to the underlying etiology? Pacing Clin Electrophysiol 2003;26:175–80.

22. Aranda JM Jr, Woo GW, Conti JB, Schofield RS, Conti CR, Hill JA. Use of cardiac resynchronization therapy to optimize beta-blocker therapy in patients with heart failure and prolonged QRS duration. Am J Cardiol 2005;95:889–91.

23. Bardy GH, Lee KL, Mark DB, et al. Amiodarone or an implantable cardioverter-defibrillator for congestive heart failure. N Engl J Med 2005;352:225–37.

24. Aranda JM Jr., Woo GW, Schofield RS, et al. Management of heart failure after cardiac resynchronization therapy: integrating advanced heart failure treatment with optimal device function. J Am Coll Cardiol 2005;46:2193–8.

25. Leon AR, Greenberg JM, Kanuru N, et al. Cardiac resynchronization in patients with congestive heart failure and chronic atrial fibrillation: Effect of upgrading to biventricular pacing after chronic right ventricular pacing. J Am Coll Cardiol 2002;39:1258–63.

26. Breithardt OA, Sinha AM, Schwammenthal, et al. Acute effects of cardiac resynchronization therapy on functional mitral regurgitation in advanced systolic heart failure. J Am Coll Cardiol 2003;41:765–70.

27. St John Sutton MG, Plappert T, Abraham WT, et al. Effect of cardiac resynchronization therapy on left ventricular size and function in chronic heart failure. Circulation 2003;107:1985–90.

28. Auricchio A, Stellbrink C, Block M, et al. Effect of pacing chamber and atrioventricular delay on acute systolic function of paced patients with congestive heart failure. Circulation 1999;99:2993–3001.

29. Van Gelder BM, Bracke FA, Meijer A, et al. Effect of optimizing the VV interval on left ventricular contractility in cardiac resynchronization therapy. Am J Cardiol 2004;93:1500–1503.

30. Leon AR, Abraham WT, Brozena S, et al. Cardiac resynchronization with sequential biventricular pacing for the treatment of moderate to severe heart failure. J Am Coll Cardiol 2005;46:2298–304.

31. Bordachar P, Lafitte S, Reuter S, et al. Echocardiographic parameters of ventricular dyssynchrony validation in patients with heart failure using sequential biventricular pacing. J Am Coll Cardiol 2004;44:2157–65.

32. Bax JJ, Bleeker GB, Marwick TH, et al. Left ventricular dyssynchrony predicts response and prognosis after cardiac resynchronization therapy. J Am Coll Cardiol 2004:441834–40.

33. Pitzalis MV, Iacoviello M, Romito R, et al. Cardiac resynchronization therapy tailored by echocardiographic evaluation of ventricular asynchrony. J Am Coll Cardiol 2002;40:1615–22.

34. Adamson PB, Abraham WT, Love C, Reynolds D. The evolving challenge of chronic heart failure management: A call for a new curriculum for training heart failure specialists. J Am Coll Cardiol 2004;44:1354–7.

Index